# FAMILY VIOLENCE

## A Clinical and Legal Guide

# FAMILY VIOLENCE

## A Clinical and Legal Guide

### Edited by
### Sandra J. Kaplan, M.D.
Associate Chairman
Department of Psychiatry for Child
and Adolescent Psychiatry
North Shore University
Hospital-Cornell University Medical College
Manhasset, New York
Associate Professor of Clinical Psychiatry
Cornell University Medical College
New York, New York

### With legal commentary by
### Howard A. Davidson, J.D.
Director, ABA Center on Children and the Law
American Bar Association
Washington, D.C.

Washington, DC
London, England

Copyright © 1996 American Psychiatric Press, Inc.
ALL RIGHTS RESERVED
Manufactured in the United States of America on acid-free paper
99   98   97          4   3   2
First Edition

American Psychiatric Press, Inc.
1400 K Street, N.W., Washington, DC   20005

**Library of Congress Cataloging-in-Publication Data**
Family violence : a clinical and legal guide / edited by Sandra J. Kaplan. — 1st ed.
    p.   cm.
   Includes bibliographical references and index.
   ISBN 0-89042-010-6
   1. Victims of family violence.   2. Family violence—Prevention.
3. Family violence—Law and legislation—United States. I. Kaplan, Sandra J., 1941-
RC569.5.F3F35   1995
616.85′822—dc20                                                                     95-628
                                                         CIP

**British Library Cataloguing in Publication Data**
A CIP record is available from the British Library.

# CONTENTS

Contributors . . . . . . . . . . . . . . . . . . . . . . . vii

Preface . . . . . . . . . . . . . . . . . . . . . . . . ix
   *Sandra J. Kaplan, M.D.*

Introduction . . . . . . . . . . . . . . . . . . . . xiii
   *Sandra J. Kaplan, M.D.*

**1  Physical Abuse of Children and Adolescents** . . . . . 1
   *Sandra J. Kaplan, M.D.*

**2  Child and Adolescent Neglect and Emotional
    Maltreatment** . . . . . . . . . . . . . . . . . . . 37
   *Hershel D. Rosenzweig, M.D.*
   *Sandra J. Kaplan, M.D.*

**3  Overview of Child Sexual Abuse** . . . . . . . . . . 73
   *Arthur H. Green, M.D.*

**4  Treatment and Prevention of Child Sexual Abuse** . . 105
   *Christine B. L. Adams, M.D.*

**5  Domestic Violence** . . . . . . . . . . . . . . . . 139
   *Mary Lystad, Ph.D.*
   *Matilda Rice, M.D.*
   *Sandra J. Kaplan, M.D.*

**6  Elder Maltreatment** . . . . . . . . . . . . . . . 181
   *Marion Zucker Goldstein, M.D.*

**7** Adult Survivors of Child Abuse and Neglect . . . . 209
*Jean M. Goodwin, M.D., M.P.H.*

**8** Memories of Childhood Trauma: Therapeutic
Considerations for Assessment and Treatment . . . 241
*Stephen J. Ceci, Ph.D.*
*Maggie Bruck, Ph.D.*

Resource Appendixes . . . . . . . . . . . . . . . . 277
*Sandra J. Kaplan, M.D.*
*Howard A. Davidson, J.D.*

Index . . . . . . . . . . . . . . . . . . . . . . 309

# Contributors

Christine B. L. Adams, M.D., Private Practice in Child and Adult Psychiatry, Louisville, Kentucky

Maggie Bruck, Ph.D., Professor of Psychology, Department of Psychology, McGill University, Montreal, Quebec, Canada

Stephen J. Ceci, Ph.D., Helen L. Carr Professor of Developmental Psychology, Cornell University, Ithaca, New York

Howard A. Davidson, J.D., Director, ABA Center on Children and the Law, American Bar Association, Washington, D.C.

Marion Zucker Goldstein, M.D., Clinical Associate Professor, Departments of Psychiatry and Internal Medicine, School of Medicine and Biomedical Sciences, State University of New York at Buffalo, Buffalo, New York

Jean M. Goodwin, M.D., M.P.H., Professor of Psychiatry, University of Texas Medical Center, Galveston, Texas

Arthur H. Green, M.D., Clinical Professor of Psychiatry, Columbia University College of Physicians and Surgeons, and Medical Director of the Therapeutic Nursery, Columbia-Presbyterian Medical Center, New York, New York

Sandra J. Kaplan, M.D., Associate Chairman, Department of Psychiatry for Child and Adolescent Psychiatry, North Shore University Hospital-Cornell University Medical College, and Associate Professor of Clinical Psychiatry, Cornell University Medical College, Manhasset, New York

Mary Lystad, Ph.D., Consultant, Mental Health Studies of Emergencies; Former Chief, Center for Mental Health Studies of Emergencies, National Institute of Mental Health, Bethesda, Maryland

Matilda Rice, M.D., Private Practice in Psychiatry, Maple Glen, Pennsylvania

Hershel D. Rosenzweig, M.D., F.A.A.C.A.P., Senior Clinical Lecturer, University of Arizona, Tucson, Arizona

# PREFACE

---

## Overview of Book
## Contents and Focus

*Family Violence: A Clinical and Legal Guide* is intended to provide professionals in the mental health, other medical, and legal fields with assistance in practice with patients or clients who have been the victims of child physical and/or sexual abuse, child neglect, domestic violence (also known as *spouse or partner abuse*), or elder abuse and neglect, and with the families of these victims. It consists of eight chapters, on the following topics:

- Child physical abuse
- Child neglect and emotional maltreatment
- Overview of child sexual abuse
- Treatment and prevention of child sexual abuse
- Domestic violence
- Elder abuse and elder neglect
- Adult survivors of child maltreatment
- Eliciting information about memories of childhood traumas

Each of the first six chapters reviews the mental health literature, advises how to do a physical and mental health assessment, and discusses treatment methods as well as prevention and legal advocacy needs. Chapters 1–7 also contain discussions of various laws, plus commentary on the legal responsibilities of mental health and other medical professionals. There are also eight resource appendixes, which include, among other topics, the following:

- References for clinical protocols for case recognition and clinical management
- Advocacy, referral, and educational resources

> Examples of clinical guidelines and position statements about family violence put out by professional organizations
> Suggestions for improving the legal and judicial process with regard to the work of health and mental health care professionals

## Book Sponsorship and Authorship

The idea for this book came from the Committee on Family Violence and Sexual Abuse of the American Psychiatric Association's Council on Children, Adolescents, and Their Families. Portions of chapters have been prepared as a collaborative effort between members of the Committee on Family Violence and Sexual Abuse of the American Psychiatric Association and others who were invited. It presents the individual perspectives, experiences, and points of view of the authors and is not official policy of the American Psychiatric Association. The legal commentary in the chapters has been prepared by Howard A. Davidson, J.D., Director of the ABA Center on Children and the Law of the American Bar Association, Washington, D.C.

The editor wishes to thank Christine Adams, M.D., Elaine Hilberman Carmen, M.D., Marion Zucker Goldstein, M.D., Arthur H. Green, M.D., Kathryn Kotrla, M.D., Mary Lystad, Ph.D., Cynthia Pfeffer, M.D., Matilda Rice, M.D., Hershel Rosenzweig, M.D., and Karen Taylor-Crawford, M.D., all 1990–1993 members of the Committee on Family Violence and Sexual Abuse; and Maggie Bruck, Ph.D., Stephen J. Ceci, Ph.D., and Jean M. Goodwin, M.D., for their participation in the preparation of this book.

The editor also wishes to thank her son Lawrence Kaplan for his patience, support, and affection regarding the development of her careers as mother, psychiatric administrator, family violence investigator, clinician, and educator.

In addition, the editor thanks her secretary Sandra Valli and the North Shore University Hospital-Cornell University Medical College, Division of Child and Adolescent Psychiatry, Department of Psychiatry staff, including Harriet Urgo, Office Manager, and her Editorial Assistants, Aliza Septimus, M.A., Leah Friedman, and Rachel Epstein, M.B.A., for their encouragement and assistance in the preparation of this manuscript and for their friendship and career development support.

The editor is grateful to her professional mentors for their inspiration and support: Jack Katz, M.D., Chairman, Department of Psychiatry, North Shore University Hospital-Cornell University Medical College, and John S. T. Gallagher, President and Chief Executive Officer, North Shore Health System; Stella Chess, M.D., Emeritus Professor of Psychiatry, New York University School of Medicine; David Pruitt, M.D., Mohammad Shafii, M.D., and Larry Silver, M.D., former Chairpersons of the American Psychiatric Association's Council on Children, Adolescents, and Their Families; Lawrence Stone, M.D., also a former Council Chairperson, and current President of the American Academy of Child and Adolescent Psychiatry; Elissa Benedek, M.D., former President of the American Psychiatric Association; and Mary Jane England, M.D., current President of the American Psychiatric Association. The editor is also grateful for the comments and suggestions of Donald Gair, M.D., and Elva Poznanski, M.D., reviewers of this manuscript for the Council on Children, Adolescents, and Their Families of the American Psychiatric Association, and for the comments and suggestions of the various manuscript reviewers for the Joint Reference Committee of the American Psychiatric Association.

*Sandra J. Kaplan, M.D.*

# INTRODUCTION

Family violence was recognized as a major public health problem by *American Medicine* in 1962 when an article entitled "The Battered Child Syndrome" was published in the *Journal of the American Medical Association* (Kempe et al. 1962).

Twenty-three years later, in 1985, the Surgeon General of the United States, C. Everett Koop, M.D., convened a national conference to study violence, including family violence, as a public health problem. In 1987 the American Psychiatric Association initiated the Committee on Family Violence and Sexual Abuse as a Committee of the Council on Children, Adolescents, and Their Families. However, despite a 30-year medical history and increasing awareness and advocacy by the Public Health Service and the Centers for Disease Control (CDC), as well as by the American Psychiatric Association, the American Medical Association, the American Academy of Pediatrics, the American College of Obstetrics, and the American College of Emergency Room Physicians, as well as other distinguished groups and organizations, family violence is still often underdiagnosed, and resources for both treatment and research are either inadequate or lacking.

Less than 5% of the injuries resulting from domestic violence are recognized as such by emergency room staff (Stark and Flitcraft 1988). There are government-documented treatment programs available for only 5% of indicated cases of child abuse (U.S. Advisory Board on Child Abuse and Neglect 1991), and even fewer available for cases of domestic violence and elder abuse.

Medical education on domestic violence was not provided in 53% of American medical colleges surveyed by the New Jersey Medical College (Holtz and Hanes 1989). Injury research, including that on injuries caused by family violence, is also underfunded (Rice, MacKenzie, and Associates 1989), and research is urgently needed to further inform and direct family violence prevention.

---

## Definitions and Prevalence

*Family violence,* as the term is used in this book, includes physical or sexual injury inflicted by a family member on another family member. According to "The Cost of Injury in the United States," a 1989 congressional report, over one-third of injury deaths in the United States are intentional (Rice, MacKenzie, and Associates 1989). Family violence is often the cause of these deaths, frequently ending in homicide (Mercy and Saltzman 1989) and preceding suicide (Deykin 1989). *Child abuse* refers to the physical or sexual abuse of children under 18 years of age. In 1993, 1,018,692 children were substantiated or indicated as victims of maltreatment. Twenty-four percent of these cases involved physical abuse, and 14% involved sexual abuse (U.S. Department of Health and Human Services 1995). The 1995 National Center on Child Abuse Study of the Prevalence of Child Abuse in America reported that there were 1,028 deaths from child abuse and neglect in 1993 (U.S. Department of Health and Human Services 1995). *Domestic violence* refers to the injury of adults by their significant others. It has been estimated to occur in 16%–25% of American couples (Gelles and Straus 1988). Domestic violence is the leading cause of injury to women (Stark and Flitcraft 1988) in the United States, and 1.8 million women are severely assaulted by their partners each year (Straus 1991). During 1992, 3.9 million women were physically abused by their partners (Commonwealth Fund 1993). The CDC reported that between the years 1976 and 1985 there were 16,595 deaths in the United States resulting from domestic violence (Mercy and Saltzman 1989). *Elder abuse* refers to the injury of elderly people and is estimated to affect 3.2% of the elderly population in the United States (Pillemer and Finkelhor 1988). It has been estimated that approximately 818,000 elders became victims of elder abuse during 1994 (National Center on Elder Abuse 1995).

---

## Cost

Because victims of intentional injury, including that caused by domestic violence or by child abuse, are often young (National Committee for Injury Prevention and Control 1989), the loss of productive years by victims, and therefore the financial cost of injury, is enormous. The lifetime cost of injury sustained from child abuse and domestic violence by 57 million people was $158 billion in 1985 and had risen to $188 billion by 1988 when inflation was taken into account (Rice, MacKenzie, and Associates 1989).

## Roles of Mental Health and Other Health Care Providers

Family violence is repetitive, increases in severity as it persists (Stark 1990), and is transmitted across generations and toward society by those exposed to it in their homes (Straus 1991). The efforts of physicians and other mental health professionals are required if we are to contain this epidemic. Steps that must be taken include

➤ Increased recognition and diagnosis of the problem
➤ Collaboration with legal and community resources to ensure protection of victims
➤ Increased facilities and resources for treatment of the physical and psychological injuries of the victims, witnesses, and perpetrators of family violence
➤ Advocacy for increased prevention and research

References for specific protocols designed for the assessment of victims of each type of family violence, including both interview and observation protocols, are included in Appendix C. These protocols will help in recognition and management of cases and documentation of physical findings.

## Risk Factors

Risk factors for committing any of the various types of family violence include

➤ Exposure to family violence
➤ Stressful events (Egeland et al. 1980)
➤ Young or single parenthood (Gelles 1992; Goodman and Rosenberg 1987; Hotaling and Sugarman 1986; Kaufman and Zigler 1987; Steinmetz 1977; Widom 1989)
➤ Four or more children closely spaced (U.S. Department of Health and Human Services 1985)

➤ A female as the target of anger (Earls et al. 1991)
➤ Social isolation (Anetzberger 1987; Salzinger et al. 1983)
➤ Victim-perpetrator power imbalance, such as that resulting from
   victim dependency due to age or illness (Wolf et al. 1984)
➤ A lack of empathy and of nonviolent conflict resolution strategies
   (Pagelow 1984)
➤ Substance abuse (Goldstein 1987)
➤ Depression (Carmen et al. 1984; Steinmetz 1977)

In addition, those raising young children have an increased risk of using the most abusive forms of violence toward their children (Gelles 1992).

Wolfner and Gelles (1993) found that the highest rates of abusive violence occurred in families that resided in the East, families in which the father was unemployed, families in which the caretakers held blue-collar occupations or whose annual income was below the poverty line, families in which the caretakers used drugs at least once, and families with children 3–6 years old.

An additional risk factor for homicide or suicide associated with family violence is the presence of firearms within a home (Fingerhut and Kleinman 1990; Kellerman and Reay 1986). There will be specific examples of risk factors according to type of family violence in each chapter of the book.

## Protection

After a clinician makes a diagnosis of family violence, advocacy for protection of victims is desirable. The ability to advocate for this protection will be enhanced by a thorough knowledge of local family violence reporting requirements and procedures for making reports to law enforcement agencies, legal resources, and social service departments. The appendixes and each chapter of this book contain information on resources for victim protection and legal action.

## Assessment and Treatment Efficacy

Training in family violence case recognition and diagnoses is effective. McLeer and Anwar (1989) reported that training emergency room staff in domestic violence recognition leads to increases in the number of patients correctly diagnosed as having traumatic injuries from domestic violence assaults. The writers hope that this book will enhance the ability of the clinician and the legal professional to provide accurate medical and legal case assessments, case management, and protection of and for their patients and clients. We also hope that this book will stimulate additional advocacy for enhanced prevention, intervention, and research efforts.

Although they are expensive and complex, there are mental health programs that have been able to rehabilitate violent families. These programs provide the following care: interdisciplinary teams, outreach, 24-hour on-call coverage, and evening hours available for treatment.

Services provided by these programs include 1) mental health and substance abuse evaluation and treatment (including individual, group, and family therapy for parents and children), 2) assessment and remediation of child educational and adult vocational status, 3) training in social skills, parenting, and nonviolent conflict resolution, and 4) financial, housing, and homemaking assistance referral capacity (Cohn and Daro 1987; Kaplan et al. 1981). Programs such as the Family Crisis Program of the Division of Child and Adolescent Psychiatry, Department of Psychiatry, North Shore University Hospital-Cornell University Medical College, Manhasset, NY, and the Therapeutic Nursery and Family Center at Presbyterian Hospital, New York, may serve as models to be emulated by all those who seek to develop mental health treatment programs to reverse the growing incidence of family violence. (See the appendixes for sample program resource references.)

## Education and Prevention

This book is also intended to stimulate the development of effective curricula for the public and for physicians, including psychiatrists, and for other mental health professionals. These courses of study will include individual, family, and gender development, nonviolent and empathic communication skills, parenting, and human sexuality. We believe such education will reduce the incidence of family violence.

We also hope that this book will inspire mental health and other health care professionals to advocate for prevention programs. Such advocacy will be enhanced by addressing the need for control of firearms and other weapons and the need to collaborate with the media to control public violence exposure (Heath et al. 1986). Because there is evidence that violence reported in great detail by the media is contagious, a vitally important advocacy goal is the promotion of programs that teach empathy and emphasize nurturing role models and nonviolent interpersonal conflict resolution. It is also important to enhance the value of those most likely to be victims of family violence: women, elderly people, and children. Advocacy for the abolishment of corporal punishment in schools will serve to strengthen the value society puts on children and will prevent children from learning violence as a behavior control strategy (National Committee for Injury Prevention and Control 1989; U.S. Department of Health and Human Services 1985).

Advocacy by psychiatrists and other mental health professionals for community education, plus their participation in that education, will contribute to the prevention of family violence. This education could begin in elementary school as an essential part of health education for all children and should continue as a component of health education throughout the life span.

Victims of family violence and their families have great needs for mental health services and legal advocacy. The development of clinical skills and the acquisition of knowledge needed for case identification, for the protection of victims and witnesses of family maltreatment, and for the assessment and treatment of victims and perpetrators will enable clinicians to help meet those needs. In addition, research and prevention efforts by practitioners will give them more power to combat family violence.

The contents of this book are intended as a springboard resource for the reader. Assessing and treating victims and witnesses of family violence provides an opportunity to help halt the cycle in which violence perpetuates more violence.

*Sandra J. Kaplan, M.D.*

## References

Anetzberger G: The Etiology of Elder Abuse by Adult Offspring. Springfield, IL, Charles C. Thomas, 1987

Carmen E, Ricker P, Mills T: Victims of violence and psychiatric illness. Am J Psychiatry 3:378–383, 1984

Cohn AH, Daro D: Is treatment too late: what ten years of evaluative research tell us. Child Abuse Negl 11:433–442, 1987

Commonwealth Fund: First Comprehensive National Health Survey of American Women. New York, The Commonwealth Fund, July 1993

Deykin EY: The utility of emergency room data for record linkage in the study of adolescent suicidal behavior. Suicide Life Threat Behav 19:90–98, 1989

Earls F, Slaby RG, Spirito A, et al: Position Paper, Panel on Violence Prevention (draft). Third National Injury Control Conference, Denver, CO, April 1991

Earls G, Slaby RG, Spirito A, et al: Prevention of violence and injuries due to violence. Position papers from the Third National Injury Control Conference, U.S. Department of Health and Human Services, Public Health Service, Centers for Disease Control. Washington, DC, Government Printing Office, 1992

Egeland B, Breitenbucher M, Rosenberg D: Prospective study of the significance of life stress in the etiology of child abuse. J Consult Clin Psychol 48:195–205, 1980

Fingerhut LA, Kleinman JC: International and interstate comparisons of homicides among young males. JAMA 263:3292–3295, 1990

Gelles RJ: Poverty and violence toward children. Special issue: the impact of poverty on children. American Behavioral Scientist 35:258–274, 1992

Gelles RJ, Straus MA: Intimate Violence: The Definitive Study of the Causes and Consequences of Abuse in the American Family. New York, Simon & Schuster, 1988

Goldstein PJ: Targeting interventions at substance abuse problems—impact of drug related violence. Public Health Report 102:625–627, 1987

Goodman GS, Rosenberg MS: The child witness to family violence, in Domestic Violence on Trial: Psychological and Legal Dimensions of Family Violence. Edited by Sonkin DJ. New York, Springer, 1987

Heath L, Kruttschnitt C, Ward D: Television and violent criminal behavior: beyond the bobo doll. Violence and Victims 1:177–190, 1986

Holtz H, Hanes CA: Evaluation of medical student training in women abuse. Abstracts of the Eighth Mid-Atlantic Regional Society of General Internal Medicine Conference, 1989

Hotaling GT, Sugarman DB: An analysis of risk makers in husband to wife violence: the current state of knowledge. Violence and Victims 1:101–124, 1986

Kaplan S, Samit C, Pelcovitz D, et al: The family crisis program: an overview. North Shore University Hospital 4:19–24, 1981

Kaufman J, Zigler E: Do abused children become abusive parents? Am J Orthopsychiatry 57: 186–192, 1987

Kellerman A, Reay D: Protection or peril? An analysis of firearm related deaths in the home. N Engl J Med 314:1557–1560, 1986

Kempe CH, Silverman FS, Steele BF, et al: The battered child syndrome. JAMA 181:17–24, 1962

McLeer S, Anwar R: A study of battered women presenting in an emergency department. Am J Public Health 79:65–66, 1989

Mercy JA, Saltzman LE: Fatal violence among spouses in the United States. Am J Public Health 79:595–599, 1989

National Center on Elder Abuse: Understanding the Nature and Extent of Elder Abuse in Domestic Settings. Washington, DC, National Center on Elder Abuse, 1995

National Committee for Injury Prevention and Control: Injury Prevention: Meeting the Challenge. New York, Oxford University Press, 1989, pp 252–260

Pagelow MD: Family Violence. New York, Praeger, 1984

Pillemer K, Finkelhor D: The prevalence of elder abuse: a random sample survey. Gerontologist 28:51–57, 1988

Rice DP, MacKenzie E, and Associates: Cost of Injury in the United States. A Report to Congress. San Francisco, CA, Institute for Health and Aging, University of California/San Francisco; and Injury Prevention Center, School of Hygiene and Public Health, Johns Hopkins University, 1989

Salzinger S, Kaplan S, Artemyeff C: Mother's personal social network and child maltreatment. J Abnorm Psychol 22:253–256, 1983

Stark ED: Rethinking homicide. Int J Health Serv 20:3–26, 1990

Stark E, Flitcraft A: Violence among intimates: an epidemiological review, in Handbook of Family Violence. Edited by Van Hasset VB, Morrison RL, Bellack AS, et al. New York, Plenum, 1988, pp 293–317

Steinmetz S: The Cycle of Violence: Assertive, Aggressive and Abusive Family Interaction. New York, Praeger, 1977

Straus MA: Discipline and deviance: physical punishment of children and violence and other crime in adulthood. Social Problems 38:133–154, 1991

U.S. Advisory Board on Child Abuse and Neglect: The Continuing Child Protection Emergency: A Challenge to the Nation. Washington, DC, U.S. Department of Health and Human Services, 1991

U.S. Department of Health and Human Services: Report on the Surgeon General's Workshop on Violence and Public Health, Leesburg, VA, October 1985. Washington, DC, U.S. Government Printing Office, 1985

U.S. Department of Health and Human Services, National Center on Child Abuse and Neglect: Child Maltreatment 1993: Reports from the States to the National Center on Child Abuse and Neglect. Washington, DC, U.S. Government Printing Office, 1995

Widom CS: Does violence beget violence? A critical examination of the literature. Psychol Bull 106:3–28, 1989

Wolf R, Godkin M, Pillemer K: Elder Abuse and Neglect: Final Report From Three Model Projects. Worcester, MA, University Center on Aging, University of Massachusetts Medical Center, 1984

Wolfner GD, Gelles RJ: A profile of violence toward children: a national study. Child Abuse Negl 17:197–212, 1993

# CHAPTER 1

## Physical Abuse of Children and Adolescents

*Sandra J. Kaplan, M.D.*

The physical abuse of children and adolescents is a major United States public health problem. The 1993 Reports from the States to the National Center on Child Abuse and Neglect estimated that 1,018,692 children in the United States were documented victims of maltreatment and that 1,028 children died that year as a result of maltreatment (U.S. Department of Health and Human Services 1995). Abused children often exhibit aggressive behavior toward society (Alfaro 1978; Lewis 1985; Lewis et al. 1979; Widom 1989), toward other family members (Kaufman and Zigler 1987; Straus et al. 1980; Straus and Gelles 1986), and toward themselves (Deykin et al. 1985; Green 1978b; Pfeffer 1986; Rotheram and Bradley 1987).

Child abuse psychiatric studies and treatment programs are still in the early stages of development. Kempe, a pediatrician, and his psychiatric colleague Steele, of the University of Colorado, who with others wrote "The Battered Child Syndrome" in the *Journal of the American Medical Association* in 1962 (Kempe et al. 1962), were largely responsible for medicine's (including psychiatry's) beginning to focus on child abuse in the United States (Steele and Pollack 1968).

1

# Definitions

The Child Abuse Prevention, Adoption, and Family Services Act of 1988, Public Law (P.L.) 100-294, defines physical abuse as "the physical injury of a child under 18 years of age by a person who is responsible for the child's welfare, under circumstances which indicate that the child's health or welfare is harmed or threatened thereby, as determined in accordance with regulations prescribed by the Secretary of Health and Human Services." According to that law, a person responsible for a child's welfare includes an employee of a residential facility, any staff of a facility, or any staff person providing out-of-home care. The Family Court Act (1976) of New York State defines physical abuse as "the situation which results when a parent or other person legally responsible for a child less than 18 inflicts or allows to be inflicted upon such child physical injury by other than accidental means" (Garbarino and Ebata 1983). Straus and Gelles, the principal investigators of the National Incidence Studies of Violence in America, define child abuse as the use by a parent of any of the acts on the Severe Violence Index of the Conflict Tactics Scale. This scale defines severe violence as kicking, biting, or hitting with a fist; hitting or trying to hit with an object; battering; or using or threatening to use a gun or a knife (Straus and Gelles 1986).

# Prevalence

Straus and Gelles (1986), in their 1985 study of violence in the United States, found that the incidence of physical abuse of children and adolescents was 19/1,000 for children ages 3–17 years. This compares with the same authors' 1975 study of violence in the United States, which found that 36/1,000 children ages 3–17 years were abused. The two studies differed in that the earlier study used in-person interviews with the Conflict Tactics Scale (Straus et al. 1980), whereas 10 years later the researchers used telephone interviews. Methodological differences in interviewing, increased public awareness, and legislation regarding child abuse may have accounted for the decrease in rates reported by the 1985 study. The latest national incidence and prevalence study of the National Center on Child Abuse and Neglect estimated that of the 1,018,962 children documented in the United States as maltreated during 1993 (U.S. Department of

Health and Human Services 1995), approximately 51% were 7 years or younger and 20% were 13 years or older. Females were documented to have been maltreated more often than males (U.S. Department of Health and Human Services 1995).

Despite these statistics, the exact incidence of child abuse in the United States is unknown. Reporting biases and investigatory procedural constraints exist. Reporting probability is increased for ethnic minorities, urban residents, low-income people, and those who use public rather than private sources of health care. The documentation and substantiation provided by child protective services (CPS) agencies vary with the source of the reporter. The reports most likely to be substantiated by investigatory agencies (Eckenrode et al. 1988) are those made by physicians.

## Age at Onset

The National Incidence Study reported in 1988 that the severity of abuse varied inversely with the age of the child victim, with most fatalities occurring in younger children (U.S. Department of Health and Human Services 1988). Prepubertal child abuse most often involves single-parent, ethnic-minority, and low-income families. On the other hand, abuse of adolescents, as reported in a study conducted in 1977, usually involved white, intact two-parent families earning more than $11,000 per year (U.S. Department of Health and Human Services 1981). The documented physical abusers of adolescents are usually fathers, whereas mothers are more often the documented physical abusers of younger children (Straus et al. 1980). Most studies of abuse involving adolescents report that although the abuse sometimes begins in early childhood and continues into adolescence, the majority of cases begin during adolescence (Libbey and Bybee 1979; Lourie 1979; Straus et al. 1980).

Garbarino et al. (1984), Libbey and Bybee (1979), Lourie (1979), and Pelcovitz et al. (1984) explain the adolescent onset of abuse as relating most often to interpersonal conflicts around adolescent developmental tasks and to parental midlife crises rather than to the socioeconomic stress that often triggers the abuse of prepubertal children (Pelcovitz et al. 1984). Parental psychopathology has been hypothesized by Pelcovitz and Kaplan as an additional risk factor for abuse in the families of abused adolescents.

## Fatalities

The number of child abuse fatalities reported in the United States has increased, ranging from 1,179 in 1987 to 1,199 in 1988 to 1,237 in 1989. The number of child abuse fatalities increased more than 38% between 1985 and 1990. The 1990 estimate was that three children a day were reported as fatal victims of child abuse, of whom, according to the 15 states that mentioned age of the child at time of death (and on whose statistics the national estimate is based), more than 50% were less than 1 year old (Daro and Mitchel 1990).

However, because of the variances in cause-of-death categorizing procedures by states, these statistics may underestimate the problem (Daro and Mitchel 1990). Some child homicide, accidental deaths, and sudden infant death syndrome (SIDS) deaths might have qualified as child abuse deaths if more comprehensive investigations had been conducted (Kempe et al. 1962). Many states are beginning to address this problem by establishing *death review committees*. Establishing more accurate procedures for the recognition of child abuse fatalities should help reduce their number as experts begin to learn with precision the factors that lead to death.

## Etiology

The most widely accepted model of the etiology of abuse is the ecological model (Belsky 1980), which views child abuse as the consequence of the interactions of parental vulnerabilities, such as young age, mental illness, or substance abuse; child vulnerabilities, such as low birth weight, difficult temperament, a particular developmental stage (adolescence, toddler); social stressors, such as lack of social supports, poverty, single parenthood, minority ethnicity, lack of acculturation, four or more children in a family; stressful events; and exposure to extrafamilial and intrafamilial violence (Belsky 1980; U.S. Department of Health and Human Services 1988).

## Psychopathology and Other Effects in Abused Children and Adolescents

There have not yet been standardized psychopathology studies comparing abused children or adolescents who have been referred for treatment with those not so referred. However, those studies of psychiatric disturbance in abused children and adolescents who have been referred for treatment have found these children and adolescents to be impulsive, hyperactive (Martin and Beezley 1977) or depressed (Green 1978a; Kaplan et al. 1986); to have conduct disorders (Kaplan et al. 1986; Kinard 1980), learning disabilities (Kline and Christiansen 1975; Salzinger et al. 1984); and frequently to be substance abusers (Kaplan et al. 1986). Cuddy and Belicki (1992) report that individuals who were physically abused experience higher nightmare and night terror frequency than those who were not abused. Histories of physical child abuse have been reported in child and adolescent psychiatric patient populations (Kashani et al. 1987a, 1987b). Lewis (Lewis 1985; Lewis et al. 1979) and Alfaro (1978) found that delinquent and violent adolescents also frequently had histories of physical abuse. The experience of physical child abuse has an impact on the expression of violent behaviors. Truscott (1992) reported that violent behaviors in adolescent males were found to be associated with physical abuse inflicted by fathers.

Salzinger et al. (1984) found that referred maltreatment victims, and to a lesser extent their siblings, showed significantly more hyperactivity, conduct disturbance, anxiety, and tension than did a nonmaltreated comparison group. In Salzinger et al.'s (1993) study comparing physically abused children with nonabused children, abused children were found to have lower peer status. Their peers rated them as less cooperative and more aggressive, and their teachers and parents rated them as more disturbed. In an analysis of data using the Diagnostic Interview for Children and Adolescents (DICA) (Herjanic and Reich 1982; Reich et al. 1982) on a referred sample, abused children and adolescents were diagnosed significantly more often than nonmaltreated children and adolescents as suffering from depression, alcohol abuse, and conduct and attention deficit disorders (Kaplan et al. 1986).

Analyses of commonly suggested risk factors for child psychopathology such as parental psychopathology (Weissman et al. 1984; Wolkind and Rutter 1985), family cohesion or adaptability (Wolkind and Rutter 1985), child perception of parental supportiveness (Keller et al. 1986), marital discord (Illfeld 1977), prolonged separation of child from parent (Rutter 1971; Wolkind and Rutter 1973) or head trauma (Rutter et al. 1983) were *not* included in any of the above-mentioned studies. Only the study by Kaplan et al. (1986) included an analysis of psychiatric illness in parents who abused their children. It found that abused children of parents with psychiatric disorders were more often diagnosed as having psychiatric disorders themselves than were nonabused children of parents with psychiatric disorders. Because multiple risk factors for child mental illness are frequently present in child abuse, future research on the association of child mental illness and abuse will be improved by the inclusion of analyses that adjust for the presence of these risk factors.

## Suicide

An association between suicide and abuse has been found in studies of adolescents who attempt suicide, and in studies of mothers who attempt suicide. Deykin et al. (1985) found that adolescents who attempted suicide had more often been reported as abuse victims than adolescents who had not attempted suicide. Pfeffer (1986) reported frequent child abuse in families of children who attempted suicide, and Farber (Farber et al. 1984), Kaplan (1986), and Rotheram and Bradley (1987) reported that adolescent runaways had high rates of suicide attempts. Garbarino and Farber (Garbarino et al. 1984; Farber et al. 1984), reported that runaway youth had high rates of adolescent abuse. Green (1978b) reported self-mutilation in abused and neglected children.

Shaffer (1987), in a preliminary report on adolescent suicide in the New York metropolitan area, found that substance abuse, conduct disorders, and—less frequently—depression, family discord, family histories of suicide, and other exposure to suicide appeared to be risk factors for adolescent suicide. These same psychiatric disorders and family histories have also been reported in child and adolescent abuse victims (Kaplan et al. 1986). Mothers who attempted suicide exhibited child abuse behaviors more often than a comparison group of non-suicidal mothers (Hawton et al. 1985). Suicide attempts by parents are known to be major risk factors for adolescent suicide (Shaffer 1989).

The etiology of the association of physical abuse and suicidal behavior remains to be further studied. The abuse may be secondary to exposure to the suicidal modeling of aggressive behavior within the family, or to the behavior of family members. It may also be secondary to increased biological risk in these families for disorders that have been highly associated with suicide: substance abuse, affective disorders, and impulsive conduct disorders (Kaplan et al. 1983, 1986; Shaffer 1987). Finally, the frequent social isolation of the abused adolescent, as well as that of his or her parents and family, may also increase the risk for suicide ( Salzinger et al. 1983; Shaffer and Fisher 1974; Spinetta and Rigler 1972).

## Psychopathology of Parents

Comparative studies have reported an increased incidence of psychopathology in abusive parents but have been limited by the failure to use structured diagnostic interviews (Estroff et al. 1985; Paulson et al. 1976; Smith et al. 1973); the study of populations inadequately defined as abusive (Bland and Orn 1986); the fact that cases studied had been referred for treatment; and the fact that study samples of parents of child and adolescent abuse victims were often combined. These studies have reported maltreating parents as aggressive (Kaplan et al. 1983; Wolfe 1985), depressed (Bland and Orn 1986; Breiner 1992; Kaplan et al. 1983; Wolfe 1985), having low self-esteem (Breiner 1992), having more physically and verbally aggressive behaviors when interacting with the child, having increased somatic concerns, exhibiting an imbalance in the proportion of negative to positive and more aversive control behaviors when interacting with the target child, and having increased arousal and reactivity to aversive child stimuli when compared to nonmaltreating parents (Wolfe 1985).

In research that used diagnostic structured interviews and distinguished between parents of abused children and adolescents and parents of children and adolescents who were not abused, significantly more parents of abused children and adolescents than nonmaltreating parents were diagnosed as having psychopathology. Fathers—usually the perpetrating parents in the abusive families studied—were more often diagnosed as having antisocial personality disorders or labile personalities or as abusing alcohol, whereas mothers in these families were more frequently diagnosed as having depressive disorders. Mothers of maltreated adolescents were found to have diagnoses of drug abuse less often than were mothers of maltreated children under 12 years of age (Kaplan et al. 1983).

## Intergenerational Transmission

Abuse during one's childhood increases the risk for becoming an abusive parent (Kaufman and Zigler 1987; Straus et al. 1980). Kaufman and Zigler (1987) suggested in a critical review that approximately *one-third* of those who were physically abused, sexually abused, or severely neglected will maltreat their offspring. It is important to note that this risk was reduced by the presence of one supportive parent during childhood, a supportive spousal relationship, and fewer stressful events during adulthood (Kaufman and Zigler 1987).

## Social Functioning and Isolation of Abusive Families

Both child abuse victims and their parents (Salzinger et al. 1983; Salzinger et al. 1984) have been found to have impaired social competence. Mothers of abused children and adolescents were reported as employed outside their homes less often and as being more socially isolated, particularly with respect to peers, than the mothers of nonmaltreated children (Salzinger et al. 1983). This type of social isolation from peers may be hypothesized to lead to a lack of child-rearing acculturation of the abusive parent (Salzinger et al. 1983).

## Ritualistic Abuse

Ritualistic abuse has been reported both by clinicians caring for abused children (Hudson 1989; Jonker and Jonker-Bakker 1991) and by adults who recalled such abuse during their childhoods (Braun 1986; Kluft 1988; Young et al. 1991). Ritualistic abuse has also been an issue in legal proceedings involving the alleged abuse of children in day care settings (Finkelhor et al. 1988). Satanic or ritualistic abuse of children, according to the President's Child Safety Partnership (1987), has begun to appear in the United States.

Ritualistic abuse has been defined by Finkelhor et al. (1988) as that occurring in a context of symbols or group activities with a religious, magical, or supernatural connotation, and where repeated invocation of these symbols or activities, is employed to frighten the children. Kelly (1988) defined ritualistic abuse as repeated, systematic sexual, physical, and psychological abuse of children in cult or satanic worship.

Finkelhor et al. (1988) have also proposed three subtypes of ritualistic abuse: *true cult based,* in which the abuse is part of the child's immersion in cult rituals and belief; *pseudoritualistic,* in which the abuse is the primary activity and the cult rituals are less prominent; and *psychopathological ritualism,* in which a psychiatrically disordered perpetrator practices idiosyncratic rituals during abuse.

## ▌ Prevalence

Looking back to 1983, according to Lanning (1991), legal investigations of child abuse cases with allegations of ritualistic abuse, have found little or no corroborative evidence of this type of abuse. Therefore, meaningful estimates of its actual prevalence cannot be made. However, in an analysis of 270 United States day care child abuse cases, 13% (35) included *allegations* of ritualistic abuse (Finkelhor et al. 1988). In California, police have investigated reports of cases of day care center abuse involving 900 children in which ritualistic child abuse was alleged to have been part of the problem (Hudson 1989).

## ▌ Effects

Aggressive behavior; dissociative amnestic behavior, anxiety (particularly at bedtime with nightmares), nighttime enuresis, separation concerns, and regression in bowel training have been reported in children alleged to have been ritualistically abused (Hudson 1989). E. Poznanski (personal communication, October 1991) has observed that such children exhibit sexualized behavior, severe regression, and apparently unprovoked episodic violent behavior. She has stressed the importance of physical assessment of these children in order to detect physical evidence of physical and sexual abuse, such as skin tattoos of cult symbols on the shoulders or other areas. Dissociative disorder diagnoses, including multiple personality disorder, have been reported to occur in adults who have alleged ritualistic abuse during their childhoods (Braun 1986; Gould and Cozolino 1992; Kluft 1988; Young et al. 1991).

## ▌ Need for Caution

Pediatric (Krugman 1991), psychiatric (Jones 1991), and forensic (Lanning 1991) child abuse experts have urged caution regarding the care of children or adults in cases involving allegations of ritualistic abuse because, as Lanning pointed out, legal investigation and prosecution of alleged ritualistic abuse have usually not found substantiating corroborative evidence. Krugman (1991), Jones (1991), and Putnam (1991) urged that when dealing with these cases in clinical practice, assault details and type-of-abuse histories be obtained from the alleged victim, and that treatment be designed to deal with the effects of the reported abuse rather than focusing exclusively on the alleged ritualistic aspect of the case. Jones (1991) also urged that in assessing and treating these cases, attention be paid to the fact that most allegedly involve multiple victims from different families abused by the same perpetrator.

## Assessment in Cases With Allegations of Physical Abuse

### ▮ History Taking

Specific histories from parents and children, interviewed separately, regarding child disciplinary methods and family conflict resolution strategies will enhance the ability of a clinician to diagnose child abuse. References for sample interviews and guidelines for diagnosing child abuse are included in Appendix C.

### ▮ Physical Examination Findings

A physical examination is an important component of the assessment of the child or adolescent who may have been physically abused. The American Medical Association (AMA) Diagnostic and Treatment Guidelines Concerning Child Abuse and Neglect (Council on Scientific Affairs, American Medical Association 1985) report the following with regard to diagnostic physical findings:

> Characteristically, the injuries are more severe than those that could reasonably be attributed to the claimed cause. Physical signs of abuse include: bruises and welts of the face, lips, mouth, ears, eyes, neck, or head, trunk, back, buttocks, thighs, or extremities on multiple body surfaces or soft tissue forming regular patterns, often resembling the shape of the article used to inflict the injury (e.g., hand, teeth, belt buckle, or electrical cord); burns inflicted with cigars or cigarettes, especially on the soles, palms, back, or buttocks; immersion burns (stocking or glovelike on the extremi-

ties, doughnut-shaped on buttocks or genitals), or patterned burns resembling an electrical appliance (e.g., iron, burner, or grill); fractures of the skull, ribs, nose, facial structure, or long bones, frequently with multiple or spiral fractures in various stages of healing; lacerations or abrasions; rope burns on wrists, ankles, neck, or torso, palate, mouth, gums, lips, eyes, or ears or external genitalia; bruises of the abdominal wall; intramural hematoma of duodenum or proximal jejunum; intestinal perforation; ruptured liver or spleen; ruptured blood vessels, kidney, bladder, or pancreatic injury; and central nervous system injuries including subdural hematoma (often reflective of blunt trauma or violent shaking); retinal hemorrhage; or subarachnoid hemorrhage (often reflective of shaking).

## Treatment

Parental psychopathology and substance abuse often present risk factors for child or adolescent psychopathology, as well as for continued child abuse, in violent families. Comprehensive programs for abused children and their families require assessment and treatment for parental mental illness and substance abuse as well as assessment and treatment for the abused child or adolescent.

There is considerable literature on the diagnosis of child abuse and initial phases of management. However, there is a dearth of information regarding long-term psychotherapeutic management, and few empirical studies evaluating the effectiveness of therapeutic modalities or techniques with this population.

Most child abuse treatment programs have focused on treatment of the abusing parent, offering little treatment for the maltreated child. This treatment model views abuse and neglect as a consequence only of parental psychopathology and child-rearing difficulties. The "ecological" or multidimensional view of child abuse defines treatment needs as broader than this parental psychopathological model. Main and Goldwyn (1988) and Wolfe (1987) have stressed the importance of focusing on the interactional aspect of the cycle of maltreatment and the importance of changing negative modes of parent-child interactions. Other variables are seen as contributing to abuse and neglect. These include family dysfunction, environmental stress factors such as parental unemployment, parental emotional disturbances, the degree to which social support systems exist and operate for parents, and the vulnerability of the target child. This model emphasizes that child abuse results as a function of the degree to which the parents' environment tends to enhance or to undermine good parenting. If support is adequate, parental propensities toward violence are controlled. If, however, there is little social support, violent propensities are expressed.

Treatment programs that are effective in stopping child abuse address the multidimensional and individual nature of the etiology of family violence. These programs have multidisciplinary treatment teams equipped to use interventions based on individual psychopathology, family dysfunction, stress, and lack of social supports.

Individual psychotherapy for the child victim needs to address low self-esteem, identification with and imitation of aggressive behavior (or, conversely, the development of extreme passivity) as a conflict resolution strategy, self-blame for the abuse, and a sense of being damaged. Therapists also must address depressive and frequently suicidal ideations and self-destructive behaviors, including substance abuse.

Individual psychotherapy for parents and therapy for families must include the addressing of parental knowledge of child development and must present conflict resolution strategies that can serve as alternatives to violence during child rearing.

## ▌ Treatment Outcome

In the study done from October 1979 to October 1981, Daro looked at 19 child maltreatment clinical demonstration programs funded by the National Center on Child Abuse and Neglect that served 1,000 families. She found that clinicians rated families who received 13–18 months of treatment in family therapy or group therapy as having made the most progress and as being the least likely to have a relapse of child maltreatment necessitating re-reporting (Daro 1988). Parental substance abuse was associated inversely with treatment progress (Daro 1988), as was the presence of multiple types of maltreatment exhibited by a family prior to referral (Straus and Gelles 1986).

In a study of physically abusive families with a child in out-of-home placement resulting from abuse, Barth et al. (1985–86) found that low socioeconomic status, older age of child, greater severity of abuse, and victim school behavioral problems predicted a poor outcome of social service agency rehabilitative effort and the consequent need for permanent out-of-home care for abused children.

# ▌ Parent Treatment

When abusive parents are referred to traditional community mental health clinics, there is an unusually high dropout rate. Because abusive parents were frequently reared in a family environment where their needs for nurturance and dependency were often met with rejection and violence, it is not surprising that these parents often view authority figures with suspicion and mistrust. Resistance and missed appointments during initial treatment phases are almost inevitable components of the treatment engagement process. To get beyond the parents' lack of basic trust, outreach to these families is often necessary in a manner not usually needed with nonabusive parents. This outreach includes staff's being available to the families on a 24-hour basis, plus treatment hours in the evening and the use of home visits.

Parental psychotherapy has two primary components. The first component is providing the parents with intense emotional support as well as positive models of parenting. The parents must be taught appropriate developmental expectations so they can stop making unrealistic demands on their children. They also must learn effective, nonpunitive child-rearing techniques. The second component is psychotherapy aimed at insight and conflict resolution. This usually begins as individual psychotherapy during which the therapist endeavors to establish a solid, trusting therapeutic relationship with the parent. In later stages, conjoint family sessions deal with interactional issues, such as marital conflict and the scapegoating of the abused child (Kaplan 1981).

# ▌ Child Treatment

Abused children and adolescents are at risk for serious behavioral and emotional disorders, developmental disorders, and learning problems. Complete medical, developmental, and psychiatric evaluations are needed as screening procedures for all abused and neglected children. School records should provide information regarding school performance, behavior, attendance, cognitive capacity, and achievement. Referral for more appropriate educational placement is frequently indicated, as is referral for individual psychotherapy. The goal of psychotherapy is not only to overcome the emotional problems of abuse, but also to facilitate emotional development in a manner that will break the intergenerational cycle of abuse.

## Hospital Management

Hospitals frequently diagnose and report child abuse and neglect. Children are often routinely hospitalized following these reports. Interdisciplinary and interdepartmental child protection teams have been developed by many hospitals to assess cases of child abuse and neglect. These teams cooperate with the state agencies responsible for receiving and investigating child abuse reports, assist in formulating treatment recommendations, and consult with and educate hospital staff. The following case example shows cooperative case management:

### ➤ Case Example

Six-year-old Tom was referred for an evaluation by a child and adolescent psychiatrist when his teacher made a child abuse complaint to the State Central Register for Child Abuse Reports. An evaluation of Tom, his parents, and his sister revealed the following:

Tom is the older of two children, both of whom live with their parents in a two-bedroom apartment. His problems began with the birth of his sister 3 months ago when his teachers noticed a change in his behavior. He began pushing other children and hit a classmate with a metal truck, causing a laceration of the classmate's scalp. When Tom's teacher talked privately to him about his behavior, she noticed what seemed to be cigarette burn marks on Tom's forearms. Tom's sister was "colicky," slept for only short periods of time throughout the day and night, and stopped crying only when her mother held her. Tom's mother became depressed and had little time for Tom. Tom's father, who chain-smoked, took over his care on evenings after day care and on weekends. Tom's father began to drink more than usual, a half bottle of wine each evening, and became increasingly irritable. He argued with his wife over her attention to the infant and the requirement that he take care of Tom. Tom, a bright, curious, active, talkative 6-year-old, asked constant questions and often asked to carry the baby. When his parents said no, he would cry and throw his toys. Since his sister's birth, he also began to wet his pants while playing, to have difficulty falling asleep, and to awake repeatedly during the night with nightmares.

Tom's father was unable to cope with his demands for attention. When Tom persisted with questions, his father would yell, and if drinking and smoking, he would grab Tom and put out his lit cigarette on Tom's arms or chest.

When interviewed, Tom presented as a lively and attractive blue-eyed blond boy dressed in jeans, a T-shirt, and sneakers. He related appropriately and warmly to the interviewer and easily separated from his parents in the waiting room. His intelligence appeared above average, as indicated by his fund of knowledge, vocabulary, and drawings of a person and of geometric forms. About his sister, Tom said, "She's a bad girl. She cries all the time. I get hit and burnt when I cry, but no one hits or burns the baby." When asked about fights at school, he said, "I hit John [his playmate] because he takes my toys." He said he was afraid to go to sleep because he had bad dreams of an old man killing him and of his house being on fire.

Tom's changed behavior included temper tantrums at home, fighting with other children at school, having trouble falling asleep, and wetting himself while playing. These few symptoms are not indicative of a syndrome that would justify the diagnosis of a disorder. Therefore, Tom was given the residual diagnosis of Adjustment Disorder with Mixed Disturbance of Emotions and Conduct.

## ➤ DSM-IV Diagnoses (American Psychiatric Association 1994)

| | |
|---|---|
| Axis I | Adjustment disorder of emotions and conduct |
| Axis II | None |
| Axis III | None |
| Axis IV | Psychosocial Stressors: Physical Abuse |
| | Severity: 5—Extreme (predominantly acute events) |
| Axis V | Current Global Assessment of Functioning (GAF) 50, highest GAF 80 |

## ➤ Treatment Follow-Up

Tom, along with his mother, father, and infant sister, began a family therapy program, coordinated with his school, that included behavioral therapy for Tom and parent training for his mother and father. His father was persuaded to join Alcoholics Anonymous, has stopped drinking, and has been able to control his anger at his son. Tom's mother was treated with antidepressant medication and individual psychotherapy. Four months later, Tom's aggressive behavior ceased. He was doing well with peers and in his academic work, sleeping throughout the night and had stopped having temper tantrums and wetting himself during play. His father and his mother no longer argued over his mother's attention to the infant and the requirement that his father take care of Tom.

## Prevention

There are three types of primary prevention strategies in current use for child maltreatment. The first type is parental competency enhancement such as that provided in parent education programs. The second is the prevention of the onset of maltreating behaviors, by such methods as media campaigns, crisis hotlines, and community and school socialization programs for parents and for adolescents (Prothrow-Stith 1987). The third type is targeting families for programs that increase parent-child contact concomitant with providing family support such as visiting nurses or home-visiting parent aides (Rosenberg and Repucci 1985). The effectiveness of these programs still needs to be adequately studied. There is little prevention outcome research using comparison groups.

A methodologically sophisticated study of high-risk mothers did indicate that simply providing visiting nurses reduced the rates of maltreatment, enhanced the parents' positive perceptions of their infants, improved the health of high-risk mothers, and reduced subsequent prematurity rates, in comparison with the outcomes for those who did not receive these services (Rosenberg and Repucci 1985).

## Role of the Psychiatrist and Other Mental Health Care Providers

Psychiatrists and other mental health care providers are also able to make important contributions to case management in child abuse and neglect by consulting with social service agencies, hospitals, and courts and by establishing and participating in treatment programs designed for these families.

Because children and parents in child maltreatment cases are not routinely screened for psychopathology and substance abuse, the prevalence of psychopathology and substance abuse have probably been frequently underestimated and untreated. In a survey of hospitals with pediatric beds and of CPS in the New York City metropolitan area, Kaplan and Zitrin found that the majority of abused and neglected children and their parents were *not* being assessed by psychiatrists or psychologists (Kaplan and Zitrin 1983a, b). Psychiatrists or psychologists were *not* members of child protection committees in most hospitals surveyed (Kaplan and Zitrin 1983b). In a study of maltreated children and their parents in cases reaching Manhattan Family Court, more than half of these children and more than half of their parents had *not* had diagnostic mental health evaluations by psychiatrists, psychologists, or social workers prior to court proceedings, despite having been known to multiple social and health service care agencies prior to court referral. The initial custody plans of legal guardians for maltreated children in family court proceedings were modified following psychiatric consultations in 21 of 40 cases (Kaplan 1981). Psychiatrists and other mental health care providers are urged to become involved as members of hospital child protection committees. It is also important that psychiatric consultations consisting of evaluations of parents and children, psychological testing of children to screen for developmental and learning disabilities, and regular review of maltreated children's school records be provided routinely by agencies and attorneys involved in planning for these families.

Because child and adolescent mental health treatment compliance depends on parental as well as child and adolescent motivation, the coordination of treatment advocacy efforts by all agencies, including those of social service and health care providers, will often enhance treatment compliance.

## Corporal Punishment

Corporal punishment has been defined by the American Academy of Child and Adolescent Psychiatry (AACAP) as the discipline method in which a supervising adult deliberately inflicts pain upon a child in response to a child's unacceptable behavior and/or inappropriate language. Straus (1991a, 1991b) demonstrated an association between the infliction of corporal punishment and of physical abuse. Prevention of corporal punishment is an important step in violence and abuse prevention. AACAP, the National Congress of Parents and Teachers, the American Medical Association, the American Bar Association, the American Academy of Pediatrics, the National Education

Association, and the National Association of School Psychologists have joined together in calling for an end to this form of punishment by schools. All of these groups oppose teaching children to resolve conflicts by the use of physical force and recommend distrust of those in supervisory or nurturing roles who use violence to control child behavior (American Academy of Child and Adolescent Psychiatry 1988/1990).

## Conclusion

Mental health efforts directed at understanding, preventing, and intervening in child abuse are still in an early stage. Maltreated children, their parents, and their relatives are at great risk for the development of mental disorders, substance abuse, and aggressive behaviors. Psychiatric and other health provider advocacy will enhance prevention efforts for the alleviation of environmental stressors, the cessation of exposure of children to family violence, and an increase in education in parenting techniques and child development for parents and children. In addition, mental health and other health care providers need to advocate for an increase in mental health services and research for child maltreatment. Less than 5% of abused children have treatment resources available in their communities (U.S. Advisory Board on Child Abuse and Neglect 1990).

## Legal Commentary

### ▌ Issues Related to Victims, Other Family Members, and Offenders

The infliction of physical injuries upon children by their parents emerged as a major policy issue only in the 1960s. Following the lead of Dr. C. Henry Kempe and his colleagues, who wrote a seminal article in 1962 on the "battered child syndrome" in the *Journal of the American Medical Association,* the U.S. Children's Bureau convened early in that decade a group of experts who helped develop a model law on the reporting of child abuse.

By 1967 all 50 states had enacted a fairly unique statutory concept: a legal mandate for certain professionals (especially physicians, teachers, and social workers) to report mere suspicions that a child with whom they had professional contact was abused by his or her parents or legal guardian. Few novel state legislative proposals have ever been as quickly or as universally endorsed as these laws. The mandatory reporting laws in place by the late 1960s were progressively strengthened in the 1970s and later by affirming the immunity of professionals who reported their suspicions of child maltreatment in good faith and by extending the reporting obligations to other professionals who come into contact with children and parents, such as psychologists and child care workers.

The intent of the mandatory child abuse reporting laws was to identify maltreated children so that they, and their abusers, could receive proper attention. As the volume of reported cases skyrocketed from about 60,000 in 1974 to approximately 2.5 million by the end of the 1980s (U.S. Advisory Board on Child Abuse and Neglect 1990), the public social service agencies generally responsible for receiving and acting on those reports, known as child protective services (CPS), became the key actors in legal and judicial intervention on behalf of abused children.

The federal Child Abuse Prevention and Treatment Act of 1974 (CAPTA) (42 U.S.C. Sec. 5701 et seq.), has played a modest role over the past 20 years in supporting innovative state activities on behalf of maltreated children, but certainly had little, if any, impact on the rise of reported cases or the strengthening of the basic CPS response to reports. CAPTA funds to the states have simply been too small to make any significant difference in how child welfare agencies have responded to the huge increase in case volume.

In many states, professionals who suspect child abuse have always had the option of reporting to either CPS or a local law enforcement agency (e.g., the police). Today, about half the states require that initial reports of intrafamilial abuse be made directly to a CPS agency, and the other half allow reporting to either a law enforcement agency or CPS agency.

When the reporting obligation can only be legally fulfilled through a report to CPS, many state laws now require that CPS promptly forward information on reports of serious physical and sexual abuse to the police or a prosecutor so that 1) a criminal investigation can ensue, 2) a joint coordinated police-CPS investigation can take place, and 3) assistance can be provided to CPS in determining whether children are in imminent danger of death or serious bodily harm as a result of parental maltreatment, so that, if necessary, the children can be removed from their home on an emergency basis (no court order).

Generally, however, if a CPS case worker determines that a child is in such imminent danger, that worker—without police assistance—has the legal authority to remove the child from the home. With increased fear of violent responses by adults in the child's home, however, CPS workers increasingly seek police assistance for such a removal.

It is important to remember that true child abuse, as defined by law, is always a crime and thus is an appropriate matter for consideration by the criminal justice system. However, that system is not always able or prepared to deal effectively with intervention in sensitive family matters.

Much of the content of a child abuse investigation involves skills that are within the expertise of an appropriately trained police officer. These include the gathering of relevant facts, the observation of the alleged crime scene, the preservation of evidence, and the taking of victim, witness, and occasionally offender statements. However, few law enforcement personnel are specifically trained to understand dysfunctional family dynamics, child development, parent-child bonding and separation issues, or the operation of the foster care system. Police may have the authority to take a child out of his or her home against a parent's wishes and to bring that child to a hospital or protective care setting, but they are unlikely to have appropriate understanding of or direct access to services that can *prevent* the need to remove the child from home.

Social services intercession related to child abuse has become quite complex; CPS investigation and intervention actions are governed both by specialized state statutes and by detailed agency regulations and practice manuals. There are also federal laws, most notably the 1980 Federal Adoption Assistance and Child Welfare Act (Public Law 96-272), that affect the response by CPS. As this book was going to press, Congress was considering action that would either repeal or substantially modify these laws.

Professionals and the general public must realize that CPS has become overwhelmed with the responsibility for investigating child maltreatment reports, particularly in urban areas. There has been documentation of CPS failures to promptly investigate even serious abuse allegations (especially cases in which one parent accuses the other of child abuse). There have also been many cases in which CPS has removed children from their home, school, or neighborhood improperly (or at least without an adequate investigation). In some cases in which CPS had already been involved with a family, a child was re-abused to the point of death or severe bodily harm despite the fact that CPS was supposed to be providing the child with in-home protective supervision.

Most CPS caseworkers are overworked, undertrained, and underpaid. The U.S. Advisory Board on Child Abuse and Neglect, established in 1988, has described the CPS system as being on the verge of collapse, and the problem of child maltreatment in the United States as being a "national emergency" (U.S. Advisory Board on Child Abuse and Neglect 1990). With the public child protection system in such a state of chaos, mistakes are more likely—and negligence by CPS agency staff in their child protection responsibilities is more possible. However, in 1989 the U.S. Supreme Court held in the case of *DeShaney v. Winnebago County Department of Social Services* that a federal court action cannot be brought on the basis of the alleged violation of a child's constitutional rights when a state fails to protect him or her from abuse by a "private actor" (e.g., a parent or stepparent).

Child abuse can, in a way, be viewed on a continuum. At one end is the situation in which a child, on only one occasion, is corporally punished for misbehavior, resulting in the child's suffering some minor physical injury that the parent did not intend. In the middle of the continuum are cases in which parents bring a child to a hospital or a physician's office with head injuries, broken bones, burns, or severe bruises. In such situations, depending upon how parents explain what happened, a reasonable suspicion of child abuse may be raised. At the furthest extreme is the situation in which a child appears to have been repeatedly and systematically beaten or tortured, to the extent that the child is severely harmed, permanently disabled, or dies of those injuries. Most substantiated child abuse falls within the two extreme polarities.

Generally, child abuse reporting laws require the reporting of *any* physical injuries of a child that are suspected of having been inflicted by other than accidental means, *or* in any situation in which a child is believed to have been "harmed" by a parent. Some laws require that the infliction of injury be "willful" and that the child be "endangered" by the inflicted harm. The most severe forms of abuse, likely to result in the criminal prosecution of the abuser, include the torturing, maiming, disfigurement, or mutilation of children, as well as the fracturing of the child's bones, intentional burning of the child, or the causing of injuries that require the child to receive medical treatment. Some state laws also define child abuse in terms of cruelty, malicious and unjustifiable behavior, the infliction of excessive pain, or the use of unreasonable force. Other laws limit child abuse to the infliction of "serious" or "substantial" injury.

It is important to understand that *the likelihood of imminent harm* to a child from parental actions may warrant reporting and legal intervention, even when the child has not yet been physically injured by abuse. The most extreme example of this would be the situation in which a parent fires a gun at the child, but misses. Some forms of parental physical conduct toward a child may not have resulted in physical harm, yet if that behavior were to continue, the child would clearly be in danger of suffering serious injury. Even when a parent's violence is not directed against a child, but (for example) against the child's mother, CPS and/or the police may view the home situation as so dangerous to the child that intervention may be appropriate. However, in such cases, removal of the violent adult from the home (with appropriate restraining orders and criminal proceedings) would generally be preferable to placing the child in foster care.

In certain circumstances, parental physical punishment of children rises to the level of child abuse and is clearly against the law. Corporal punishment of a child typically rises to such a level when it is inflicted with great malice or cruelty, with callous disregard for the safety and well-being of the child, with a lack of regard for the child's physical vulnerability, or with a deliberate intention to cause injury to the child. A disciplinary slap on the clothed bottom of an 8-year-old by a parent is not legally child abuse, but a punch to the face of a 3-year-old by the parent most certainly *is* child abuse.

Many state laws specify that "reasonable" forms of corporal punishment inflicted by a parent (or one acting *in loco parentis*) is not child abuse. The key word in whether such a defense to child abuse will be accepted is the word "reasonable." In making the determination of reasonableness for legal purposes (for both child protective and criminal justice purposes) a court looks at the age, size, and physical build of the child as well as the parent; the type of child misbehavior that generated the parental disciplinary response (and whether one was disproportionate to the other); whether any implement was used in the punishment; the nature of the child's injuries; and whether the disciplinary action was an isolated one or was repeated over time.

In cases involving allegations of physical abuse, medical testimony will typically be critical to establishing that the child's injuries were not the result of an accident (such as a child's fall) but rather must have been the result of harm inflicted by an adult. If the judge in a child protective proceeding determines that the child was abused, it may not be necessary for anyone to establish *who* committed the abuse for the court to take protective jurisdiction over the child (e.g., declaring the child to be abused or a child in need of care). In a criminal child abuse proceeding, it will be necessary to prove beyond a reasonable doubt that the person *accused* actually committed the abuse, or assisted in its commission.

Once a civil child protective petition or criminal charges have been filed, the court may order, or the attorneys may request, mental health evaluations of the alleged perpetrator, the other parent or adults in the home, and the child. These evaluations may be paid for by the court, using its own resources or that of a mental health program associated with the court, or a public child protective service or mental health agency may absorb the costs of the evaluations. In cases in which a diagnostic workup is needed for the child, a crime victim compensation program or crime victim assistance program may be tapped to pay for these costs. In addition, the court may have the authority to order the alleged perpetrator of the abuse to pay for any costs connected with the evaluation or treatment of the child victim.

In some civil and criminal child abuse cases, a central issue for the court will be the culpability (i.e., the legal responsibility) of the child's nonabusive parent. In these cases, prosecutors may allege that a child's mother stood by and did nothing while the abuse occurred, either within or outside her immediate presence. By not stopping the abuse, calling the police, taking her child(ren) and leaving the perpetrator, or reporting her child's abuse to anyone, it may be claimed, the mother so neglected the protection of her child that she should be held partly responsible for that child's abuse.

However, in cases in which maternal culpability for the abuse of a child by another is alleged, the often simultaneous abuse of the child's mother by a battering partner—and her inability to leave the batterer— are important issues to consider and may mitigate or legally eliminate the mother's culpability in some cases. As more is learned about the connections between child abuse and domestic violence, it becomes clearer that CPS case workers and other professionals working with mothers of abused children should be providing mothers with information on where they can turn for help if they themselves are abused.

There are more likely to be witnesses to abusive acts in physical than in sexual abuse cases. Occasionally, these witnesses will be siblings of the maltreated child. Testifying against a parent, or the mother's paramour, will often be extremely difficult for a child. The decision of the prosecutor to call the abused child or a sibling to testify is one that should be made in consultation with child mental health professionals.

In all civil child protective proceedings, the court is required to appoint either a guardian ad litem (GAL) or legal counsel to represent the child. The GAL is generally responsible for protecting the best interests of the child in the court proceedings. Legal counsel is more likely to be appointed for children in certain cases, such as those involving older children, in which legally trained advocates are needed to help articulate their own wishes and needs. In some cases, the court may appoint both a GAL and an attorney for the child. As for the qualifications and background of the GAL: depending on state law, this person may be an attorney, social worker, or, increasingly, a specially trained volunteer lay citizen advocate. In hundreds of communities throughout the country, there are special Court-Appointed Special Advocate (CASA) programs that coordinate, train, and supervise the work of these volunteer child advocates.

A GAL or CASA will not be obligated to follow the strict rules for attorneys regarding the confidentiality of communications that fall under the lawyer-client privilege, but rather will have to follow whatever confidentiality rules the court has set for court-appointed GALs or CASAs. Where an attorney is appointed to represent a child, he or she will be strictly bound by the lawyer-client privilege, as well as the rules governing the professional responsibilities of lawyers generally. An increasing trend, although still generally rare, is the appointment by a judge in a criminal child abuse case of a GAL for the child victim or a child witness. Whether in juvenile court or criminal court, child mental health professionals should always work closely with court-appointed advocates for children in connection with any judicial proceedings affecting the abused child.

The mental health professional will also be likely to interact with other attorneys involved with the child abuse case. In a criminal proceeding, these will of course include the prosecutor and the defense counsel. In the civil child protective proceeding, the parents will probably be represented by counsel (possibly by two different counsels, given the potential conflicting interests between the abusing and non-abusing parent), and the CPS agency should be represented either by their own counsel or by the district attorney, county or state's attorney, or municipal attorney.

In many states, the legislature has established a broadly based multidisciplinary team that has either the discretion or the mandate to review child abuse cases. Some of these teams may be attached to hospitals; others may be based in children's advocacy centers. At one extreme, these multidisciplinary inquiries generally result when a child dies from injuries sustained from one or more assaults. In such cases, there is an emerging trend to present the known facts to a specially composed child fatality review team or committee. These review bodies will often make decisions concerning legal actions that should be taken involving the child's parents and siblings. At the other end of the continuum is review of serious, but not life-threatening, physical abuse cases by a child protection team. Multidisciplinary teams or committees will typically involve a physician, a social worker, and a representative of the criminal prosecutor.

It is not inappropriate for a mental health professional who has been involved with the child's family to be consulted during these multidisciplinary review processes. When a team of professionals from various public and private agencies seeks to get information from a mental health professional who has worked with a child and family, the issue of breach of confidentiality is raised. Although the therapist-patient legal privilege is generally abrogated for the purposes of mandatory reporting, as well as when the therapist is called to testify in a child abuse court proceeding, the sharing of confidential client information with team members may be more of a problem. Clinicians should consult with an attorney about how their state laws address the issue of privacy of client information and patient records. The trend in the law is to promote, rather than inhibit, the sharing of relevant personal history and family information among professionals and agencies seeking to protect children from abuse and neglect.

Once a case of child abuse is before the court, a mental health professional who has evaluated the child, an alleged perpetrator, or other family members may be called to testify by the prosecutor or petitioning agency's attorney, the parent's attorney, or the child's attorney or GAL. The testimony can be sought at a variety of stages of the case.

The first stage is a preliminary hearing, where the juvenile court might need expert testimony related to a party's mental status and parenting capacity to determine whether the child should be temporarily placed in foster care. The second stage is the trial itself (called the adjudicatory hearing in juvenile court), where the testimony might focus on an admission of abuse made to the mental health professional or information concerning a parent's state of mind that might be relevant to whether an injury was intentionally inflicted. The third stage is the disposition hearing (called the sentencing hearing in criminal court), where the testimony might focus on treatment recommendations and prognosis, as well as the extent to which the perpetrator presents a danger to the community and thus should be incarcerated. Finally, the mental health professional might be asked to testify at a postdisposition review hearing, or a termination of parental rights proceeding, where the issue could be the progress (or lack thereof) of the treatment of the parents and child and the likelihood that a parent will have the capacity in the foreseeable future to provide adequate care for the child.

## ▌ Guidance for Mental Health Professionals and Practitioners

The term *child abuse* has cultural/social, professional, and, of course, legal meaning. What a diagnostician or therapist considers acts of child maltreatment may not correspond with how a state legislature or the courts have defined or construed those acts. Clinicians must obtain a copy of the state child abuse reporting law for every state in which they practice, as well as the juvenile court law that defines child abuse for child protective intervention purposes, and the criminal law that defines child abuse.

In some states, the trigger of a child abuse reporting requirement is the examination or observation of a child in one's professional capacity (e.g., the child has been brought into a hospital emergency room or the school nurse's office). In many other states, it will be *any* information—from whatever source—that would lead a reasonable person to suspect that child abuse has occurred. Furthermore, some states will narrowly define child abuse to cover only maltreatment allegedly committed by a family member, while other states do not limit the reporting of child abuse to that which occurred in intrafamilial settings. Thus, in the latter states, information related to a child's abuse by someone in a child care, school, or recreational setting, or by a neighbor, may have to be reported. Again, because the facts that precipitate a reporting obligation vary so much, it is essential for mental health professionals to consult with legal experts on child protection in their states.

The failure to report child abuse as required by state law may subject the professional to civil liability. The California case of *Landeros v. Flood* (1976) is commonly cited as a leading judicial precedent for holding professionals liable for damages pursuant to their failing to properly diagnose and report child abuse. In most states, laws also provide criminal misdemeanor penalties for professionals covered by the mandatory child abuse reporting law who fail to exercise their statutory reporting obligation. There is at least one appellate court decision, the Florida case of *Fischer v. Metcalf* (1989), affirming the conviction of a psychiatrist for failure to report.

Many professionals who are required to report suspected child abuse fear legal reprisals from parents who claim that their privacy was invaded and/or that they were wrongfully accused and exposed to public humiliation. Generally, reporters of abuse are protected by state law that provides immunity related to child abuse reporting.

Many states qualify that immunity is predicated on the report's being made in good faith and on a reasonable suspicion that abuse occurred. This has not been a difficult standard for professionals to meet when they have been sued. Some states go even further and protect the reporter from liability even if the report was false or was made in bad faith. However, because of a growing consciousness that some reports are made willfully and maliciously—and are therefore knowingly false—a number of states have created new criminal offenses for the intentionally false reporting of child abuse.

There are some questions about the extent to which immunity laws protect designated mandatory reporters for actions beyond the initial making of the report. For example: 1) a mental health professional may be asked to serve on a multidisciplinary child protection team that discusses information relevant to a child's case, 2) the professional may be asked to provide information from psychiatric records to aid in a CPS or law enforcement investigation of a child abuse allegation, 3) the professional may be asked by CPS or the police to question the child or conduct a diagnostic evaluation, and 4) the professional may be asked to testify in a court proceeding that results from the initial making of the report. Again, state laws and court decisions vary in the scope of immunity protections, and individual legal consultation on this subject is very important. As a rule, however, the trend in the law is to construe immunity protections broadly as an integral part of state child abuse policy.

A potential area of child abuse liability, where there is as yet little litigation, involves harm to third parties related to the professional's involvement in a child abuse case. For example, a mental health professional may be treating an adult child abuse offender and be aware of facts suggesting the continued danger that this adult poses to certain children specifically—or children in general. The failure to provide this information to the parents affected, or to the proper authorities, can result in liability if the adult later abuses other children. Likewise, the treatment of an abused child who may, for example, present a physical danger to other children in a school or foster home can warrant certain protective disclosures to the school principal or foster care agency. This duty to warn, although legally speculative, is a natural extension of the principle of liability described in the seminal California case of *Tarasoff v. Regents of the University of California* (1976).

Under the laws of many states, a statutory psychotherapist-patient privilege may prevent a mental health professional from testifying in court as to facts disclosed in the course of the privileged relationship. However, the child abuse reporting laws of most states specifically eliminate (i.e., abrogate) most legally privileged communications. The common exceptions to this abrogation rule are the priest-penitent and attorney-client privileges, which few state laws abrogate for any reason. It is important to stress that the law on abrogation of privileged communications is a different law from that requiring mandatory reports of suspected child maltreatment (although these laws generally can be found in close proximity in most state collections of statutes).

Given the variations in state laws related to privileged communications and their abrogation, it is essential for mental health professionals to get specific legal advice about the effects of the laws of the states in which they practice. If the professional's testimony is sought concerning the outcome of a court-ordered mental health evaluation, the issue of privileged communications should not be relevant. Many state laws give judges the authority to order that parties to a judicial proceeding undergo a psychiatric or psychological evaluation. When such an examination has been court-ordered, the written report and oral testimony related to it should be admissible without regard to the existence of a statutory privilege in that state.

When the privileged communications are deemed abrogated, or do not apply to the testimony at all, the scope of what can be disclosed is likely to be very broad, including not merely the mental health professional's testimony, but also his or her written records and reports. The reason for this is that in cases of child abuse, the parent's and child's right to privacy and confidentiality must yield to the greater public interest in the protection of the safety and well-being of the child.

Another way in which state laws encourage the reporting of child abuse is to tie training on child abuse and compliance with reporting obligations to professional licensing and peer disciplinary actions. Some states require certain licensed professionals to be educated in child abuse reporting. Others specify that nonreporting may lead to a referral to the state professional disciplinary board.

(See Appendix H for legal resources.)

# References

Alfaro J: Summary report on the relationship between child abuse and neglect and later socially deviant behavior. New York, Select Committee on Child Abuse, 1978

American Academy of Child and Adolescent Psychiatry: Guidelines for the Clinical Evaluation of Child and Adolescent Sexual Abuse. Washington, DC, American Academy of Child and Adolescent Psychiatry, 1988/1990

American Psychiatric Association: Diagnostic and Statistical Manual of Mental Disorders, 4th Edition. Washington, DC, American Psychiatric Association, 1994

Barth R, Snowden L, Broeck E, et al: Contributors to reunification or permanent out of home care for physically abused children. Journal of Social Service Research, 9:31–45, Winter1985/Spring 1986

Belsky J: Child maltreatment: an ecological integration. Am Psychol 35:320–335, 1980

Bland R, Orn H: Psychiatric disorders, spouse abuse and child abuse. Acta Psychiatr Belg 86:444–449, 1986

Braun BG: Issues in the psychotherapy of multiple personality disorder, in Treatment of Multiple Personality Disorder. Edited by Braun BG. Washington, DC, American Psychiatric Press, 1986, pp 1–28

Breiner SJ: Observations on the abuse of women and children. Psychol Rep 70:153–154, 1992

Caffey J: Multiple fractures in the longbones of infants suffering from chronic subdural hematoma. American Journal of Roentgenology 56:163–173, 1946

Council on Scientific Affairs, American Medical Association: AMA diagnostic and treatment guidelines concerning child abuse and neglect. JAMA 254:796–800, 1985

Cuddy MA, Belicki K: Nightmare frequency and related sleep disturbance as indicators of a history of sexual abuse. Dreaming Journal of the Association for the Study of Dreams 2:15–22, 1992

Daro D: Confronting Child Abuse: Research for Effective Program Design. New York, The Free Press, 1988

Daro D, Mitchel L: Current Trends in Child Abuse Reporting and Fatalities: The Results of the 1989 Annual Fifty State Survey. Chicago, IL, National Center on Child Abuse Prevention Research, 1990

DeShaney v Winnebago County Department of Social Services, 489 U.S. 189 (1989)

Deykin E, Alpert J, McNamarra J: a pilot study of the effect of exposure to child abuse or neglect on suicidal behavior. Am J Psychiatry 142:1299–1303, 1985

Eckenrode J, Powers J, Doris J: Substantiation of child abuse and neglect reports. J Consult Clin Psychol 56:9–16, 1988

Estroff T, Herrera C, Gaines R, et al: Maternal psychopathology and perception of child behavior in psychiatrically referred and child maltreatment families. J Am Acad Child Psychiatry 23:649–652, 1985

Family Court Act. McKinney's Consol. Laws Book 29A, Part 1. St. Paul, MN, West Publishing Co., 1976

Farber E, Kinast C, McCord W: Violence in families of adolescent runaways. Child Abuse Negl 8:295–299, 1984

Finkelhor D, Williams L, Burns N, et al: Sexual Abuse in Day Care: a National Study, Final Report. Durham, NH, Family Research Laboratory, University of New Hampshire, March 1988

Garbarino J, Ebata A: The significance of ethnic and cultural differences in child maltreatment. Journal of Marriage and the Family 11:733–783, 1983

Garbarino J, Sebes J, Schellenbach D: Families at risk for destructive parent-child relations in adolescence. Child Dev 55:174–183, 1984

Gould C, Cozolino LJ: Ritual abuse, multiplicity, and mind control. Special Issue: Satanic ritual abuse: the current state of knowledge. Journal of Psychology and Theology 20:194–196, 1992

Green A: Psychopathology of abused children. J Am Acad Child Psychiatry 17:92–97, 1978a

Green A: Self-destructive behavior in battered children. Am J Psychiatry 135:579–582, 1978b

Hawton K, Roberts J, Goodwin G: The risk of child abuse among mothers who attempt suicide. Br J Psychiatry 146:486–489, 1985

Herjanic B, Reich W: Development of a structured psychiatric interview of children: agreement between child and parent on individual symptoms. J Abnorm Psychol 10:307–324, 1982

Hudson PS: Therapy with children who have been ritualistically abused. Paper presented at annual meeting of the Child Abuse Prevention Council, Contra Costa, CA, May 1989

Illfeld F: Current social stressors and symptoms of depression. Am J Psychiatry 134:161–166, 1977

Jones DP: Ritualism and child sexual abuse. Child Abuse Negl 15:163–170, 1991

Jonker F, Jonker-Bakker P: Experiences with ritualist child sexual abuse: a case study from the Netherlands. Child Abuse Negl 15:191–196, 1991

Kaplan S: Child psychiatric consultation to attorneys representing abused and neglected children. Bull Am Acad Psychiatry Law 9:140–148, 1981

Kaplan S, Zitrin A: Psychiatrists and child abuse, I: case assessment by CPS. J Am Acad Child Psychiatry 22:253–256, 1983a

Kaplan S, Zitrin A: Psychiatrists and child abuse, II: case assessment by hospitals. J Am Acad Child Psychiatry 22:257–261, 1983b

Kaplan S, Pelcovitz D, Salzinger S: Psychopathology of parents of abused and neglected children. J Am Acad Child Psychiatry 22:238–244, 1983

Kaplan S, Montero G, Pelcovitz D: Psychopathology of abused and neglected children. Paper presented at International Congress of Child Psychiatry and Allied Professions, Paris, France, July 1986

Kaplan W: Runaway youth: psychiatric aspects. Child Psychiatry Grand Rounds Presentation, North Shore University Hospital, February 1986

Kashani JH, Hoeper EW, Beck N: Personality, Psychiatric disorders, and parental attitude among a community sample of adolescents. J Am Acad Child Adolesc Psychiatry 26:879–885, 1987a

Kashani J, Beck N, Hoeper E, et al: Psychiatric disorders in a community sample of adolescents. Am J Psychiatry 144:584–588, 1987b

Kaufman J, Zigler E: Do abused children become abusive parents? Am J Orthopsychiatry 57:186–192, 1987

Keller M, Beardslee W, Dorer D: Impact of severity and chronicity of parental affective illness on adaptive functioning and psychopathology in the children. Arch Gen Psychiatry 43:930–937, 1986

Kelly SJ: Ritualistic abuse of children: dynamics and impact. Cultic Studies Journal 5:228–236, 1988

Kempe CH, Silverman FN, Steele BF, et al: The battered child syndrome. JAMA 181:17–24, 1962

Kinard E: Emotional development in physically abused children. Am J Orthopsychiatry 50:689–696, 1980

Kline D, Christiansen J: Educational and Psychological Problems of Abused Children, Final Report. ERIC (Educational Resources Information Center [microfiche]), No ED121041, 1975

Kluft RP: On giving consultations to therapists treating MPD. Dissociation 1:23–29, 1988

Krugman RD: Editorial. Child Abuse Negl 15:161, 1991

Lanning K: Commentary, ritual abuse: another view. Child Abuse Negl 15:171–173, 1991

Lewis D: Biopsychosocial characteristics of children who later murder: a prospective study. Am J Psychiatry 142:1161–1167, 1985

Lewis D, Shanok S, Pincus J, et al: Violent juvenile delinquents: psychiatric, neurological, psychological, and abuse factors. J Am Acad Child Psychiatry 18:307–319, 1979

Libbey R, Bybee R: The physical abuse of adolescents. Journal of Social Issues 35:101–126, 1979

Lloyd DW: Ritual Child Abuse: Where Do We Go From Here? (National Center on Child Abuse and Neglect publication.) Washington, DC, U.S. Government Printing Office, 1990

Lourie I: Family dynamics and the abuse of adolescents: a case from a developmental phase specific model of child abuse. Child Abuse Negl: 967–974, 1979

Main M, Goldwyn R: Predicting Rejection of her Infant Son from Mother's Representation of her Own Experience: Implications for the Psychopathology. Newbury Park, Sage Publications, 1988

Martin H, Beezley P: Behavioral observations of abused children. Dev Med Child Neurol 13:373–387, 1977

Paulson MJ, Schwemer FT, Bendel RB: Clinical application of the P, Ma, and (PH) experimental MMPI scales for further understanding of abusive parents. J Clin Psychol 32:558–564, 1976

Pelcovitz D, Kaplan S, Samit C, et al: Adolescent abuse: family structure and implications for treatment. J Am Acad Child Psychiatry 23:85–90, 1984

Pfeffer CR: The Suicidal Child. New York, Guilford, 1986, p 61

President's Child Safety Partnership: a Report to the President. Final Report (190-893-814/70170). Washington, DC, U.S. Government Printing Office, 1987

Prothrow-Stith D: Violence Prevention Curriculum for Adolescents. Newton, MA, Educational Development Center, 1987

Putnam FW: Dissociative phenomena, in Review of Psychiatry, Vol 10. Edited by Tasman A, Goldfinger S. Washington, DC, American Psychiatric Press, 1991, pp 159–174

Reich W, Herjanic B, Weiner Z, et al: Development of a structured psychiatric interview for children: agreement on diagnosis comparing child and parent interviews. J Abnorm Child Psychol 10:302–306, 1982

Rosenberg M, Repucci ND: Primary prevention of child abuse. J Consult Clin Psychol 53:576–585, 1985

Rotheram MJ, Bradley R: Evaluation of imminent danger for suicide among youth. Am J Orthopsychiatry 57:102–110, 1987

Rutter M: Parent-child separation: psychological effects on the children. J Child Psychol Psychiatry 12:233–260, 1971

Rutter M, Chadwick O, Shaffer D: Head Injury in Developmental Neuropsychiatry, Edited by Rutter M. New York, Guilford, 1983

Salzinger S, Kaplan S, Artemyeff C: Mother's personal social network and child maltreatment. J Abnorm Psychol 22:253–256, 1983

Salzinger S, Kaplan S, Pelcovitz D, et al: Parent teacher assessment of children's behavior in child maltreating families. J Am Acad Child Psychiatry 23:58–64, 1984

Salzinger S, Feldman R, Hammer M, et al: The effects of physical abuse on children's social relationships. Child Dev 64:169–187, 1993

Shaffer D: a critical look at suicide prevention in adolescence. Address to the Society for Adolescent Psychiatry, New York, April 1987

Shaffer D: Youth suicide, epidemiology, risk factors, prevention and biology. Presentation, North Shore University Hospital-Cornell University Medical College, December 1989

Shaffer D, Fisher P: The epidemiology of suicide in children and adolescents. J Child Psychol Psychiatry 15:275–291, 1974

Smith S, Hanson R, Nobel S: Parents of battered babies: a controlled study. BMJ 4:388–391, 1973

Spinetta J, Rigler D: The child-abusing parent: a psychological review. Psychol Bull 77:296–304, 1972

Steele BF, Pollack C: a psychiatric study of parents who abuse infants and small children, in The Battered Child. Edited by Heifer RE, Kempe CH. Chicago, IL, University of Chicago Press, 1968

Straus M: Discipline and deviance: physical punishment of children and violence and other crime in adulthood. Social Problems 38:133–154, 1991a

Straus M: New theories and old canards about family violence research. Social Problems 38:180–197, 1991b

Straus M, Gelles R: Societal change and change in family violence from 1975 to 1985 as revealed by two national surveys. Journal of Marriage and the Family 48:465–479, 1986

Straus M, Gelles R, Steinmetz S: Behind Closed Doors: Violence in the American Family. New York, Anchor Press, 1980

Tarasoff v Regents of the University of California, 551 P.2d 334 (CA 1976)

Truscott D: Intergenerational transmissions of violent behavior in adolescent males. Aggressive Behavior 18:327–335, 1992

U.S. Advisory Board on Child Abuse and Neglect: Child Abuse and Neglect: Critical First Steps in Response to a National Emergency. Washington, DC, U.S. Government Printing Office, 1990

U.S. Department of Health and Human Services: National Study of the Incidence and Severity of Child Abuse and Neglect (OHDS 81-30325). Washington, DC, U.S. Government Printing Office, 1981

U.S. Department of Health and Human Services: Study Findings: Study of National Incidence and Prevalence of Child Abuse and Neglect. Washington, DC, U.S. Government Printing Office, 1988

U.S. Department of Health and Human Services, National Center on Child Abuse and Neglect: Child Maltreatment 1993: Reports from the States to the National Center on Child Abuse and Neglect. Washington, DC, U.S. Government Printing Office, 1995

Weissman M, Prusoff B, Gammon G, et al: Psychopathology of the children (ages 6–18) of depressed and normal parents. J Am Acad Child Psychiatry 23:78–84, 1984

Widom CS: Child abuse, neglect, and adult behavior: research design and findings on criminality, violence, and child abuse. Am J Orthopsychiatry 59: 355–367, 1989

Wolfe D: Implications for Child Development and Psychopathology. Newbury Park, CA, Sage, 1987, p 12

Wolfe D: Child abusive parents: an empirical review and analysis. Psychol Bull 97:462–482, 1985

Wolkind S, Rutter M: Children who have been "in care": an epidemiological study. J Child Psychol Psychiatry 14:97–105, 1973

Wolkind S, Rutter M: Separation, loss and family relationships, in Child and Adolescent Psychiatry: Modern Approaches, 2nd Edition. Edited by Rutter M, Hersov L. Oxford, England, Blackwell Scientific, 1985

Young WC, Sachs RG, Braun BG, et al: Patients reporting ritual abuse in childhood: a clinical syndrome. Child Abuse Negl 15:181–189, 1991

# CHAPTER 2

# Child and Adolescent Neglect and Emotional Maltreatment

*Hershel D. Rosenzweig, M.D.*
*Sandra J. Kaplan, M.D.*

Child and adolescent neglect and emotional maltreatment overlap in many areas. In this chapter, although we discuss the topics separately, we are aware of the importance of the interaction of all types of neglect and maltreatment.

## Neglect

### ▋ Definition

Giovannoni (1988) said of child neglect that, whereas abuse was an act of commission, neglect was one of omission. Neglect is perpetrated by caretakers who fail to fulfill their obligations to children. Neglect occurs primarily 1) when there is a parenting or caretaker problem, 2) when there is social deviance—such as substance abuse, mental retardation, mental illness, or criminality—that is secondary to parenting or caretaker problems, and 3) when physical abuse or sexual abuse of the child exists.

Neglect has been categorized further as physical neglect, educational neglect, and emotional neglect (U.S. Department of Health and Human Services 1988).

# ■ Types

## *Physical*

**Refusal of health care.**   Failure to provide or allow needed care in accord with recommendation of a competent health care professional for a physical injury, illness, medical condition, or impairment.

**Delay in health care.**   Failure to seek timely and appropriate medical care for a serious health problem that any reasonable layperson would recognize as needing professional medical attention.

**Abandonment.**   Desertion of a child without arranging for reasonable care and supervision. This category includes cases in which children are not claimed within two days, and cases in which children are left by parents or parent substitutes who give no (or false) information about their whereabouts.

**Expulsion.**   Other blatant refusals of custody, such as permanent or indefinite expulsion of a child from the home without adequate arrangement for care by others, or refusal to accept custody of a returned runaway.

**Other custody issues.**   Custody-related forms of inattention to the child's needs other than those covered by abandonment or expulsion. For example, repeated shuttling of a child from one household to another because of apparent unwillingness to maintain custody, or chronically and repeatedly leaving a child with others for days or weeks at a time.

**Inadequate supervision.**   Child left unsupervised or inadequately supervised for an extended period of time or allowed to remain away from home overnight without the parent or parent substitute knowing (or attempting to determine) the child's whereabouts.

**Other physical neglect.**   Conspicuous inattention to avoidable hazards in the home; inadequate nutrition, clothing, or hygiene; and other forms of reckless disregard of the child's safety and welfare, such as driving with the child while intoxicated, leaving a young child unattended in a motor vehicle, and so forth.

## Educational

**Permitted chronic truancy.**   Habitual truancy averaging at least 5 days a month was classifiable under this form of maltreatment if the parent or guardian had been informed of the problem and had not attempted to intervene.

**Failure to enroll/other truancy.**   Failure to register or to enroll a child of mandatory school age, causing the child to miss at least one month of school; or a pattern of keeping a school-age child home for nonlegitimate reasons (e.g., to work, to care for siblings, etc.) an average of at least 3 days a month.

**Inattention to special educational need.**   Refusal to allow or failure to obtain recommended remedial educational services, or neglect in obtaining or following through with treatment for a child's diagnosed learning disorder or other special educational need without reasonable cause.

## Emotional

The National Center of Child Abuse Study (U.S. Department of Health and Human Services 1988) defined emotional neglect as a parent's providing a child inadequate nurturing and affection, exposing the child to chronic or extreme abuse of the parent's partner, allowing the child to misuse drugs or alcohol, allowing other maladaptive behavior, or refusing psychological care to the child.

# ▍ Incidence

The 1993 Child Maltreatment Reports from the States to the Naitonal Center on Child Abuse and Neglect stated that nearly half the 1,018,692 children documented as maltreated were neglected (U.S. Department of Health and Human Services 1995).

# ▍ Psychopathology of Neglected Children and Adolescents

The emotional and behavioral sequelae of neglect have been studied even less than has child abuse. Egeland (1985), in one of the few studies of child neglect, reported that physically neglected children at 12 months are more likely than nonneglected children to have insecure attachments. At 24 months, they are more likely to be noncompliant and easily frustrated, as compared to controls. When they reach 42 months they are rated as more likely to have low self-esteem and self-assertion, less flexibility, and less self-control, and to have a difficult time dealing with frustration. They also lack enthusiasm on educational tasks and are more dependent. Other problems surface in elementary school such as attentional problems and greater internalizing behaviors than children in control groups. Neglected children are also more socially isolated and in general experience more daily stress than nonmaltreated children (Williamson et al. 1991). The neglected children were also found more than the control-group children to show declines in cognitive testing, insecure attachment, avoidance of emotional contact, depression, and aggressive behavior.

In another study, Ethier et al. (1992) asserted that neglected children often assume a parental role in relation to their parents. Eckenrode et al. reported that maltreated children perform significantly below their nonmaltreated peers on standardized tests and receive lower grades. They are also more likely to repeat a grade. Moreover, neglected children have a high amount of discipline referrals and suspensions. Of the various types of maltreated children studied, neglected children showed the poorest outcomes on academic performance, and physically abused children demonstrated the most discipline problems (Eckenrode et al. 1993).

## ▮ Psychopathology of Neglectful Parents

There have been few studies of the mental health of neglectful parents. Williamson et al. (1991) contend that adolescent neglect is primarily associated with extrafamilial difficulties. Nay et al. (1992) attribute poor parental care to a number of general factors: marital problems, immaturity, alcohol abuse, unemployment, drug abuse, and financial problems. Aragona and Eyberg (1981) found that neglectful mothers use more direct commands, use less verbal praise or acknowledgment, and are more critical when interacting with their children than nonneglectful mothers. Ethier et al. (1992) found neglectful mothers to be socially isolated women who are even more financially disadvantaged than are physically abusive parents.

Maternal depression was reported by Zuravin (1988) to be associated more often with physical child neglect than with physical child abuse, whereas Williamson et al. (1991) found adolescent physical abuse strongly linked to rigid family relations and poor maternal understanding of child development and to adolescent externalizing behaviors. Taylor et al. (1991) showed that neglectful parents tend to have intellectual impairments, as revealed by low IQ scores.

Spouse abuse, to which children are often exposed, has been redefined as a form of emotional neglect (U.S. Department of Health and Human Services 1988). Parents who abuse their spouses also have been found frequently to abuse drugs or alcohol (Kaplan 1989). Their nonviolent spouses usually have depressive disorders (Kaplan et al. 1988).

## ▌ Assessment of Neglected Children and Adolescents

### *Physical Examination Findings*

The following have been suggested by the Council on Scientific Affairs of the American Medical Association (1985) as typical physical findings of neglected children:

1. *Physical neglect.* Malnutrition, repeated pica, constant fatigue, poor hygiene, and clothing inappropriate for weather or setting.
2. *Medical neglect.* Lack of appropriate medical care for chronic illness, absence of appropriate immunizations or medications, absence of dental care, absence of necessary prostheses such as eyeglasses or hearing aid, discharge from treatment against medical advice.
3. *Emotional neglect.* Delays in physical development and failure to thrive.

### *History*

Not all sources of neglect are obvious. Therefore, in order to ensure successful exploration of several harmful patterns, one must elicit careful histories of many specific areas that may be deficient in caretaking. This effort must go beyond seeking evidence of mental disorder and substance abuse in the children or adolescents and their parents. It includes obtaining information on family supervision schedules for the children or adolescents, on the identity of caretakers, on school attendance, on medical care history, and on personal hygiene routines. Successful exploration of harmful patterns also includes observing the adequacy of child or adolescent nutrition, growth, attire, and housing (according to parental economic ability to provide housing). Homelessness is not child or adolescent neglect if parents are financially unable to afford adequate housing.

### Protocols for Child and Adolescent Neglect Case Assessment

All agencies that provide services to children or adolescents—in health care, law enforcement, social service, and education settings—should have protocols in place to assist in the assessment and management of child or adolescent neglect. (See Appendix C for protocol resources.)

## ▌ Treatment of Neglect

### Children or Adolescents

Individual, group, or family therapy, with or without pharmacotherapy, and substance abuse treatment regimens may be appropriate for the neglected child or adolescent, depending on diagnosis and context. Poor school attendance, learning problems, and lack of home supervision of schoolwork are often problems. Therefore, attention to educational remediation is often a necessary component of a treatment plan.

### Parents

Individual, group, family, and marital therapy; pharmacotherapy; and substance abuse treatment may be appropriate for neglectful parents, depending on their diagnoses and situation. Other services are often required such as obtaining housing, food stamps, health care, transportation, financial resources, and vocational rehabilitation. Behavior modification techniques as well as child development education are necessary parts of learning and treatment for these parents. Case management with an effort to coordinate care provided by all agencies involved with each family is also required in order to provide maximum advocacy for enhanced parenting, and to avoid duplication, omission, and conflicts in agency efforts.

> **Case Example**

John, age 10, and Sam, age 8, were reported as educationally neglected to the New York State Department of Social Services by their school. They had each missed 30 days of school during a 6-month school period. Investigation by the Department of Social Services documented neglect due to failure of their widowed 44-year-old engineer father, Mr. B, to arrange for their school attendance. They and their father were referred by Social Services to an outpatient psychiatric program for assessment and treatment. Both boys were diagnosed as having separation anxiety disorders. Their father was diagnosed as having a major depressive episode.

## ➤ Treatment Plan

The following treatment plan was developed by the psychiatric team in collaboration with the Child Protective Services (CPS) of the New York State Department of Social Services:

1. Individual psychotherapy and antidepressant medication was arranged for Mr. B, the boys' father.
2. Individual psychotherapy was arranged for both Sam and John.
3. Family therapy was arranged for John, Sam, and their father. The therapy emphasized establishing appropriate times of separation for the boys from their father, enhancing their father's understanding of parenting techniques and of child development, and enriching the family's social network.
4. The Department of Social Services placed a homemaker in the home to assist the father in organizing his household and in developing a child care routine, including school attendance, for Sam and John.
5. Both boys were referred for after-school day care.

As a result of treatment, Mr. B's depression remitted. Both boys returned to school, and their separation anxiety subsided. Socialization of the boys and their father increased with the participation of John, Sam, and Mr. B in the day care center's programs for parents and children. Psychotherapy continued for 18 months.

---

# Emotional Maltreatment

## ▌ Emotional Abuse

Emotional abuse has been defined by Garbarino in a classification oriented toward child development as a pattern of psychically destructive behavior inflicted by an adult on a child. This pattern may take five forms: rejecting, isolating, terrorizing, ignoring, or corrupting (Garbarino et al. 1986).

Table 2–1, adapted from the Study of the National Incidence and Prevalence of Child Abuse and Neglect (U.S. Department of Health and Human Services 1988), provides information on the incidence of specific forms of emotional abuse in the United States in 1986.

Types of emotional abuse are defined as follows:

### Close Confinement (Tying or Binding and Other Forms)

Tortuous restriction of movement, as by tying a child's arms or legs together or binding a child to a chair, bed, or other object, or confining a child to an enclosed area (such as a closet) as a means of punishment.

### Verbal or Emotional Assault

Habitual patterns of belittling, denigrating, scapegoating, or other nonphysical forms of overtly hostile or rejecting treatment, as well as threats of other forms of maltreatment (such as threats of beating, sexual assault, abandonment, etc.).

### Other or Unknown Abuse

Overtly punitive, exploitative, or abusive treatment other than (that) specified under other forms of abuse, or unspecified abusive treat-

| Table 2–1. | Totals and incidence of specific forms of emotional abuse during 1986 in the United States | |
|---|---|---|
| Form | Rates per 1,000 children | Totals[a] |
| Close confinement | 0.1 | 11,100 |
| Verbal or emotional assault | 2.3 | 144,300 |
| Other or unknown abuse | 1.0 | 63,200 |
| Total | 3.4 | 211,100 |

[a]Total number of children rounded to the nearest 100 not adjusted by population totals.
*Source.*   Adapted from U.S. Department of Health and Human Services (1988).

ment. This form includes attempted or potential physical or sexual assault; deliberate withholding of food, shelter, sleep, or other necessities as a form of punishment; economic exploitation; and unspecified abusive actions.

# Emotional Neglect

A definition and a statement of the incidence of emotional neglect appears in the first part of this chapter under the section on types of neglect.

# Malparenting and Substance Abuse

A significant number of psychologically, physically, and sexually abusive parents have serious alcohol and drug dependency problems. For some, these chemicals are used as self-medication in an effort to assuage unhappy feelings that are difficult to tolerate. Often the use has become habitual and its origins are difficult to trace. All the abusive person knows is that life seems boring and bleak without chemical adjuncts. Alcohol serves as a depressant, initially lowering inhibitions, then impulses, and finally awareness. It also gets in the way of coordination and good judgment. Cocaine is a stimulant, initially increasing energy and drives, although chronic use results in the deterioration of both. Infants born with fetal alcohol syndrome or addicted to cocaine have become major mental health concerns. Marijuana may create a sense of well-being and self-satisfaction, but often at the price of being emotionally indifferent, unaware, and unresponsive to the needs of others. Each chemical increases the user's underlying tendencies to be more in touch with his or her own immediate needs and less attuned to the needs of others, including children. Intoxicated parents are poor role models for their children, and it is not surprising that there are many second- and third-generation drug abusers.

When operating under the influence of alcohol or drugs, parents are often more likely to insult, disparage, threaten, and coerce children than when in a chemical-free state of mind. Some may repress any recall of their noxious behaviors having occurred during blackouts and some may rationalize their conduct as obviously unintended and attribute it to "the alcohol talking." However, children respond with anxiety, sadness, and anger to the hostile comments and behaviors of parents, whatever the parents' state of mind. When the expressions of hostility and rejection are particularly intense, as is often the case when one is intoxicated, or when the ability to respond to a child's needs is particularly impaired, the child often feels worthless and desperate. When alcohol and drug abuse are contributing factors in parental maltreatment of a child, therapists must confront the addictions. This is difficult, because addicted individuals often deny the severity of their problem and are frequently oblivious to the effect of their addiction on their children. Therapists concerned about protection of maltreated children have a sense of urgency regarding parental substance abuse treatment: the children can't wait for the implementation of a 12-step program, and a period of tenuous sobriety, to be spared the insults to their psychological development that addictive parents may impose.

### Children Exposed to Substances in Utero

The United States is experiencing a virtual epidemic of children born to mothers who abused substances during their pregnancies, with crack cocaine often only one of several such abused substances.

**Prevalence.**    A nationwide survey of 36 hospitals reported an 11% incidence of substance abuse in pregnancy, based on discharge diagnosis of mother or infant after delivery (Chasnoff 1989). New York City birth certificates for 1990 indicated that 24.3/1,000 live births involved illicit drug abuse, of which 17.6/1,000 live births involved crack cocaine use, 3.1/1,000 involved heroin, and 3.9/1,000 involved methadone (Damos 1991).

**Behavioral characteristics.**    According to a study performed by Hume et al. (1989), cocaine exposure in utero disrupted central nervous system development. Hence, infants so exposed were found to have problems of hyperarousability, including crying for prolonged periods, feeding and sleeping problems, irritability, tonicity problems, and attentional problems. They were also reported to manifest low birth weight, seizures, and congenital malformations (Chasnoff 1989). Moreover, children of parents who abused drugs or alcohol scored significantly lower than did children of parents who did not on measures of depression and anxiety and in arithmetic (Johnson et al. 1990). Preschoolers who were exposed to substances in utero showed lower developmental quotients (DQs) when measured on the Bayley Scales of Infant Development, deficits in spontaneous play where self-initiation, organization, and follow-through are called for, diminished representational play, more insecure attachment behaviors, and more attentional deficits than do a comparison group of children not exposed to controlled substances. Their insecure attachments included disorganization of intentionality and absence of the expression of pleasure and delight in comparison to children not exposed to controlled substances (Rodning et al. 1989).

**Treatment.** Treatment that addresses impairments in attention, arousability, activity level, and sensory and cognitive functions often is required both for infants and children exposed in utero to substances and for the child's caretakers. Dyadic interactional treatment for caretakers and children is an important component of the treatment plan. Oppositional child behavioral, attentional, and irritability difficulties decrease when caretakers are taught behaviorally oriented child-rearing strategies. One study concluded that comprehensive prenatal care may improve outcome in pregnancies complicated by cocaine abuse (MacGregor et al. 1989). Special education services for infants, preschoolers, and school-age children exposed to such substances in utero can improve language, cognitive, and behavioral impairments. Children who were exposed in utero to controlled substances also benefit from substance abuse and mental health services delivered in individual, group, family, and parental-couple formats. Such services may be provided in inpatient, outpatient, or day care settings, depending on the specific circumstances and needs of families.

Treatment programs are needed for pregnant women with substance abuse problems and for children and the parents of children exposed to substances. Currently, there are few treatment programs for children born exposed to substances, despite the great need.

Resources for program development are facilitated by special education, child mental health, adult mental health, substance abuse, pediatric, medical, and social services departments working in collaboration to ensure implementation and funding of services.

It is noteworthy that Part H of the Education for the Handicapped Act (EHA) of 1986 requires that states provide free special education to handicapped infants and toddlers from birth through 2 years of age for developmental, cognitive, and psychosocial difficulties.

A treatment program example is outlined here.

A recently established program within the Department of Psychiatry at the North Shore University Hospital-Cornell University Medical College (Imhof and Kaplan 1990) provides for interdepartmental and interagency collaboration. It uses multiple hospital departments and county and state agencies working together with the goal of enhancing child development and child and family health, and preventing child foster placement. This program illustrates the possibilities for coordination of substance abuse and child mental health treatment. It is a comprehensive, family oriented, substance abuse day treatment program for pregnant and/or parenting women, their children, family members, and significant others. Its services include individual, group, and family therapy, parent effectiveness training, drug and alcohol prevention, prenatal and postpartum health education, medical and nursing services, infant and child psychiatric psychological assessments and therapies, and a special educational component for infants and preschoolers. (See Appendix G for program information.)

# ▌ Intervention for Emotional Maltreatment

Because child or adolescent maltreatment and other forms of family violence frequently coexist within families, treatment needs for the various types of family violence are often similar. Because siblings who witness maltreatment or who become additional targets may experience maltreatment themselves, they also require assessment and can benefit from treatment. After recognizing the type and severity of the neglect or abuse, the clinician can design a course of action to assist not only the abused person, but, whenever possible, all other members of the affected family. Because psychological maltreatment is usually multifactorial and complex in its origins, a multidisciplinary approach is sensible. If a multidisciplinary team is available, the clinician should seek its services. If a preexisting team is not available, the clinician needs to define what clinical skills are needed and who might be available to provide them in that particular clinical setting or in the community.

Often, when the coercive influence of CPS or juvenile court cannot be employed, the foremost task in intervention is to form an alliance with the family that will help them become receptive to the services offered. Layzer reported that counseling and casework were the most frequent services provided to parents (Layzer and Goodson 1992). Although most caretakers do not identify themselves as maltreating, many do recognize that they are having problems. These parents often identify their problems quite differently than the clinician might, however—complaining of poverty, unemployment, depression, and the inability to cope with a difficult, unresponsive, and unappreciative child. Forming an alliance with these parents necessitates listening to their problems (which, of course, are stressors contributing to the maltreatment), recognizing that the person committing the abuse is just as needy in his or her own right as the person being abused, and attempting to respond to those needs in concrete ways as well as with compassion and psychological understanding.

## Intervention With Neglectful Families

Less than 20% of child maltreatment cases are taken to court to legally remove children from their homes or to enforce court orders for family rehabilitation. Therefore, the number actually removed from their homes is significantly less than 20% (Kaplan 1981). This means that the clinician is called upon most often to design a plan to assist the child in his or her family setting. Any such plan requires addressing the caretaker's needs too, just as the child's needs must be presented to the caretaker. Skillful presentation of the plan can facilitate the caretaker's cooperation and decrease the chances for resentment.

Although intervention is often needed to alleviate the psychological stress on the child, it is also often necessary to package or reframe many interventions to alleviate stress on the parents. Clinicians who have become sensitive to the psychological maltreatment of children often identify with their young clients' distress and feel anger toward the parents. Such resentment may be expressed as accusations, confrontations, and blame and often is anticipated by parents who already experience a great deal of doubt about their parenting abilities, who usually already lack self-esteem, and who often have experienced just such critical and hostile attitudes from other social service or helping agencies. Consequently, it is important that clinicians listen attentively to the caretakers as well as to the children and recognize that the so-called victimizers are often themselves victims—products of their own maltreatment, of their defective environment, of pressures, and of a lack of knowledge and understanding about child development and parenting.

It is essential in cases of child neglect—whether physical, educational, or psychological—to have an appreciation of the family's role as a potentially potent curative agent in addition to its role as a contributor to the child's problems. The degree to which the family can actually be involved in the therapeutic process varies greatly depending on the child's age, the current placement of the child (whether still in the family residence or living elsewhere), the willingness of the family members—or the degree of pressure brought to bear on the family—to participate in the process, and the therapist's skill in engaging the whole family in an effort to resolve the difficulties contributing to the family's malfunctioning. How the family is to be engaged, and whether that engagement leads to the termination of the maltreatment, depends greatly on the manner in which the family is approached from the onset of intervention.

**Self-referred families.**    From the outset there are two issues that need to be clarified. The first concerns the way the child has been referred, and the second concerns the family members' perception of the problem. Ideally the adult members of the family have concluded that they are in need of some help with their parenting skills and would appreciate some guidance, direction, or treatment for those problems they have identified as contributing to ineffective rearing or maltreatment of their children. Unfortunately, such situations are relatively rare. An example would be parents who seek marital counseling in part because of conflicts over what to expect of their children, what to allow, and how to deal with emerging behaviors. Another example would be parents who are concerned about how their drinking, drug abuse, impatience, and temper outbursts may affect their children and who become motivated to seek help for these or other problems. These families are self-referred, and the parents are strongly motivated to change themselves rather than to place the focus of the problem on the child. Other families may also be self-referred but identify themselves as having a "problem child." The child's identified difficulty may be virtually any one or more of a large number of emotional or behavioral problems that have come to the parents' attention. Such families are genuinely concerned about their child's well-being but may have little or no awareness as to how their own treatment of the child has contributed to the youngster's present difficulties. Although such families may be asking the mental health professional to fix their child, they also need to be encouraged through therapy and education to understand how they can help to mitigate their child's difficulties by developing new attitudes, perspectives, skills, and techniques for parenting.

**Agency-referred families.**    When the child or family has been referred by an outside agency, particularly one that carries a great deal of power and can threaten removal of the child from the home, such as juvenile court (Landau 1980) or CPS, the task of engaging the family is more difficult. Interestingly, Taylor et al. (1991) reported that parents with low IQs have a greater tendency to accept court-ordered services concerning their neglected child. Parents diagnosed with serious emotional disorders were more likely than less disturbed parents to reject court-ordered services and to have their children permanently removed from the home. The family may recognize that they are having difficulties with their child, but may perceive their problem as how to deal with an intrusive social service system and a therapist who is seen as an extension of that system. Both the system and the therapist may be seen as threatening, coercive, and untrustworthy. While acknowledging the referral source, the therapist must establish his or her separation from the agency and demonstrate genuine concern for the welfare of the whole family as well as that of the identified child. The therapist's interest in and respect for the thoughts and feelings of each family member and his or her acknowledgment of the parents' genuine interest in doing that which is in their child's best interest (which is usually the expressed sentiment of even the most inadequate parents) may help to provide support to parents who are afraid that confiding and cooperating might serve to discredit them as parents and might provoke the removal of their child from the home.

**Diagnostic evaluations.**    When the parents perceive the problem as being primarily within their child, the mental health professional needs to approach that perspective respectfully. A detailed history should be obtained to determine what the child's symptoms or inappropriate behaviors are, when and how the problem began, and the parents' perception of why the child conducts himself or herself as he or she does. Such an exploration often provides useful information, including an understanding of the parents' thinking regarding causality. It may uncover notions of hereditary determination ("She's just stubborn like her grandfather!"); social determination ("It's those bad friends of hers"); biological causality ("He's been overactive, uncontrollable, and into everything since he was old enough to walk"); or personal guilt ("I never should have left him with my mother; she just ruined that child"), albeit obscured in this last example by projection onto others.

It is also helpful to explore what the parents have been doing to solve the problem as they see it. Parental interventions are not necessarily related to conscious perceptions of causality, but may provide valuable information regarding unconscious notions of parenting techniques. For example, a statement such as "We ignored it [child's aggressive behavior] 'cause boys do that and just grow out of it," suggests notions of sexual determinism, perhaps even sexual identity appropriateness, and states that time alone will cure the problem. It also indicates a tendency to ignore (or neglect) both a situation and a child in need of direction and guidance. It is often difficult for mental health professionals to elicit and to tolerate hearing parental descriptions of patently abusive behaviors, which the parents consider not only socially acceptable for their subculture, but would in fact consider themselves negligent as parents for not administering. For instance, "I washed her [a 7-year-old's] mouth out with soap for saying those awful things, and sent her to bed to pray that the devil won't take her" may evoke dismay in a therapist who perceives this behavior as rejecting and terrorizing, as well as physically abusive. Tolerant listening, with awareness of cultural differences and of countertransference issues, allows the parents to feel that they are respected at least for their good intentions, prior to exploring alternative approaches. When the parents continue to complain about their child's behaviors despite their (abusive) interventions, the ineffectiveness of these approaches becomes apparent, and the parents may be willing to explore less abusive, more effective, approaches.

An initial goal of the therapist is to establish an empathic therapeutic alliance with the family as well as with the child. Because this is more difficult to do when the family perceives the therapist as having been imposed on them, it consequently requires greater skill on the part of the therapist. The task is easier if the therapist sees that both the family and the child are hurting and that the situation can be altered only by establishing a bond of trust with both. It is not necessary, and may not be particularly helpful, to label established patterns of child rearing as "neglectful" or "abusive," especially when there is no viable alternative to working with the child in his or her

family milieu. Helping the family explore more effective child management techniques without making the parents feel assailed themselves
is a primary goal of treatment.

One approach, involving family, focuses primarily on immediate
change; that is, within the span of only a few therapeutic sessions. The
Mental Research Institute of Palo Alto, as described by Weakland and
Jordan (1992), focuses on families building cooperation, agreeing on
the problems, discussing solutions already attempted, taking small
yet significant steps toward change, solidifying gains, and building
a safety net and support networks as soon as possible. Many maltreating families struggle with seemingly overwhelming problems. A therapist who helps the family alleviate some of these stressors may
facilitate an alliance with the family at the same time he or she re-
duces the factors leading to abuse. Concrete as opposed to psychological action may involve helping the family to get the heat turned on, to
obtain food stamps and food supplements, to obtain public assistance,
to find adequate medical care, to obtain employment, and to get information on birth control and day care. It may also involve making
contact with support systems such as Alcoholics Anonymous (AA),
Narcotics Anonymous (NA), and Parents United (PU), and focused
therapy/support groups such as Divorce Recovery Programs, Adults
Molested as Children (AMAC), and AL ANON for children and spouses
of alcoholic parents. Therapists cannot provide these services themselves, but they can facilitate the family's access to them by passing
on their knowledge of the community's resources.

Making these connections may seem like a formidable task, one
that is often complicated by the isolated family's resistance to becoming involved in any community activities, even potentially helpful
ones. Although this resistance is frustrating to the therapist, it creates an opportunity for exploring the family's distrust of outsiders and
its anxiety about the dangers of being involved with others. Despite
the family's need for companionship, pleasurable activity, and concrete services, an isolated family may object to involvement with all
types of social organizations, from church groups to bowling leagues
to the Salvation Army. The therapist must walk a careful line between
too much encouragement and assistance, which may appear critical
and pushy, and too little, which may seem indifferent and uncaring.
However, it is clear that providing the real help needed is not a task
for the passive or timid therapist, and also requires great sensitivity
to the family's feelings of distrust, privacy, and pride.

# ▌ Intervention With Neglected and Psychologically Maltreated Children

As with the physically or sexually abused child, the initial thrust of treatment must be to halt the neglect and to ensure that the child's physical, medical, educational, and emotional needs are adequately met. The therapist also needs to terminate psychological abuse by interdicting, in whatever way necessary, the rejecting, isolating, terrorizing, ignoring, and corrupting behaviors that are inflicting the psychological injury. Severely neglected children who bear physical signs of their neglect, such as malnutrition, failure to thrive, persistence of treatable medical illnesses due to poor hygiene or failure to obtain essential medical care, or chronic failure to attend school due to parental lack of interest, may be removed from their parent's care by action of CPS and the juvenile family court. These children may then be placed in foster homes, residential treatment centers, children's shelters, or hospitals, depending on their immediate needs.

These separations from the parents may, despite the children's neglected state, inflict further trauma on them, and consequently should be implemented only in emergency situations or when all other means of providing support to the families have failed to alter neglectful situations. When social agencies can provide financial and other material assistance to responsible parents, children should not be removed from their homes. However, if a parent is unable to use such assistance (e.g., because of mental retardation; mental illness, such as profound depression or psychosis; or addiction to alcohol or drugs), temporary—and perhaps longer—removal may be essential to protect the children despite other possible negative consequences. After the children have been placed in a safe haven, further efforts can be made to assess and remediate the underlying causes of the parent's neglect in hopes of eventually reuniting the family under more favorable circumstances.

Immediate intervention with psychologically maltreated children is often much more complex and difficult except in those cases in which there is an obvious medical problem, such as the failure of an infant to thrive due to maternal deprivation, in which case immediate hospitalization is needed as a life saver. A court order may be needed to implement such intervention if the parent objects. This is similar to a situation in which parents refuse to provide appropriate medical care when a child is suffering from a potentially life-threatening ailment. However, when the parental refusal to provide care is based on a conscious decision or on religious grounds, the courts are confronted with a much more difficult challenge than when the parent is debilitated because of mental illness or addictions. In those cases in which the adult has actually violated a law by contributing to the delinquency of a minor, such as using a child to steal or run drugs, or encouraging sexual activity and prostitution, the criminal justice system may intervene to incarcerate the parent and to place the child in the care of CPS.

These situations of psychological maltreatment, however, are extremes. Intervention is much more difficult in the vast majority of cases in which the maltreatment is more insidious and chronic. If the professional can establish sufficient rapport with the parent and can address his or her need for a respite from the stresses of parenting, it is sometimes possible to facilitate the temporary and voluntary placement of the child with relatives, friends, or in an appropriate shelter while the parent obtains treatment for his or her own difficulties— physical or mental illness, alcohol or drug addiction, or merely exhaustion. More commonly, however, the professional will be obliged to treat the child within the noxious environment while at the same time trying to improve that environment and the quality of the parenting.

The psychological effects of neglect and emotional maltreatment include the whole gamut of psychiatric disorders in children, except for those that have a well-defined biogenetic origin. Even then the child who has a strong biogenetic loading or predisposition toward a psychiatric disorder may be further stressed by psychological maltreatment to manifest symptoms of that disorder. Consequently, the treatment of such children involves the entire armamentarium of psychiatric interventions, always tailored to the needs of the individual child. As a fundamental principle, however, it should be noted that the neglected and emotionally abused child, with whatever other specific diagnosis, almost always suffers from a profound and well-justified distrust of adults. Therefore, the initial thrust of all interpersonal therapies is building rapport with the child and establishing, by virtue of the therapist's kindness and consistency, the notion that at least some adults can be trusted. Howing has found that social skills training programs benefit adults and nonmaltreated children by improving interpersonal communication skills, problem-solving skills, self-control, assertiveness, and stress management. This training seems promising for intervention with maltreated children, especially when therapists endeavor to communicate with parents and children (Howing et al. 1990). In an era of increasingly biological interventions, the importance of rapport is often neglected as a powerful therapeutic tool.

Because the maltreated child's inadequate caretakers have disdained and subverted the child's thoughts and feelings, a second principle of therapy with such a youngster is the importance of respecting his or her thoughts and feelings and of encouraging the appropriate expression of ideas and emotions by the child. This is a much more difficult task than it may seem because maltreated children are frequently out of contact with their inner feelings, which they have suppressed or repressed when no one seemed at all interested in them. Such youngsters may appear blunted in their affect, indifferent, and shallow; their emotional life may be manifested only in their often unacceptable behaviors.

Some children have become so preoccupied with their efforts to read what others want of them and to accommodate to others' needs, either to avoid retribution or to obtain whatever approval they can, that they have never developed much capacity for introspection. Others may have developed a narrow repertoire of feelings, usually different degrees of anger, with which to meet the work, and some have become masters at deception and manipulation with little hope of having their needs met if they were to be straightforward and honest. Getting in touch with emotions such as sadness and longing may make them feel unbearably vulnerable. Some children have learned to adopt a tough, seemingly indifferent exterior or to display attitudes of hostility and resentment. Many may identify with the attitudes and behaviors of their maltreating parents and may engage in cruel and destructive behaviors themselves, showing little capacity for compassion or empathy, emotions with which they may have had little experience, and which may be perceived as weaknesses. Helping these youngsters get in touch with their tender and hurt feelings requires that they trust their therapist to be understanding and supportive.

Because anger has often been the most pervasive affect with which these children have been intimately familiar, they frequently express their anger quickly, both verbally and physically, and often with what seems to be very little provocation. Some of this rage may be due to the child's identification with the aggressor—the emotionally abusive parents—and some of it is a reaction to the psychological insults and injuries to which the child has been subjected. This anger may be displaced onto all authority figures, peers, and the therapist rather than being expressed toward the neglectful parent. Even when the child does turn his rage onto his parents, the therapist's support for that anger may result in the ambivalent child's sudden defense of his parents. The therapist needs to help the child find appropriate ways of expressing his or her anger and of channeling the energy so generated in constructive directions. The therapist also needs to be prepared to deal with the child's transference reactions when the anger is turned onto the therapist and with his or her own countertransference reactions if the child's anger becomes too difficult to handle. Setting and testing of limits, manipulations, and confrontations are often recurrent themes in the individual therapy of maltreated children. These occur before the child is able to accept interpretations designed to help him or her understand and control his or her often disruptive behaviors.

Many maltreated children have found ways to cope with their family situation. Some assume a passive, compliant, withdrawn stance, which hopefully avoids mistreatment. Others adopt a hostile, oppositional, defiant stance, which constantly challenges adults. The child's coping style is determined by the nature of his or her temperament, environment, and experiential history; and by his or her physical and psychological assets and weaknesses. This adaptation may be effective for the child in terms of minimizing the amount of abuse to which he or she is subjected or it may contribute to the cycle of abuse by provoking more rejection and hostility from the parents. In any case, such coping styles are rarely adaptive for the child in dealing with school, peers, and society, and frequently result in further difficulties for the youngster in making effective interpersonal adaptations. Helping the child to learn more appropriate and emotionally satisfying means of coping with his or her feelings and with the world in which he or she lives constitutes the complex task of the therapy.

In addition to individual psychotherapy, many children, and especially adolescents, may benefit from a variety of group therapies. Sometimes these may be activity groups designed to teach skills and build self-esteem and basic social skills; sometimes groups may be psychotherapeutic with a great deal of exploration and expression of feelings, peer confrontations, and interpretations; and sometimes they may be focused, such as Al-Anon for children of alcoholic and drug-addicted parents or Daughters and Sons United (DSU) for children from incestuous families. Graziano and Mills (1992) described cognitive and behavioral treatments, which include self-control training, social skills training, and contingency management programs. Psychodrama often helps children recreate their noxious family situations and learn more effective ways of dealing with the feelings evoked. One form of treatment is a contingency play strategy, which aims at reducing stress and alienation of neglected children and forming positive modes of behavior in a day treatment program. Gunsberg (1989) reports that such a program promotes contingency development, impulse control, child-initiated interaction, and child-teacher interaction. Some children with well-defined psychiatric syndromes and symptoms that interfere with their functioning may be helped by psychopharmacology. Because there is a rapidly expanding literature dealing with tailoring psychopharmacology to the specific clinical situation, no effort will be made here to elucidate the various possibilities.

## Types of Treatment for Families, Children, and Adolescents

**Respite care.**   Because forced removal of the child or adolescent is rarely an option, and may in fact produce even more psychological trauma for the child or adolescent and family, the clinician needs to be familiar with the familial and community resources that are available. If, in order to provide a respite for the stressed parents and the child or adolescent, a brief separation is needed, the clinician might recommend voluntary placement of the child in a protective children's shelter. This is as much to provide relief for the family as to assist the child directly. Such shelters have become available in many communities and may offer a variety of additional services, such as further advice on using community systems—i.e., social services, health care, food stamps, educational programs on child development and parenting, self-help groups such as Parents Anonymous, and even brief focused counseling. In some communities there may be respite care foster homes sponsored by community agencies, such as CPS or private religious and social service organizations. These temporary and voluntary foster homes may vary considerably in quality. Some may provide a unique opportunity for the overwhelmed parents to receive some parenting themselves. One creative option available in some communities is a foster grandparent program, which may provide an ongoing support system in the form of an ersatz extended family, including occasional respite child care for parents.

Shelters for runaway teenagers, or "safe houses" as they are called in some communities, also can be used by families for temporary placement of a youngster in an effort to prevent elopement or to extricate a youngster from an intolerable situation, such as intoxicated or abusive parents. Such halfway houses or shelters also may offer brief therapeutic services usually oriented toward attempting to return the youngster, whether runaway or voluntarily placed, to his or her home as quickly as possible. Sometimes "throw-away" or homeless children try to hang on to their education as a residual link with one adult system that seems to care about them. As a result, high school guidance counselors may have access to voluntary foster homes into which surrogate parents are willing to take a youngster for a time. A number of church groups provide similar services. It is not uncommon for emotionally maltreated adolescents to become actively involved in street gangs or in cults, which offer them an identity and a sense of self-worth. When such a group accepts them—albeit conditional upon their acceptance of the group's morals, rituals, and behaviors—it may also aim to convert the youth to its unhealthy purposes. Placement of a young person who has been ejected from his or her home may serve as protection against becoming initiated into such a group.

**Family therapy.**   Although establishing a therapeutic alliance with the family is essential, there are several other vital roles the therapist must assume. A therapist's effectiveness is enhanced by being attuned both to the psychodynamics of each family member and to the family dynamic—the patterns of interpersonal relationships and communications within the family. Ideally, a therapist has adequate time to spend with each family member alone: with each parent or stepparent; with the maltreated child or children; with siblings; and with other significant individuals, such as grandparents or a parent's boyfriend or girlfriend residing in the home. This ideal is often difficult to achieve. Trying to do so, however, helps to involve the individual members in seeking solutions. If a multidisciplinary team is available, it is often very helpful in meeting the specific needs of each family member. Periodic family therapy meetings, which include all or selected members of the family at the therapist's discretion, invariably shed added light on the interpersonal dynamics and family structure. Such sessions can be volatile and require the skill of a knowledgeable and adaptable family therapist. The maltreated child or adolescent is invariably part of a malfunctioning family system. Interventions that focus on the child or the parents exclusively are not likely to be as effective as interventions that also deal with the family system.

Extensive literature is available describing different types of dysfunctional family systems and different therapeutic techniques for effective intervention. Thus it would be unrealistic to attempt to discuss all the available options here. However, in dealing with psychologically maltreating families, there are several broad issues that need to be considered. Because psychological maltreatment can take so many variable, subtle, and complex forms, it is important that the therapist be flexible and adaptable and not wed to a single approach. Despite the fact that therapists have been working with maltreating families and maltreated children for generations, there is no study that substantiates one therapeutic approach as consistently more effective than others. Consequently the therapist's judgment is important in selecting the approach that seems most useful for each specific family. It is important that families learn to communicate more positively within the therapeutic experience in the hope that this will carry over into other aspects of family life. The family therapist should become a role model for positive communications, giving judicious and honest praise and support as frequently as possible and recognizing that the parents may need nurturing, which they do not know how to give either to themselves or to their family. It is also important that the therapist be comfortable with the use of humor in therapy and in family meetings. Almost all families have some form of family humor that holds them together in a mutually pleasurable way. Of course, if their primary modes of humor are sarcasm, disparaging teasing, or sadistic practical jokes, these need to be explored in the family sessions to help both the person making the joke and the person who is the target of the joke become aware of and express their feelings in more appropriate ways.

Therapists need to reinforce diminutions in defensiveness and projective blaming by praising family members when they accept personal responsibility for errors, mistakes, or personal slights. The therapist may provide a role model by apologizing for tardiness, interruptions, or unintentional hurting of others' feelings (all of which inevitably occur in family meetings), as a means of demonstrating to the family that one can acknowledge mistakes without losing face, respect, or authority. These are important issues in the treatment of maltreating families.

Of course the therapist must note family composition, ages of children, the relative explosiveness and expressiveness of family members, and so on, in order to determine the frequency and composition of family therapy sessions. For instance, when infants, toddlers, or preschoolers seem to be the focus of maltreatment, couples therapy may be most useful, although the actual presence of the infant serves to focus the treatment. When latency-age or adolescent children dominate the household and appear to be abused, the therapist—recognizing that sibling competitiveness and conflict are major themes that often provoke parental reactions and that may reflect the children's hunger for attention, need for appropriate limits, and projected hostilities and resentments—might appropriately include all siblings. With adolescents who are striving for independence and control of their own lives, sessions that exclude younger siblings but that facilitate mutually respectful dialogue between parents and teenagers may be appropriate.

There is no single formula for success, and the creativity, adaptability, and judgment of the family therapist is critical in guiding this complex process. Because family therapy is often seen merely as an elective adjunct to a variety of other therapeutic modalities, we have given considerable attention here to the role of family therapy in working with maltreating families. Whether the goal is to improve mutual understanding among family members, to improve communication between family members, or to alter the dynamic structure of the family in order to alleviate the emotional maltreatment of one or more members, family therapy should be considered a core component of the treatment of emotionally maltreating families.

## Therapy for Neglectful Parents

**Individual therapy.**     Often it is the family's difficulty in tolerating the process of a child's individuation and separation that provokes maltreatment. Consequently, the therapist needs to be able to provide individual treatment for both the adults and the children. If the primary therapist does not have the time, training, or experience to juggle all of these therapeutic tasks, which is often the case, he or she must assemble a team of colleagues who can work in collaboration. In treating the parents of maltreated children, issues of transference and countertransference emerge immediately, and the therapist must deal with them effectively for therapy to progress. Therapists by temperament and training are usually humanistic in their philosophical and emotional orientation. They are also schooled in the benefits of positive reinforcement and in the detrimental effects of disparagement, rejection, and punishment. It is often difficult for therapists to be sympathetic to victimizers of children and to recognize that these parents usually do care about their children's welfare and have often acted as they have (however misguided their actions may have been) in the belief that their "spare the rod, spoil the child" approach is in the child's best interest.

Individual therapists need to appreciate that these parents are often struggling with many psychological problems of their own in addition to the "real" difficulties cited above. Many are poorly educated in general and may have had little or no education regarding child development, behavioral management, or emotional and psychological development. Many parents are suffering from their own burden of emotional problems, from overdependency on others, low self-esteem, poor impulse control, emotional immaturity and impulsivity, a multitude of potential anxieties, social and emotional isolation, distrust of outsiders, and depressed moods. Some have full-blown psychiatric disorders, such as affective disorders, which include a variety of depressive disorders. Some have frank psychoses. Many neglectful parents fit within the diagnostic criteria for personality disorders. They often have lifelong histories of impaired interpersonal relationships and poor judgment. Their deficits often have led to relatively isolated life-styles, which lack the social support systems that even the most effective parents need to sustain them during periods of crisis (Zuravin 1988).

Many parents who maltreat their children have themselves been the victims of neglect and abuse. Despite their unhappy experiences as children, many appear to have incorporated their parents' negligent or abusive approaches into their own parenting styles. It has been suggested that because they may not have been given much love, attention, or positive feedback as children, they may have little to give to their own children as adults. Many parents seem to be curiously blocked in their ability to recall or to be in touch with their own sad feelings as a result of being rejected, isolated, terrorized, ignored, and corrupted as children. Getting in touch with these repressed feelings is often a goal of individual therapy because it is imperative that parents be able to experience and tolerate such feelings in order to experience genuine empathy for their own maltreated offspring.

**Expressive therapies.** When treating emotionally abusive and neglectful parents, it is effective for the therapist to encourage the expression of the patient's feelings and impulses, regardless of how abhorrent these may appear to be. However, the therapist needs to clearly differentiate between expressing such sentiments in individual therapy for the purpose of understanding and modifying them, and expressing and acting on these feelings and impulses in the context of the family. Unfortunately, expressive therapy may inadvertently perpetuate the notion that one should express one's feelings frankly and directly at all times in order to have honest communication. In maltreating families, there is already a tendency to "let it all hang out," "it" referring to an abundance of negative, hostile, and emotionally destructive feelings. Even many nonabusive families exercise a dismal minimum of good manners toward fellow family members, and many maltreating families appear to regress to the most primitive interactions within their family relationships, reserving refinement for putting on a good show with neighbors and strangers.

Helping adults reframe their negative feelings in constructive ways and encouraging the identification and effective expression of positive feelings become important therapeutic tasks. Because of their own insecurities and sense of vulnerability, many maltreating parents have great difficulty listening to their children's expressions of feelings. It becomes clear from listening to family interactions that many parents do not want to hear what their children think, feel, or desire, and that such expressions are perceived as threatening to the adult's authority and self-esteem. Perhaps the most common rejecting rebuke to children is the sharply stated "Shut up," a blunter version of the sentiment that "children are to be seen and not heard" and are "to speak only when spoken to." Maltreating parents may see their children as endlessly demanding or complaining, and their requests may be experienced as accusations spotlighting the parents' inadequacy in meeting their children's needs.

Reducing this sense of anxiety in parents constitutes another formidable therapeutic goal, but one that must be achieved in order for parental listening to become a meaningful part of the communication equation. Children are frequently informed that "respect must be earned," that respect is not a given when one's status is that of a child. Yet children are as human as adults and warrant as high a degree of respect for that condition. However, if there is any truth in the first dictum, then it certainly follows that parents must also earn their children's respect, which can be most effectively achieved by careful and attentive listening. Listening, however, appears to be extremely threatening to insecure parents who experience it as being cast back into the role of passive, dependent children themselves and who prefer to say, "Now look here, young man, you listen to me!"

### Intervention Issues for Clinicians

**Countertransference, candor, and confidentiality.** Although the countertransference feelings that these issues evoke need not be discussed in the therapy with the maltreating parent, the therapist must be cognizant that they can often emerge in ways that, if unrecognized, may undermine the most earnest therapeutic endeavors. Adults entering treatment because of the alleged maltreatment of their children often bring with them their own preconceived notions, which include serious doubts and suspicions about the therapist. Such parents are particularly sensitive to any suggestion or criticism on the part of the therapist. Even when parents are self-referred for concerns about their parenting abilities, they still may be exquisitely sensitive to criticism and may be desperately seeking some affirmation of their worth as individuals and as parents. If the therapist has been assigned by an agency rather than chosen freely by the adults, the parents' concern about the therapist's primary allegiance may be intensified. It is important that the therapist make it clear that he or she is concerned about the welfare of both the children and the adults in the family. It is important for the therapist to be candid with parents about his or her mandate in regard to confidentiality and reporting of suspected neglect or abuse. Although such candor may seem initially intimidating to parents, honesty on the part of the therapist often brings forth honesty from patients, whereas avoidance of any discussion of the issue may foster doubts, suspicions, and withholding of information.

## Summary

Physical and emotional neglect and emotional abuse are undoubtedly the most frequent yet also the most underreported forms of child and adolescent maltreatment. They may occur alone or together in many guises. The psychological trauma and the sequelae that invariably accompany all forms of maltreatment may ultimately have an adverse effect on personality, emotional stability, and the ability to cope with the tasks and stresses of life. Intervention depends on recognizing the many diverse forms that maltreatment takes. Psychological impact is determined by the child's preexisting temperament, by the nature of the maltreatment, by the child's age and stage of psychological development, by the acuteness or chronicity of the maltreatment, by the availability of a support system and professionals who can and will intervene therapeutically, and by the responsiveness of the child's family to change. Although removal of the child or adolescent may be necessary in the most extreme situations of neglect and emotional maltreatment, the most frequent and most difficult course of therapeutic intervention consists of developing rapport with the family and with the child or adolescent and thus bringing about changes in both while the child or adolescent remains in this less than good environment. Effective intervention requires the use of a multimodal approach; it often necessitates the diverse skills of a multidisciplinary treatment team or of separate professionals in the community working in close coordination.

# Legal Commentary

## ▌ Issues Related to Victims, Other Family Members, and Offenders

### Physical Neglect

All state civil child protective laws include provisions for intervention on behalf of children who are without certain necessary care and sustenance. Some state laws simply refer to the child who lacks "proper parental care or control" (an admittedly vague term). Others specify that a child must be deprived of adequate food, clothing, and shelter as a basis for child protective intervention. Severe neglect of a child is also a criminal offense. Evidence of a permanent or long-term relinquishment of parental responsibilities may lead to child protective intervention and criminal prosecution of the parent for the acts of child abandonment or criminal nonsupport.

One defense commonly accepted in neglect cases is that parents lack the financial resources to provide the necessities of life for their child or children. It is a general rule that parents cannot be adjudicated for child neglect simply because of their poverty status. They must have, or be provided with, the resources to adequately care for their child or children before the state can interfere with the parent-child relationship. Inadequate housing, sometimes leading to families being homeless, has in recent years become a more common ground for child protective intervention. Some laws and court decisions occasionally specify that special housing assistance must be provided before the state may involuntarily separate children from their parents.

A more common basis for state child protective intervention is the claim that a parent is inadequately supervising a child (and not assuring satisfactory alternative care), leading to the child being endangered by his or her environment. In the more egregious cases, the parent will leave an infant or toddler unattended at home for many hours, or even days, or a child will be injured in a house fire while left alone. Given the large numbers of single-parent families with young children, and the lack of affordable and accessible child care, it is not unusual to find children left unattended for some period of the day or evening. Generally, child neglect laws and public CPS agency policies do not specify at what age and for how many hours children can be left alone. This makes the legal issue of lack of supervision difficult. CPS caseworkers and police must often make on-the-spot decisions based on the need to ensure the child's immediate safety, which may result in a child's being removed from the home but later returned because the legal grounds for involuntary state intervention had not been met, or because the parent's justification for leaving their child unattended was reasonable.

One area of child neglect that has become a major concern is the inability of parents to provide adequate care for a child because of parental drug or alcohol abuse. In rare instances, decisions concerning legal child protective intervention may be made before a mother has given birth. In most cases the focus of legal decision making will be on what action to take after a prenatally substance-exposed child has been born. Some state laws have made the physical dependency or exposure of a child to drugs, or a child suffering from fetal alcohol syndrome, a basis for mandatory child neglect reporting, civil child protective intervention, or criminal prosecution of the child's mother. Other states permit a judicial finding of child neglect to be predicated on the drug- or alcohol-addicted parents' ability to provide their child with proper care or supervision.

The most controversial aspect of child protective intervention is the issue of whether any intervention can be legally justified prior to the birth of a child. What should the law permit or require in the area of child protection when a clinician becomes aware that a pregnant woman is abusing alcohol or drugs? There is a wide spectrum of opinion—but almost no settled law—on this topic. One point of view is that forcible intervention into the woman's life (including mandatory reporting, which would trigger such intervention) is completely wrong at this point—a violation of the woman's constitutional right to privacy. At the other extreme, some advocate for both mandatory reporting and court intervention (through a juvenile court or civil commitment proceeding) if it can be established that the woman's continued substance abuse will severely harm her fetus. In another controversial and unsettled area of the law, civil court intervention may also be sought prenatally when the mother refuses treatment or surgery for a medical condition that would, without such care, likely lead to the death or severe permanent disability of the newborn child.

Many child neglect cases will be predicated on allegations that parents are suffering from psychosis, severe emotional disorders, mental retardation, or physical disabilities that render them incapable of providing adequate care for their children. A common question in child protective intervention proceedings will be whether a parent's handicap affects his or her parenting abilities to the extent that the child is in need of substitute care by the state. Often, the court will need expert testimony on how the parental disability will affect the likelihood of future neglect. Thus, in such parental incapacity cases, courts may be asked to intervene when children have not yet suffered any harm but are merely deemed especially vulnerable or at-risk.

In judicial proceedings involving impaired parents, the court will be looking both at the parents' present condition and ability to care for the children and at the prognosis regarding future parental debilitation. These issues become especially troublesome in cases involving the involuntary termination of parental rights.

Because intervention by the state for alleged neglect or emotional maltreatment of a child is generally based on subjective determinations, there is a real danger that the vagueness and ambiguity of relevant laws will permit inappropriate intervention by overly zealous social workers and judges. In particular, poor and minority families, who are likely to be in greater contact with governmental authorities than other families, are very disproportionately represented among families subjected to child neglect intervention.

Often, the professionals making determinations as to adequate parental care and supervision are of a different socioeconomic and racial group than are the families affected by their decisions. Personal biases, value judgments, cultural insensitivity, and incompetency are real problems leading to occasional overintervention and the needless breakup of families. Neglect can and does harm children, just as much as (and sometimes more than) abuse, but the very imprecision of its definition should force professionals to use the utmost care in their decision-making judgments.

## Educational Neglect

One type of child maltreatment that has not yet been addressed is educational neglect. If a parent forces, or even encourages, a child to miss a substantial number of school days or otherwise interrupts the child's education, this can be the legal basis for child protective intervention by agencies and the court. However, the only issue for those who intervene will be how to get the parent to consistently send the child to school or provide an approved educational alternative. Many states also provide for such parents to be criminally prosecuted for intentionally keeping a child out of school without a valid legal reason (and the children themselves may be brought before the juvenile court on a truancy petition). Another possible basis for a complaint of educational neglect is the situation in which a parent is aware of a child's special education needs but stubbornly and irrationally refuses to allow the child to participate in a remedial special education program.

## Emotional Maltreatment

Few areas of child protective legal intervention are as controversial, as poorly defined, or as dependent on mental health expertise as are cases alleging emotional maltreatment of children. Most state laws provide for both reporting and judicial proceedings in cases in which parents have emotionally or psychologically abused their child, or have inflicted mental injury on the child. These laws are generally pretty vague, leaving it to the courts to determine what constitutes the necessary harm or impairment to a child that will permit judicial intervention to be invoked.

For example, no state has specified whether the child who is not abused herself, but who repeatedly witnesses the violent abuse of her mother, is emotionally maltreated—a condition that would provide a legal basis for child protective jurisdiction. Thus, the question of what a clinician should do when becoming aware of a violent home situation in which the children are not themselves abused—and the decision of whether this domestic violence should trigger a child abuse or neglect report leading to the involvement of a CPS agency and the juvenile court—are likely to be matters of individual subjective determination. Certainly, domestic violence experts should be consulted by clinicians in all such situations.

In some states, proof will be required that a parent actually inflicted psychological injury on the child or knowingly allowed that harm to occur in order for courts to take protective action. In other states, courts will require evidence that the child's mental injury caused by the parental maltreatment was substantial, serious, significant, or protracted. In a few states, a parent's failure to provide for a child's mental or emotional health, or to care for a child's preexisting mental or emotional condition, will be sufficient to support court intervention.

## ▌ Guidance for Mental Health Professionals and Practitioners

Especially in child neglect and parental incapacity cases, it is important for mental health professionals to understand the impact of recent federal and state laws and policies on the question of whether children should be separated from their parents. The federal Adoption Assistance and Child Welfare Act (1980) (Public Law 96-272) provides substantial federal financial support for state and county foster care systems, which is predicated on the making of "reasonable efforts" to prevent unnecessary removal of children from their homes and to facilitate their return from foster care when appropriate. Since that law was implemented, legal policies and judicial decision-making actions have been increasingly guided by an evaluation of which home-based services might be provided to the family so that their child or children need not be removed.

Given the predilection of many judges to keep families together except in the most egregious cases of abuse, expert testimony on the appropriateness of using family preservation services to permit a child to be maintained at home is likely to become increasingly common. Indeed, the federal Family Preservation and Support Services legislation (42 U.S.C. Sec. 629) had, as of 1995, the promise of providing substantial sums of new money to states for prevention of placement outside the home and reunification of families. Psychiatrists and psychologists should be involved in efforts by their state's social services agencies concerning how these funds will be spent.

Mental health professionals should become familiar with the range of in-home services that might be provided to parents of children at risk because of parental incapacity or dysfunction, and to the affected children. Court personnel are likely to ask such professionals which services they think are appropriate in specific types of child maltreatment cases and with certain categories of parents. The courts are also likely to be interested in whether the recommendations of the parents' attorney or caseworker concerning the service plan for the family are reasonably calculated to address the parental problems and, equally important, to protect the child's safety.

Child safety concerns may also emerge in cases in which parents have been ordered into, or have voluntarily sought, counseling or treatment for drug and alcohol abuse. Parents who are in treatment for drug and alcohol abuse may disclose information to therapists and counselors that raise a reasonable suspicion that their children are presently endangered because of child abuse or neglect. Despite the concern for privacy and confidentiality in substance abuse treatment programs, those professionals who are mandated reporters of child abuse and neglect under state law, and who suspect that a substance abuse patient is abusing or neglecting a child, are still obligated to report. In 1986 the federal drug and alcohol abuse treatment law (42 U.S.C. Sec. 290 dd-2) was amended to clarify that treatment providers in federally supported substance abuse rehabilitation programs, if otherwise covered under state mandatory reporting laws, are obligated to report suspected child abuse and neglect by clients in those programs.

(See Appendix H for legal resources.)

# References

Adoption Assistance and Child Welfare Act, Public Law 96-272, 1980
Aragona J, Eyberg S: Neglected children: mother's report of child behavior problems and observed verbal behavior. Child Dev 52:596–602, 1981

Chasnoff I: Drug use and women: establishing a standard of care. Ann N Y Acad Sci 562:208–210, 1989

Council on Scientific Affairs, American Medical Association: AMA diagnostic and treatment guidelines concerning child abuse and neglect. JAMA 254:796–800, 1985

Damos K: New York City Department of Health, Vital Statistics, Provisional Data. New York, New York City Department of Health, 1991

Eckenrode J, Laird M, Doris J: School performance and disciplinary problems among abused and neglected children. Developmental Psychology 29:53–62, 1993

Egeland B: The consequences of physical and emotional neglect on the development of young children. Paper presented at symposium of the National Center on Child Abuse and Neglect, Chicago, IL, November 1985

Ethier L, Palacio-Quintin E, Jourdan-Ionescu C: Abuse and neglect: two distinct forms of maltreatment? Canada's Mental Health 40:13–19, 1992

Garbarino J, Schellenbach C, Sebes J: Troubled Youth, Troubled Families: Understanding Families at Risk for Adolescent Maltreatment. New York, Aldine, 1986

Giovannoni J: Overview of issues on child neglect, in Child Neglect Monograph: Proceedings from a Symposium. Washington, DC, Clearinghouse on Child Abuse and Neglect Information, 1988, pp 1–6

Graziano A, Mills J: Treatment for abused children: when is a partial solution acceptable? Child Abuse Negl 16:217–228, 1992

Gunsberg A: Empowering young abused and neglected children through contingency play. Childhood Education 66:8–10, 1989

Howing PT et al: The empirical base for the implementation of social skills training with maltreated children. Social Work 35:460–467, 1990

Landau HR: Child protection: the role of the courts. Washington, DC, U.S. Government Printing Office, 1980

Hume RF et al: In utero cocaine exposure: observations of fetal behavioral state may predict neonatal outcome. Am J Obstet Gynecol 161:685–690, 1989

Johnson JL, Boney TY, Brown BS: Evidence of depressive symptoms in children of substance abusers. Int J Addict 25:465–479, 1990

Kaplan S: Child psychiatric consultation to attorneys representing abused and neglected children. Bull Am Acad Psychiatry Law 9:140–148,1981

Kaplan S, Pelcovitz D, Ganeles D, et al: Psychopathology of parents in violent families. Paper presented at the 141st annual meeting of the American Psychiatric Association, Washington, DC, 1988

Kaplan S, Pelcovitz D, Spitzer R: Victimization sequelae disorder. Paper presented at the 142nd annual meeting of the American Psychiatric Association, San Francisco, CA, May 1989

Layzer J, Goodson B: Child abuse and neglect treatment demonstrations. Special issue: reforming child welfare through demonstration and evaluation. Children and Youth Services Review 14:67–76, 1992

MacGregor SN et al: Cocaine abuse during pregnancy: correlation between prenatal care and perinatal outcome. Obstet Gynecol 74:882–885, 1989

Nay P, Fung T, Wickett A: Causes of child abuse and neglect. Can J Psychiatry 36:401–405, 1992

Rodning C, Beckwith L, Howard J: Prenatal exposure to drugs: behavioral distortions reflecting CNS impairment? in Drug Abuse and Brain Development. Edited by Cranmer J, Wigginis R. Arkansas, Intox Press, 1989

Taylor C et al: Diagnosed intellectual and emotional impairment among parents who seriously mistreat their children: prevalence, type, and outcome in a court sample. Child Abuse Negl 15:389–401, 1991

U.S. Department of Health and Human Services: Maltreatment 1993: Reports from the States to the National Center on Child Abuse and Neglect. Washington, DC, U.S. Government Printing Office, 1995

U.S. Department of Health and Human Services: Study Findings: Study of the National Incidence and Prevalence of Child Abuse and Neglect. Washington, DC, U.S. Government Printing Office, 1988, p 4-10

Weakland JH, Jordan L: Working briefly with reluctant clients: child protective services as an example. Journal of Family Therapy 14:231–254, 1992

Williamson J, Bordwin C, Howe B: The ecology of adolescent maltreatment: a multilevel examination of adolescent physical abuse, sexual abuse, and neglect. J Consult Clin Psychol 59:449–457, 1991

Zuravin S: Child abuse, child neglect and maternal depression: is there a connection? in Child Neglect Monograph: Proceedings from a Symposium. Washington, DC, Clearinghouse on Child Abuse and Neglect Information, 1988, pp 20–45

# CHAPTER 3

## Overview of Child Sexual Abuse

*Arthur H. Green, M.D.*

## Definition

Child sexual abuse may be defined as the use of a child under 18 years of age as an object of gratification for adult sexual needs and desires. Incest refers to the sexual exploitation of a child by a family member. The legal definition of incest is cohabitation between persons related to a degree where marriage would be prohibited by law. Sexual abuse ranges in intensity from exhibitionism and gentle fondling to forcible rape resulting in physical injury. Girls are reported as victims of sexual abuse five times more often than boys (American Humane Association 1981). The most common forms of sexual victimization encountered by girls are exhibitionism, fondling, masturbation, and intercourse (vaginal, oral, or anal) by a male perpetrator. Boys are also typically abused by a male offender and are usually subjected to fondling, mutual masturbation, fellatio, and anal intercourse. About half of the child victims are involved in repeated incidents of sexual abuse; in many cases the molestation takes place over a period of years.

## Intrafamilial and Extrafamilial Child Sexual Abuse

Incest by a parent, grandparent, older sibling, or other relative, as well as by a nonrelated adult caretaker living in the home (steppar-

73

ent, parent's paramour) is referred to as intrafamilial child sexual abuse. These cases are usually reported to and investigated by Child Protective Services (CPS), and they may ultimately be referred to the family or juvenile court for a determination of abuse or neglect.

Extrafamilial child sexual abuse refers to a wide range of sexual abuse occurring outside of the family. These include single-episode molestation by an adult stranger, single or multiple molestations by an adult acquaintance, sexual victimization in groups (schools, day care centers, clubs, and youth organizations), and involvement in pornographic sex rings. Extrafamilial sexual abuse is usually reported to the police and these cases are tried in the criminal court. According to the American Humane Association (1981), 86% of the perpetrators of sexual abuse against boys and 94% of the sexual offenders against girls were males.

## Prevalence

The National Incidence Study carried out in 1986 by the National Center on Child Abuse and Neglect estimated that 155,900 children, or 2.5/1,000 in the population, were sexually abused that year. This figure is over 3 times the estimate of 44,700 for 1980 (U.S. Department of Health and Human Services 1988). Finkelhor and Hotaling (1984) projected the annual number of new cases to be 150,000 to 200,000 if extrafamilial sexual abuse cases and unreported cases were included. During 1993, a total of 142, 537 child sexual abuse cases were documented (U.S. Department of Health and Human Services 1995).

Retrospective surveys of women estimate a higher prevalence of sexual abuse during their childhood than are reported during childhood. Russell (1983) interviewed a randomly selected group of women in San Francisco, and reported that 38% had experienced sexual contact with an adult during childhood. Wyatt (1985) discovered that approximately 45% of a community sample of white and African-American women in Los Angeles had unwanted sexual contact during childhood. The majority of these women were victims of extrafamilial abuse (Russell, 83%; Wyatt, 76%). Bagley and Ramsey (1986) found that 22% of women surveyed in Calgary, Alberta, were molested during childhood. The higher estimates of victimization obtained from these retrospective surveys, compared to the number of sexual abuse reports during childhood, suggest that most cases of child sexual abuse are never reported. In Russell's study (1983) only 2% of the intrafamilial and 6% of the extrafamilial sexual abuse cases were reported to the police or CPS.

Surveys of college students report a somewhat lower incidence of sexual abuse than those reported by Russell and Wyatt. Finkelhor's (1979) survey of 530 female college students documented a 19% incidence of sexual abuse during childhood and adolescence. Nine percent of a population of 266 male students had also been abused. Fifty-seven percent of the female students and 83% of the male students were abused outside the family. (The lower incidence of sexual abuse among the college students might be due to a sampling bias reflected by predominantly white, middle-class populations.) On the basis of eight random sample community surveys that interviewed both men and women, Finkelhor and Browne (1986) determined a ratio of 2.5 women abused for every man abused. This corresponds to percentages of 71% females and 29% males who were abused.

# Psychodynamics and Psychopathology of the Incestuous Family

The incestuous family has usually been regarded as disturbed and dysfunctional. Although there is considerable variation in the psychopathology of families in which incest occurs, some typical characteristics of the parents and children have been widely observed. A rigid, patriarchal family structure has been most frequently described, and the father often maintains his dominant position through coercion and occasional violence (Weinberg 1955). Alcohol abuse by the father is often associated with incestuous activity (Cavallin 1966; Kaufman et al. 1954). Aarens et al. (1978) reported that alcohol is involved in 30% to 40% of all cases of child sexual abuse. The family system in cases of incest is usually closed, and outsiders may be viewed with suspicion. The mothers are typically excessively dependent on their domineering spouses, and they often have histories of deprivation and rejection during their own childhood (Meiselman 1978), which compromises their parenting. Mothers in families in which incest occurs are also more likely to have been sexually abused during childhood than mothers in the general population. Mothers in such families are often sexually and emotionally unavailable to their husbands (Lustig et al. 1966), which may trigger the incestuous behavior. "Puritanical" incestuous fathers prefer to use their children as sexual outlets instead of seeking extramarital sexual relationships. Some incestuous fathers may have a pedophilic component to their sexuality and are more sexually aroused by their children than by their spouse (Groth 1982). These individuals may display additional paraphilias, such as exhibitionism, voyeurism, and sexual masochism, and may be sexually aroused by young children outside the family.

A variant of the patriarchal family structure associated with incest has been reported in which the mother is domineering and the father is passive. This type of father feels powerful only in the sexual relationship with the child. There is a significant imbalance of power in each type of parental configuration in most incestuous families.

Role confusion and a blurring of physical and psychological boundaries are common areas of dysfunction in incestuous families. The mother often delegates the marital and homemaking responsibilities to the daughter (Meiselman 1978). The father often assumes the nurturing, caretaking role, but he provides this in a sexual context (Mrazek et al. 1981). The incestuous relationship might represent the major source of intimacy and dependency gratification for the child. The father may use his daughter as a surrogate wife, expecting her to supply him with sexual gratification and emotional support. The child's fixation on her father as a sexual object usually precludes her achieving normal adolescent heterosexual peer relationships. Besides the confusion in intergenerational boundaries, there is little respect for privacy and physical space in the family in which incest occurs. There is often a lack of modesty regarding nudity and bathroom activities and poor limit setting. On the other hand, some incestuous families might be very puritanical regarding dress and modesty. The rigid boundaries between this type of family and the outside world is in sharp contrast to the blurred intergenerational boundaries (Sgroi et al. 1982).

Denial is the most common defense mechanism used by incestuous family members. The father denies and rationalizes the sexual contact with his daughter as "sex education." The mother cannot accept the incest as a reality because to do this would jeopardize the highly dependent relationship she has with her husband. The denial by some mothers may be the result of their own unacknowledged sexual victimization during childhood. The child's denial of the incest experience and her constriction of affect permits her to maintain the fantasy of having normal parents and preserves the equilibrium of the family. Some children are reluctant to relinquish their special sense of power, derived from being the father's favorite. Persistence of the denial used by all the family members complicates the assessment and treatment of the sexually abused child and the family.

## Psychological Sequelae of Child Sexual Abuse

Until the mid-1980s the literature dealing with the impact of child sexual abuse was limited to anecdotal clinical observations and uncontrolled studies. Some observers (Landis 1956; Yorukoğlu and Kemph 1966) maintained that the sexual molestation of a child by an adult may not be psychologically damaging, but the majority of mental health professionals working in this area described the presence of various psychological symptoms. A critical review of the sexual abuse literature up to this point reveals the following methodological deficiencies: 1) failure to employ comparison or control groups, 2) small sample size, 3) failure to control for psychological impairment antedating sexual abuse, 4) confounding independent variables, e.g., physical abuse in addition to sexual abuse, 5) lack of differentiation between short- and long-term sequelae, and 6) failure to use standardized assessment instruments.

Despite these methodological deficiencies, there appears to be some consensus among the clinical observations concerning immediate and long-term sequelae of sexual abuse. Data from recent methodologically sound research studies are beginning to confirm some of the earlier clinical observations concerning the impact of sexual abuse. The first major controlled study of the impact of child sexual abuse was carried out by Gomez-Schwartz et al. (1985), who assessed levels of emotional distress in 156 sexually abused children evaluated and treated at an outpatient clinic over a 2-year period. The children were ages 4–18, and the emotional distress was measured by the Louisville Behavior Checklist. The sexually abused children were divided into preschool (ages 4–6), school age (ages 7–13), and adolescent groups (ages 14–18). The sample consisted of 78% girls and 22% boys. Only 17% of the preschoolers met the criteria for clinically significant psychopathology, whereas 40% of the school-age children and 24% of the adolescents demonstrated significant impairment. Common psychopathology in these children included anxieties, fears, depression, angry and destructive behavior, neurotic symptoms, phobic reactions, and deficits in intellectual, physical, and social development. Each group of sexually abused children manifested more behavioral problems than their nonabused peers but fewer problems than children attending a child psychiatry outpatient clinic. For children of all ages, the children who suffered physical injuries exhibited the greatest impairment.

In another controlled study, Conte and Schuerman (1987) studied 369 sexually abused children and compared them with nonabused and psychiatric outpatient controls on measures of psychopathology derived from a parent-completed behavior rating scale. Again, the abused children demonstrated more impairment than their normal peers but less than the child psychiatric outpatients.

More rigorous and sophisticated research is now being carried out with victims of child sexual abuse in an attempt to identify immediate and long-term sequelae of the molestation. A careful review of these recent research findings and of the older clinical observations suggests that the following areas of psychological impairment have been consistently documented in sexually abused children.

Fearfulness and anxiety-related symptoms have been frequently described as immediate and short-term sequelae of sexual abuse. Sleep disturbances, insomnia, and nightmares have been reported by Camp and Camp (1978), Lewis and Sarrell (1969), and Sgroi et al. (1982). Somatic symptoms and psychosomatic complaints have been described by Adams-Tucker (1982), Browning and Boatman (1977), and Lewis and Sarrell (1969). Sgroi et al. (1982) observed fear reactions in sexually abused children, extending to phobic avoidance of all males. These children were afraid of physical injury as a consequence of the sexual contact and feared retaliation by the perpetrator. Goodwin (1985) has frequently observed in sexually abused children some symptoms of posttraumatic stress disorder (PTSD), including fear, startle reactions, flashbacks, sleep disturbance, reenactment of the trauma, and depressive symptoms.

Kiser et al. (1988) documented PTSD in 9 of 10 children between the ages of 2 and 6 who were molested in a day care setting. The most frequently observed symptoms were fear of the traumatic event's recurring because of environmental stimuli, avoiding activities reminiscent of the traumatic event, and intensification of symptoms on exposure to events resembling the molestation. Other symptoms were visualizing the trauma (in neutral situations), sexual acting out, and nightmares related to the molestation.

McLeer et al. (1988) documented PTSD in 48% of sexually abused children evaluated at a child psychiatry outpatient clinic according to DSM-III-R (American Psychiatric Association 1989) criteria. The symptoms included reexperiencing phenomena, avoidance behavior, and autonomic hyperarousal. Seventy-five percent of children abused by biological fathers, 67% abused by strangers, and 25% abused by trusted adults met PTSD criteria, as opposed to none of the children abused by an older child.

## ▌ Paranoid Reactions and Mistrust

Herman (1981), Knittle and Tuana (1980), and Sgroi et al. (1982) described the inability of sexually abused children to establish trusting relationships with adults because of the father's breach of his parental role and the mother's failure to protect the child. Through the process of generalization, other adults and potential love objects are viewed as unpredictable and exploitative. The inability to establish trusting relationships and intimacy with others eventually causes problems with future sexual partners and spouses.

## ▌ Poor Self-Image

The strong sense of stigmatization experienced by sexually abused children contributes to a loss of self-esteem. This is often reinforced by critical comments by peers and family members blaming the child for the victimization. Sgroi et al. (1982) described the "damaged goods syndrome" in which the sexually abused child feels physically damaged and permanently altered by the molestation. The child's shame and guilt may be intensified by the experience of some pleasure associated with the gratification of phase-specific sexual fantasies. A study by Tong et al. (1987) reported that sexually abused children scored significantly lower on the Piers-Harris Self-Concept Scale than nonabused controls.

## ▌ Depression and Suicidal Behavior

Depressive symptoms are among the most frequently described in sexually abused children (Kempe and Kempe 1978; Nakashima and Zakins 1977; Sgroi et al. 1982). MacVicar (1979) observed that sexually abused adolescents are the most vulnerable to depression. Kaufman et al. (1954) and Lukianowicz (1972) described suicidal behavior in sexually abused adolescents, and Anderson (1981) reported case histories of four adolescent girls who attempted suicide following the disclosure of incest.

Two recent studies of sexually abused children admitted to psychiatric inpatient facilities confirmed the link between sexual abuse and depression. Livingston (1987) documented major depressive disorder with psychotic features in sexually abused child inpatients using the Diagnostic Interview for Children and Adolescents (DICA) as a standardized psychiatric interview. The mean age of these children was 9.7 years. Sansonnet-Hayden et al. (1987) reported a 71% incidence of major depression in sexually abused adolescents who had been admitted to a psychiatric hospital. These sexually abused adolescents had a much higher incidence of suicide attempts than their nonabused hospitalized peers.

Friedrich et al. (1986) reported that 46% of a sample of 61 sexually abused girls had significantly elevated scores on the internalizing scale of the Child Behavior Checklist, which includes behaviors described as fearful, inhibited, depressed, and overcontrolled.

## ▌ Hysterical and Dissociative Symptoms

Gross (1979) reported hysterical seizures in four incest victims, and Goodwin et al. (1989) described six cases of hysterical seizures occurring in adolescents who experienced incest. The hysterical symptoms were felt to represent the child's attempt to wall off traumatic memories of the incest through primitive defenses of denial, isolation of affect, and splitting. Multiple personality disorder (MPD) is the most extreme form of dissociation. MPD has been described in sexually abused children by Kluft (1985) and Putnam (1984). Goodwin et al. (1989) observed MPD in adult incest survivors. Child sexual abuse is the most frequent antecedent of MPD. Signs of early dissociation in children are forgetfulness with periods of amnesia, excessive fantasizing and daydreaming, the presence of an imaginary companion, sleepwalking, and blackouts.

## ▌ Impaired Peer Relationships

Adams-Tucker (1982), Knittle and Tuana (1980), and Tsai and Wagner (1981), reported inadequate social skills, social withdrawal, and difficulties in interpersonal relationships in young sexually abused children. Sgroi et al. (1982) described how incestuous families discourage peer relationships and separation-individuation in the child who is abused. Herman (1981) reported runaway behavior in sexually abused adolescents, and Reich and Gutierres (1979) described truancy and runaway behavior as sequelae of sexual abuse.

## ▌ Poor School Performance

A sudden deterioration in academic performance and behavior has been frequently observed in sexually abused children (DeFrancis 1969; Goodwin et al. 1989; Sgroi 1982). The abused child, preoccupied with the incest and with family problems, is unable to concentrate in the classroom or while doing homework. If the abused child's social withdrawal extends to the classroom, refusal to attend school might ensue. The sexually abused child may disrupt the class by attempting to reenact his or her victimization with classmates, or by displacing aggression into the school setting.

There has been research interest in the relationship between incest experiences and eating disorders. Oppenheimer et al. (1985) found that two-thirds of their sample of 78 patients with eating disorders reported a history of sexual abuse. Kearny-Cooke (1988) reported that 58% of 75 bulimic patients had been sexually abused during childhood. Sloan and Leighner (1986) documented a history of sexual abuse in 5 of 6 inpatients on an eating disorders unit. Goodwin et al. (1989) inferred a relationship between habitual vomiting in patients with eating disorders and conflicts regarding oral sex.

## ▌ Substance Abuse

Drug and alcohol abuse have been frequently reported as long-term sequelae of sexual abuse that first appear during adolescence and early adulthood. Briere (1984), Herman (1981), and Kearney-Cooke (1988) reported that 27% of sexual abuse victims had a history of alcohol abuse and 21% had a history of substance abuse. Clinical experience with adolescents and young adults with a history of sexual abuse reveals that these substances help to blot out the painful memories and affects associated with the victimization.

## ▌ Disturbances in Sexual Behavior

Disturbances in sexual behavior are among the most striking and dramatic symptoms exhibited by sexually abused children, and these appear to be specifically linked to the sexual trauma. Yates (1982) described the eroticization of preschool children by incest with the degree of eroticization proportional to the duration and intensity of the sexual contact. The sexually abused preschoolers were orgasmic and maintained a high level of sexual arousal. These preschoolers were frequently unable to differentiate affectionate from sexual relationships and were aroused by routine physical or psychological closeness. Sexual hyperarousal and sexual acting out with a tendency to repeat and reenact the incest experience have also been observed in older children and adolescents. Brandt and Tisza (1977) postulated that these children provoked further sexual contact as a means of obtaining pleasure and soothing and as a technique for mastering the original trauma. MacVicar (1979) described compulsive masturbation and promiscuity in sexually abused girls of latency age. Browning and Boatman (1977) and Sloane and Karpinski (1942) theorized that the promiscuity in sexually abused adolescents represented the acting out of conflicts in lieu of the development of neurotic symptoms. James and Meyerding's (1977) retrospective study of adult female prostitutes revealed that 36% were incest survivors.

At the other end of the spectrum, many observers describe phobic reactions and sexual inhibition in sexually abused children, and sexual dysfunction in adult incest survivors (Bess and Janssen 1982; Brooks 1982; Tsai and Wagner 1978).

In essence, there appear to be two contrasting adaptive styles in sexually abused persons: one seeking mastery through active repetition of the trauma, and the other coping by avoidance of sexual stimuli.

Studies on long-term effects of sexual abuse in adult survivors are presented in Chapter 7. Borderline personality and sexual behavioral development are discussed in this chapter.

## Assessment of Child Sexual Abuse

### ▮ Physical Evaluation

#### *History*

A detailed history concerning the molestation should be taken from the parent or caretaker, and from any person or family member to whom the child disclosed the abuse. A history should also be taken from the child in order to document his or her account of the sexual abuse. The examiner should also determine the child's preabuse medical history and psychological functioning and should observe any physical and behavioral changes in the child following the alleged molestation. The examiner should also identify the child's name for his or her body parts and genitalia. A sample interview follows.

1. "What are some things you like to do with Daddy? (Mommy?) (don't like to do?)"
2. "What are some games you like to play with Grandpa? (Grandma?) (don't like to play?)"
3. "Does your Grandpa (Grandma) do some things that you don't like? (that make you feel sad or scared?)"
4. "Do you and Daddy (Mommy) have any secrets? Are they good secrets or yucky secrets?"
5. "Has anyone touched your _____ ?"
6. "Has anyone hurt your _____ ?"
7. "Have you seen anybody else's _____ ?"
8. "Has anyone asked you to touch their _____ ?"
9. "Has anyone asked you to let them touch your _____ ?"
10. "Has anyone taken pictures of you with your clothes off?"

If the child responds "yes" to any of these questions, ask these follow-up questions:

1. "Who? What was that person's name?"
2. "Show me where _____ _____ you?" (using the child's identifying name and action)
3. "Show me with the dolls what happened."

Additional sexual abuse history formats have been developed that use semistructured interviews and discuss use of anatomically correct or detailed dolls (White et al. 1986). These interviews assist the clinician in avoiding leading questions when interviewing children.

## Examination

The physical examination should be performed immediately if the alleged molestation took place within 72 hours, or if the history suggests the presence of a sexually transmitted disease, or if there is a possibility of pregnancy in a postmenarchal female. If disclosure occurs more than 72 hours after the alleged sexual abuse, there is less urgency about scheduling the examination. If the examination takes place within 72 hours of the alleged assault, clothing, hair, and debris should be saved and child's clothing, vagina, and anus should be inspected for the presence of semen.

A parent or family member should be present along with the nurse to allay the child's anxiety regarding the examination. The child should be informed about the purpose of the examination, and be reassured that it will not hurt. If the child is uncooperative, resistant, or panicky, he or she should never be forced to submit to the examination. If there is a question of serious trauma, the frightened or resistant child may be examined under general anesthesia.

The examination may be facilitated by the use of a colposcope, which provides magnification from 5 to 30 times. This instrument permits better visualization of scar tissue and vascular changes in hymenal and perihymenal tissues and anus. The examination should include observation of the labia majora, labia minora, and vaginal vestibule encompassing the urethra, periurethral glands, hymenal membrane, hymenal orifice, Bartholin's glands, and the fossa navicularis. The anus and rectum should be examined together with the penis and scrotum in males.

As described by Finkelhor (1988), typical findings of acute trauma are lacerations, hematomas, petechiae, edema, and contusions. Signs of penile penetration include hymenal tears extending upward into the posterior vaginal wall and downward to involve the skin of the perineum. Trauma may produce scar tissue and adhesions, which distort the shape of the hymenal membrane. Other signs of chronic sexual abuse are clefts or bumps of the hymenal membrane, labial adhesions, alteration or widening of the hymenal orifice, and rounding of the hymenal edge. Signs of anal trauma include hematomas, prolapse of anal tissue, fissures, pigmentation, anal skin tags, hemorrhoids, and scar tissue. Chronic anal penetration may produce changes in the tone of the anal sphincter. Dilation of the anal sphincter may occur when the buttocks are separated or when the sphincter is touched with a Q-tip or examining finger.

Cultures of vagina, anus, and throat should be taken routinely to detect the presence of sexually transmitted diseases such as gonorrhea, chlamydia trachomatis, and herpes simplex. One must also check for the presence of venereal warts (condyloma acuminatum) and serology should be obtained for the diagnosis of syphilis. The presence of a sexually transmitted disease is usually a reliable indicator of genital contact because nonsexual transmission of these diseases is rare. However, venereal warts are more frequently transmitted nonsexually, and chlamydia may be transmitted from an infected mother to the neonate passing through the birth canal, and the organism may remain in the vagina or rectum for several years. It is the physician's duty to report any suspicions of sexual abuse to the local child abuse registry.

# ▌ Clinical Evaluation of Child Sexual Abuse

## Qualifications of the Evaluator

The American Academy of Child and Adolescent Psychiatry (1988) has formulated guidelines for the clinical evaluation of child sexual abuse. The following recommendations regarding evaluators are presented in these guidelines:

The assessment of a potential case of child sexual abuse should be carried out by a mental health professional specializing in children: a child psychiatrist, a child psychologist, or a psychiatric nurse or social worker trained to evaluate and treat children. The evaluator should also be an expert on child sexual abuse and on testifying in court and should be knowledgeable about child development and child psychopathology. Familiarity with the psychopathology and dynamics of the incestuous family is also indispensable, as well as familiarity with the characteristics of sexual offenders against children. The evaluator should be aware of the phenomenon of false allegations of sexual abuse. Finally, the evaluator should be aware of his or her feelings and biases concerning sexual behavior and sexual abuse of children so as to minimize countertransference reactions.

## Assessment of the Child

A detailed history of the child should be obtained prior to the first interview, including a developmental survey, information regarding the child's sexual interests and behavior, family attitudes toward sex and modesty, and a description of his or her typical coping mechanisms. The history should also be designed to elicit information regarding typical signs and symptoms associated with child sexual abuse, and an overview of the child's pretraumatic psychological functioning. Sexual abuse evaluations may require a slightly longer period of time than routine child psychiatry diagnostic assessments because sexually abused children are often very defensive and resistant to questioning. In some cases, several sessions might be required to establish initial rapport and trust before pursuing the sexual abuse allegations. If the child is able to talk about the molestations, detailed descriptions of the events should be obtained where possible, e.g., the type of molestation, frequency, location, and the nature of the sexual acts, and any threats used by the perpetrator to maintain secrecy. Adams-Tucker and Adams (1984) recommend exploring sensory modalities such as taste, smell, noises, and how the abuse felt.

If the child is unable to verbalize his or her memory and feelings regarding the molestation, his or her perception of the events may be obtained indirectly through play, fantasies, and dreams. Terr (1985) describes the persistence of memory in children who were traumatized prior to the acquisition of verbal skills. These children demonstrated a "perceptual memory" of their traumas through their play despite the absence of any verbal memory of the events. The child will often reveal aspects of the molestation in spontaneous drawings, which may include genitalia and exaggeration of or avoidance of sexual features. Hibbard et al. (1987) reported that sexually abused children were 6.8 times more likely to draw genitalia than were nonabused children.

It is important to assess the credibility of the child's account of the molestation by determining the accuracy of memory, the consistency of the description of the molestation, the degree of suggestibility, the sense of time, and the ability to differentiate reality from fantasy and the truth from a lie.

Young children's memories are good for events that are personally meaningful and salient. However, they recall information less spontaneously than do older children and adults (Cole and Loftus 1987). Because they have not mastered the memory strategies used by older children to trigger recollections, young children provide less information during spontaneous recall of an event. Therefore, it might be necessary to ask young children questions to elicit what they know. These same children are susceptible to being misled, so the evaluator has to avoid using leading questions.

The communications of children lack the consistency of adult communications, because children have difficulty in evaluating them for errors, inconsistencies, or contradictions (Singer and Flavell

1981). Because they have difficulty assuming another person's perspective, young children also fail to perceive that they are being mis-
understood. Nevertheless, children are capable of describing a major
event in a relatively consistent manner over time. During the assessment, the evaluator observes the consistency of the child's description
of the molestation. Grossly inconsistent and contradictory statements decrease the child's credibility, and should be gently challenged.

Studies have shown that children 10 to 11 years old are no more
suggestible than adults, but that children 4 to 9 years old are more
suggestible than older children (Cole and Loftus 1987). There is evidence that young children may be vulnerable to social pressures to say
what they think adults want to hear (Ceci et al. 1987). Even if children
are influenced by suggestions during an interview, their original memory of the event is not changed. The degree of the child's suggestibility
can be assessed during the evaluation by contradicting his or her views
on a subject unrelated to the sexual abuse to see whether he or she
persists in his or her belief or capitulates to the interviewer's expectations.

Most children are able to differentiate fact from fantasy, and seem
to know that they are pretending in their play. It is important for the
evaluator to be aware of the universality of sexual fantasies in children.
However, they are rarely used by a child to initiate a complaint against
the fantasied object, because they are pleasurable and often tinged
with self-induced guilt and secrecy. When children mistakenly believe
that their sexual fantasies are real, they are usually unable to provide
details regarding the alleged sexual contact, and their accounts of the
events are inconsistent and lack credibility. One usually finds evidence
of impaired reality testing in other major areas in these children. They
might also elaborate and act out nonsexual fantasies—for example,
that they are superheroes who have superhuman or magical powers.

Young children do not share the adult's sense of time or the ability
to measure time. Many children cannot order the months accurately
until the age of eight or nine. It is not until that age that most children can perceive a constant flow of time that applies to everyone,
independent of their own activities. Children may be quite accurate
with regard to frequency of occurrence or temporal order of events
(Brown 1975) if they are allowed to describe them in relation to holi-
days, birthdays, seasons, meals, or TV programs. Terr (1983) observed
that distortions of time and time-related phenomena may occur in

children following psychic trauma. The actual duration of the traumatic experience may be lengthened, and the sequencing of events is often confused.

### Reliability of the Child's Disclosure

The child's spontaneous disclosure of sexual activity with an adult must be taken seriously. Factors enhancing a child's credibility in describing sexual abuse include a consistent reporting of the details over time with an affect (usually painful) appropriate to the allegations. The disclosure is often delayed and difficult. The presence of the previously described signs and symptoms of sexual abuse—fearfulness, abnormal sexual behavior and seductiveness, and reenactment of the molestation through traumatic play—increase the likelihood that there has been sexual abuse. The child's ability to differentiate fact from fantasy, use age-appropriate vocabulary, and distinguish between the truth and a lie also strengthens the child's credibility.

Denial of the sexual abuse allegations by the child, on the other hand, has limited validity, because this is easily prompted by threats and coercion by the perpetrator and internally produced shame and guilt. Therefore, false denials are common, and false disclosures are rare.

## ▌ False Allegations of Child Sexual Abuse

False allegations of sexual abuse have been frequently observed during marital disputes over child custody and visitation. Benedek and Schetky (1985) were unable to document charges of sexual abuse in 10 of 18 children (56%) during disputes over custody and visitation. This is comparable to Green's (1986) determination of 4 false allegations in 11 children (36%) reported to be molested by the noncustodial parent during custody disputes. Yates and Musty (1988) indicated that 15 of 19 allegations of sexual abuse in custody and/or visitation cases (79%) involving preschool children could not be substantiated. In a study of 129 cases of alleged sexual abuse occurring during custody disputes gathered from 8 domestic relations courts throughout the country, Thoeness and Tjaden (1990) found that 50% of the allegations could not be substantiated.

### Unintentional False Allegations

Intentional false allegations of sexual abuse designed to exclude an ex-spouse or lover from the child's life are relatively uncommon. Most adults who make false allegations believe that the child is being molested. Their convictions are usually based upon misperceptions and misinterpretations of ambiguous events, associated with excessive reliance on defenses of denial and projection. In extreme cases, these individuals may be frankly delusional. Parents or caretakers with histrionic or paranoid personality disorders or paranoid psychoses are prone toward misperceiving certain types of interactions or behaviors. These behaviors may become the nucleus of a false allegation (Green 1986).

**Misinterpretation of normal caretaking practice.**   Mistrustful and/ or sexually preoccupied parents might misperceive innocent bathing or toileting of the child by the estranged spouse as evidence of sexual molestation. Washing, powdering, or drying of the child's genital or anal area may be mistaken for genital or anal fondling. Parents who innocently bathe or shower with young children might be accused of having sexual intent. In these situations, the child might be asked if the caretaker touched his or her private parts, and an affirmative answer might confirm the suspicions of the accusing parent (Green 1991).

**Misinterpretation of normal sexual behaviors in children.**   Normal children of all ages, including infants and toddlers, exhibit sexual activities consisting of direct and indirect genital stimulation, which may be associated with erections in boys and vaginal lubrication in girls (Kinsey et al. 1948, 1953). Preschool children often engage in genital handling and fondling, sex play, genital exploration, and exhibitionistic and voyeuristic activities (Gundersen et al. 1981). Rosenfeld et al. (1986) reported that 45% of boys 8 to 10 years old had touched their mothers' breasts and genitals and that 30% of girls up to age 10 had touched their fathers' genitals. These data were obtained during a survey of child-rearing practices in upper-middle-class families.

These types of normal sexual behavior in children directed toward an estranged spouse may be misperceived as evidence of sexual abuse. These behaviors may be also confused with the erotic and seductive behavior of sexually abused children, and regarded as symptoms of sexual abuse. Although sexually conflicted parents relying heavily on projective defenses will tend to misperceive these developmentally appropriate expressions of sexuality, even "normal" parents might find these behaviors puzzling.

**Misinterpretation of common psychological symptoms in children.**
Nonspecific symptoms of psychological distress in children, such as
separation anxiety, regressive behavior, sleep disorders, and phobic
symptoms, often occur during parental separation and divorce. However, these may be misperceived as fear of the noncustodial parent,
especially if they occur prior to or following visitation, and may ultimately be presented as evidence of molestation. The potential for misinterpretation is further enhanced by the frequent presence of these
symptoms in children who have been sexually abused.

**Confusion with sexual overstimulation by a parent.**   Some parents
engage in sexually overstimulating practices such as excessive hugging,
kissing, or lap sitting, or they allow the child to sleep in the parental
bed, or to bathe or shower with an older child. A parent might also
permit a child to view pornographic magazines and films. Many parents who do these things are unaware of the adverse impact of these
practices on the child. These parents usually deny sexual intent or
excitement, but they might experience unconscious sexual pleasure
from these encounters. The impact of the sexual behavior resembles
the sequelae of actual sexual abuse, which creates a problem in differential diagnosis. However, these parents are guilty of inappropriate or
improper child-rearing practices rather than sexual abuse. It is important to note that in some cases, sexual overstimulation might be
a prelude to frank genital contact by a sexual abuser. A thorough psychiatric evaluation of parent and child should help differentiate the
naively overstimulating parent from the molesting parent.

**Misinterpretation of physical signs and symptoms in the child.**
Physical signs and symptoms such as vaginal irritation or vaginal discharge resulting from a nonspecific vulvovaginitis are common in
young girls and may be mistakenly attributed to sexual contact and
used to initiate a report of sexual abuse. Similarly, nonspecific rectal
irritations or fissures may be regarded as a sign of anal penetration.
The overinterpretation of equivocal physical findings as evidence of
sexual abuse might be influenced by the persuasiveness of the accusing parent or of his or her attorney, or might reflect the physician's
own bias, and can easily lead to the substantiation of an allegation of
sexual abuse deemed unlikely by the comprehensive clinical assessment of the child and family.

## Intentional False Allegations by a Parent

A vindictive parent will sometimes fabricate incest in order to punish the child's other parent by excluding him or her from further contact with the child. The false allegation is often supported by the presence of nonspecific physical or psychological symptoms in the child, as previously described. The vindictive parent may brainwash the child by repetitively discussing the alleged molestation and deprecating the "perpetrator" in the child's presence. This type of parent rewards the child for talking about the "molestation" and displaying hostility toward the accused. This behavior in the vindictive parent is congruent with the parental alienation syndrome described by Gardner (1987).

## False Allegations by a Child

**Allegations induced by parents or other adults.**    A child can be brainwashed by a vindictive parent, as described above, or influenced by a delusional parent, who projects his or her own unconscious sexual fantasies onto the spouse. Both vindictive and delusional parents reinforce compliance by withholding love and approval if the child denies the molestation or demonstrates positive feelings toward the accused parent. In cases such as this, there is often a history of previous accusations of sexual misconduct by the spouse.

**Allegations based on fantasy.**    Fantasied incest is most common in preadolescent or adolescent girls who project their sexual wishes onto the parent, usually the father or father surrogate. These girls usually exhibit hysterical personality traits; more rarely they are frankly paranoid and delusional.

Children with severe ego impairment or children who have been sexually traumatized or overstimulated are more likely to confuse sexual fantasies with reality. Jones and McGraw (1987) observed false allegations of sexual abuse by children who were prior victims of a molestation. These children exhibited PTSD and displaced their memories of traumatization onto a new person.

**Allegations based on revenge or retaliation.**    Older children or adolescents may falsely accuse a parent of incest because of a desire for retaliation or revenge. Often the underlying motivation for this type of fictitious allegation is anger over a recent punishment or deprivation, or a wish to remove the father or stepfather from the home.

**Allegations spread by contagion.**   Children attending nursery school, day care, or any other organized program for children in which widespread sexual abuse is suspected may be influenced by descriptions of sexual activity given by other children who may or may not have been molested. These children might also be pressured into "disclosing" sexual abuse that never occurred by detectives or district attorneys using leading questions and coercive interview techniques.

**Characteristics of false allegations by children.**   Accounts of the sexual activity may be obtained rather easily, or even spontaneously, from the child without significant changes in mood and affect. The child might describe the molestation in a rote manner, often using adult terminology to describe the genitals. Descriptions of the event will usually be lacking in detail, and gross inconsistencies will be observed with repeated interviewing. There is often a marked discrepancy between the child's angry accusations toward the alleged perpetrator and the apparent closeness and affectionate behavior in his presence. In cases of brainwashing and coaching, the child will often visually check with his or her parent before responding to the interviewer (Green 1986).

Genuine incest victims, on the other hand, are secretive and distressed about the molestation; their disclosure is usually delayed and conflicted, and may be retracted. Direct questioning about the molestation usually intensifies negative affect. When the child is able to describe the molestation, he or she is often capable of providing a consistent, detailed account of the events. These children use age-appropriate sexual terminology, and may be fearful or emotionally constricted in the perpetrator's presence.

The following case illustrates several of the topics discussed here.

➤ **Case Example**

Shortly after Mrs. A initiated divorce proceedings and left her husband, Mr. A, their 3½-year-old daughter Cindy began to exhibit sexually provocative behavior at her nursery school. She tried to touch the genitals of other children and told her teacher that one of the boys in her class put a pencil in her "tushy" (vagina). Mrs. A also reported that Cindy exhibited similar sexualized behavior at home, consisting of frequent masturbation and attempts to touch her mother's genitals. The pediatrician who examined Cindy discovered an enlarged hymenal opening and vaginal tears consistent with a sexual molestation. Mr. A vehemently denied the allegations and accused Mrs. A of brainwashing Cindy. His psychotherapist issued a report stating that Mr. A could not have molested his daughter. In addition, Mr. A passed a polygraph test, which was submitted as proof of his innocence. Nevertheless, Mr. A's contact with Cindy was sharply curtailed and was limited to weekly supervised visits by the child protective agency.

Cindy, Mr. A, and Mrs. A were each interviewed by an evaluator as a part of the clinical investigation and assessment of the case.

## ➤ Evaluation of Cindy

Cindy was initially shy and cautious during the first meeting with the evaluator, but she warmed up rapidly and became more spontaneous during the subsequent sessions. When asked about her family, she mentioned that she lived with her mother, that her father had his own apartment, and that she liked to go to McDonald's with him. Later in this first interview, Cindy played with puppets and depicted the clown hurting a baby, but she couldn't provide details. When asked if anyone had ever hurt her, she appeared tense, and then replied that it hurt her when she made "doody" (a reference to her frequent constipation and abdominal cramps). During the next appointment, the evaluator initiated a pretend phone call to her father. Cindy demonstrated an eagerness to see her father at first, but then she changed her mind and mentioned that her father had scared her. Cindy became anxious and changed the subject when the evaluator asked her what her father did to frighten her.

During the third session, Cindy made a snake out of clay that "hissed," and then a menacing crocodile, and then a rabbit, described as a "good animal that doesn't bite." Then she shifted to playing with puppets and referred to the baby's "tush" hurting. The evaluator then asked Cindy if her father had done anything that hurt her "tushy," but the child turned away and resumed her play. The baby with a hurt "tush" theme continued during the next two sessions, with the cause of the hurt attributed to the chicken pox, and then to Billy, the nursery school classmate whom Cindy had originally accused of sticking a pencil in her vagina. At this point the evaluator provided Cindy with anatomically detailed dolls so that she could demonstrate this. The child put the boy's hand into the little girl's vagina. During the next session, Cindy demonstrated how the clown pushed the baby down and how the policeman punched the clown and threw him in jail. Cindy was finally able to tell the evaluator that her father hurt her "tushy" but added, "You take a bath and it gets better." She spontaneously requested the anatomical dolls, and she depicted the father putting his finger in the girl's vagina.

## ➤ Evaluation of Mr. A

Mr. A is a slightly balding 39-year-old man. His behavior was alert and well oriented. His speech was articulate, coherent, and goal directed, with no evidence of a thinking disorder, delusions, or hallucinations. His mood was labile, ranging from mildly to moderately depressed. Mr. A exhibited considerable anxiety, which he expressed by getting up from his chair and pacing around the office. He vehemently denied the sexual abuse allegations and stated his belief that Cindy was coached by her mother and told to say that he hurt her vagina. He suggested that Cindy's description of her "tushy" hurting could be attributed to her painful defecation or to his taking her rectal temperature. Mr. A claimed that Mrs. A was angry enough to make a false accusation because he had rejected her during their marriage. When Mr. A was confronted by the physical evaluation demonstrating medical evidence of sexual abuse, he claimed that Cindy might have been molested by Mrs. A or one of her nursery school teachers. Mr. A cited his passing of the polygraph test and the lack of positive findings on the penile transducer (plethysmograph) as additional proof of his innocence. He appeared greatly disturbed by his lack of access to Cindy, which was limited to weekly supervised visits.

Mr. A admitted to having had a lack of sexual desire for Mrs. A during their marriage, which had led him to augment his sexual arousal by using pornography and mechanical aids such as dildos and vibrators, and by "swinging," during which he was aroused by witnessing other couples having sex, or by others watching his sexual activity. Mr. A claimed to have experienced a normal, happy childhood and family life. He denied any physical or sexual abuse in his childhood, but admitted to having some conflicts with a domineering father.

## ➤ DSM-IV Diagnosis
### (American Psychiatric Association 1994): Mr. A

Axis I:   Adjustment disorder with anxiety
Voyeurism
Pedophilia

> ### Evaluation of Mrs. A

Mrs. A is an attractive 31-year-old woman who related in a spontaneous manner. She was alert and fully oriented. Her speech was coherent and goal directed with no evidence of a thinking disorder or psychotic symptoms. Mrs. A was very preoccupied with Cindy's alleged molestation by her father. She was certain that Cindy had been abused by Mr. A because of the child's remarks about her father hurting her, and also because of Mr. A's unusual sexual proclivities. Mrs. A was also very angry with her husband because of his physical and emotional withdrawal from her during their marriage. She was outspoken in her desire to protect Cindy; she stated her belief that Mr. A would continue to molest the child if he had access to her. Mrs. A seemed distressed as she described some of Cindy's unusual behavior at home—masturbating with a candy cane, exposing her buttocks, and attempting to fondle Mrs. A's genitals. Mrs. A had experienced difficulty in controlling Cindy's behavior, as the child had recently been prone to tantrums and oppositional behavior. Mrs. A also recognized Cindy's strong positive feeling toward her father. When she punished Cindy, the child often cried for her father.

Mrs. A described a happy childhood and denied having been physically or sexually abused in the past. Her affect was rich and appropriate to her ideation; her mood was neutral to slightly depressed.

> ### DSM-IV Diagnosis: Mrs. A

Axis I:   Adjustment disorder with anxious mood

> ### Evaluation of Mr. A and Cindy

After assessing Cindy and her parents separately, the evaluator met with Cindy and her father together. During their first encounter, Cindy was initially silent when Mr. A entered the office; then she began to whisper. After about 10 minutes she warmed up and responded positively to her father's present of a coloring book. Mr. A then asked Cindy, "How come you don't talk to me on the phone?" The child replied, "I like Mommy better than you." Cindy then became affectionate and told her father that she missed visits with him at his apartment. When Mr. A asked Cindy if she would like to resume the visits with him, the child replied that she would like to go to his house that evening. Mr. A then began to question

Cindy about his alleged molestation. He asked if "Daddy ever hurt you," to which Cindy answered in the negative. He then asked if anyone had hurt her "tushy," and she answered "no." When he asked about Billy, Cindy told him that Billy had put a pencil in her "tushy." Toward the end of the session, Cindy was given a ride on her father's back and she walked on his shoes with glee. During their next and final session together, Cindy's enthusiasm was readily apparent from the moment she saw her father. They interacted affectionately while blowing bubbles. Mr. A brought a tape recorder and tried to get Cindy to sing into it so that he could record her voice. She then took a ride on her father's back with much enjoyment. After her father left, I reminded Cindy that she told me that her father hurt her tushy. She replied "It didn't happen; I want to see Daddy."

## ➤ *Formulation*

The following observations and findings are consistent with a diagnosis of sexual abuse:

1. Cindy made a gradual and conflicted disclosure of a consistent story of having been genitally fondled by her father (in her own unique language). This information was elicited with considerable difficulty and was accompanied by a sad and painful affect. Cindy's disclosure was spontaneous and quite credible.
2. Cindy exhibited sexualized behaviors often associated with child sexual abuse. Her attempts to sexually fondle classmates and adults in an inappropriate manner and her excessive masturbation and sexual preoccupation are consistent with sexual traumatization.
3. The physical examination indicated genital trauma and changes in the vagina that are associated with sexual abuse.
4. The possibility of brainwashing by Mrs. A is unlikely; Cindy's descriptions of molestation seemed spontaneous and unrehearsed, and Mrs. A did not use defenses of denial and projection to excess. These defenses often permit individuals to misperceive ambiguous events and escalate them into sexual abuse allegations. Mrs. A never attempted to monitor or control Cindy's language or behavior during their interaction.
5. Mr. A's sexual inhibitions and difficulties with intimacy within the marriage, and his deviant sexual interests—voyeurism, exhibitionism, use of vibrators, interest in sadomasochism—are often characteristic of pedophiles.

The following observations tend to decrease the credibility of the sexual abuse allegations:

1. Mr. A was willing to submit to many tests and procedures in order to prove his innocence, such as the penile transducer and the polygraph, and he passed the polygraph test.
2. Mr. A interacted very well with Cindy, and she did not exhibit fear or anxiety in his presence. Cindy derived pleasure from their relationship.
3. Mr. A's psychiatrist stated that it was unlikely that Mr. A would sexually abuse Cindy.

When all of the observations are weighed carefully, the credibility of Cindy's disclosure of fondling and her inappropriate precocious sexual behaviors along with the positive physical findings suggest that this child was molested by her father. Although there is a slim possibility that Cindy might have been sexually abused by another person, there is little evidence for it.

## Legal Commentary

### ▌ Issues Related to Victims, Other Family Members, and Offenders

In order to prevent recurrence of child sexual abuse by identified perpetrators, many states have developed or refined their central CPS and criminal justice record repositories to help ensure that offenders are not permitted to secure employment or volunteer positions where they will have access to children. Many states have police registration requirements for convicted child sex offenders, so that if an offender moves to a new community, law enforcement officials will be advised of his or her presence. In Washington State, legislation provides for mandatory secure treatment for offenders who present a sexual danger to children, and several other states have enacted mandatory treatment laws for offenders—both outside and inside prison. Other novel legislative directions include authority for judges to impose employment-related restrictions on convicted child molesters and the required notification of children and parents when molesters are being given parole consideration or are released from prison.

There has been increased interest in special coordination of the legal response in cases of sexual offenses against young children that are committed by juveniles. Potential legislative and legal policy improvements have been recommended in four basic areas: 1) case identification and referral, 2) record keeping and access, 3) judicial intervention options, and 4) multidisciplinary cooperation in evaluation and treatment. The National Council of Juvenile and Family Court Judges has recognized the importance of mandating treatment for juvenile offenders by recommending that judges be given the authority to order treatment for youthful sexual offenders (Revised Report from the National Task Force on Juvenile Sex Offending 1993)

New legal and programmatic mechanisms to enhance multidisciplinary cooperation regarding adolescent sex offenders are beginning to be developed in an increasing number of communities across the country. For example, California has passed special legislation to design treatment programs for juvenile sex offenders and has appropriated funds for pilot projects to coordinate case referral, case management, and service delivery to juvenile sex offenders. In Minnesota a special statewide adolescent sex abuse treatment program has been established with standards, training, dispositional options, pilot program, and evaluation requirements.

The U.S. Department of Health and Human Services has also encouraged the development of projects targeted at adolescent sex offenders. One demonstration project funded during the past decade reported significant gains in accomplishing four goals: 1) increasing cooperation and communication by child abuse agencies through interagency agreements and multidisciplinary training, 2) reducing system-induced trauma to sexually abused children and their families through improved delivery of services, 3) providing quality legal intervention through greater prosecution of juvenile sex offenders, and 4) encouraging the enhancement of community-based programs to treat juvenile sex offenders.

## ▌ Guidance for Mental Health Professionals and Practitioners

Some professionals who receive disclosures of child sexual abuse work in rape crisis programs. Even if these individuals are not covered under the privileged communications laws applicable to psychotherapists and patients or to social workers and clients, the privacy of the information received from sexually abused children may be protected by the increasing number of state laws that provide protection for the confidential communications between these children and their counselors. However, depending on the language of the state reporting law and their professional background, rape crisis counselors may still be required to report suspected child abuse and neglect.

Mental health professionals may find themselves asked to assist a court in modifying its procedures for taking testimony from children alleged to have been sexually abused. For example, a child psychiatrist may be asked to testify as to why a child would experience trauma if not permitted to testify by means of closed-circuit television, rather than having to appear in the physical presence of the defendant. Some attorneys may also seek to have a child evaluated by a mental health professional for an assessment of the child's competence as a witness and capacity to withstand the rigors of cross-examination in court. The professional may also be asked to help the court or attorneys understand if or how the use of anatomical dolls or drawings may assist the child in communicating what happened to him or her.

It is also likely that mental health professionals will be asked by the court or the attorneys to aid in the development of a treatment plan for the abused child and for the person who abused the child. In juvenile sex offender cases, a juvenile court may need information about the amenability to and availability of treatment for an adolescent offender (possibly at a hearing to determine whether to transfer the case to criminal court, where the juvenile would be tried as an adult). Mental health testimony will be important to help educate judges on the importance of seriously dealing with offenders in cases of sexual molestation of children, even when the perpetrator is a young child. After offenders enter treatment programs, assistance will be required by courts, probation departments, and parole agencies to gauge the success of this intervention, and mental health professionals may be called upon to evaluate both the treatment programs themselves and the offender's treatment progress. Clinicians may be required to promptly report "treatment failures," or relapses of sex offenders, to the judge or probation department.

(See Appendix H for legal resources.)

---

# References

Aarens M, Camern T, Roizen J, et al: Alcohol, Casualties and Crime. Berkeley, CA, Social Research Group, 1978

Adams-Tucker C: Proximate effects of sexual abuse in childhood: a report on 28 children. Am J Psychiatry 139:1252–1256, 1982

Adams-Tucker C, Adams PL: Treatment of sexually abused children, in Victims of Sexual Aggression: Treatment of Children, Women, and Men. Edited by Stuart IR, Greer JG. New York, Van Nostrand Reinhold, 1984, pp 57–74

American Academy of Child and Adolescent Psychiatry: Guidelines for the clinical evaluation of child sexual abuse. J Am Acad Child Adolesc Psychiatry 28:655–657, 1988

American Humane Association: National Study on Child Neglect and Abuse Reporting. Denver, CO, American Humane Association, 1981

American Psychiatric Association: Diagnostic and Statistical Manual of Mental Disorders, 3rd Edition, Revised. Washington, DC, American Psychiatric Association, 1987

American Psychiatric Association: Diagnostic and Statistical Manual of Mental Disorders, 4th Edition. Washington, DC, American Psychiatric Association, 1994

Anderson L: Notes on the linkage between the sexually abused child and the suicidal adolescent. Journal of Adolescence 4:157–162, 1981

Bagley C, Ramsay RL: Sexual abuse in childhood: psychosocial outcomes and implication for social work practice. Journal of Social Work and Human Sexuality 4:33–47, 1986

Benedek E, Schetky D: Allegations of sexual abuse in child custody and visitation disputes, in Emerging Issues in Child Psychiatry and the Law. Edited by Schetky D, Benedek E. New York, Brunner/Mazel, 1985, pp 145–156

Bess BE, Janssen Y: Incest: a Pilot Study. Hillside Journal of Clinical Psychiatry 4:39–52, 1982

Brandt R, Tisza V: The sexually misused child. Am J Orthopsychiatry 47:80–90, 1977

Briere J: The long-term effects of childhood sexual abuse: defining a post-sexual abuse syndrome. Paper presented at the Third National Conference on Sexual Victimization of Children, Washington, DC, April 1984

Brooks B: Familial influences in father-daughter incest. Journal of Psychiatric Treatment and Evaluation 4:117–124, 1982

Brown AK: The development of memory: knowing, knowing about and knowing how to know, in Advances in Child Development and Behavior, Vol. 10. Edited by Reese HW. New York, Academic Press, 1975, pp 105–152

Browning D, Boatman B: Incest: children at risk. Am J Psychiatry 134:69–72, 1977

Cavallin H: Incestuous fathers: a clinical report. Am J Psychiatry 122:1132–1138, 1966

Ceci SJ, Ross DF, Toglia MP: Age differences in suggestibility: narrowing the uncertainties, in Children's Eyewitness Memory. Edited by Ceci SJ, Toglia MP, Ross DF. New York, Springer-Verlag New York, 1987

Cole CB, Loftus EF: The memory of children, in Childen's Eyewitness Memory. Edited by Ceci SJ, Toglia MP, Ross DF. New York, Springer-Verlag New York, 1987

Conte J, Schuerman J: Factors associated with an increased impact of child sexual abuse. Child Abuse Negl 11:201–211, 1987

DeFrancis V: Protecting the Child Victim of Sex Crimes Committed by Adults. Denver, CO, American Humane Association, 1969

Finkelhor D: Sexually Victimized Children. New York, Free Press, 1979

Finkelhor D, Browne A: Initial and long-term effects: a conceptual framework, in Sourcebook on Child Sexual Abuse. Edited by Finkelhor D. Beverly Hills, CA, Sage, 1986

Finkelhor D, Hotaling G: Sexual abuse in the national incidence study of child abuse and neglect. Child Abuse Negl 8:22–32, 1984

Friedrich WN, Urquiza SJ, Beilke R: Behavioral problems in sexually abused young children. Journal of Pediatric Psychology 11:47–57, 1986

Gardner RA: The Parental Alienation Syndrome and the Differentiation Between Fabricated and Genuine Child Sex Abuse. Cresskill, NJ, Creative Therapeutics, 1987

Gomez-Schwartz B, Horowitz J, Sauzier M: Severity of emotional distress among sexually abused preschool, school-age and adolescent children. Hosp Community Psychiatry 36:503–508, 1985

Goodwin J: Post-traumatic symptoms in incest victims, in Post-traumatic Stress Disorder in Children. Edited by Eth S, Pynoos RS. Washington, DC, American Psychiatric Press, 1985, pp 155–168

Goodwin J, Zouhar MS, Bergman R: Hysterical seizures in adolescent incest victims, in Sexual Abuse: Incest Victims and Their Families. Edited by Goodwin J. Chicago, IL, Year Book Medical, 1989

Green AH: True and false allegations of sexual abuse in child custody disputes. J Am Acad Child Psychiatry 25:449–456, 1986

Green AH: Factors contributing to false allegations of child sexual abuse and custody disputes. Child and Youth Services 15:177–189, 1991

Gross M: Incestuous rape: a cause for hysterical seizures in four adolescent girls. Am J Orthopsychiatry 49:704–708, 1979

Groth AN: The incest offender, in Handbook of Clinical Intervention in Child Sexual Abuse. Edited by Sgroi S. Lexington, MA, Lexington Books, 1982

Gundersen B, Melas P, Sklar J: Sexual behavior of preschool children: teacher's observations, in Children and Sex. Edited by Constantine L, Martinson F. Boston, MA, Little, Brown, 1981

Herman J: Father-Daughter Incest. Cambridge, MA, Harvard University Press, 1981

Hibbard RA, Roghmann J, Hoekelman RA: Genitalia in children's drawings: An association with sexual abuse. Pediatrics 79:129–137, 1987

James J, Meyerding J: Early sexual experiences as a factor in prostitution. Am J Psychiatry 134:1381–1385, 1977

Jones D, McGraw JM: Reliable and fictitious accounts of sexual abuse to children. Journal of Interpersonal Violence 2:27–45, 1987

Kaufman I, Peck A, Tagiuri L: The family constellation and overt incestuous relations between father and daughter. Am J Orthopsychiatry 24:266–279, 1954

Kearney-Cooke A: Group treatment of sexual abuse among women with eating disorders. Women and Therapy 7:5–22, 1988

Kempe R, Kempe C: Child Abuse. Cambridge, MA, Harvard University Press, 1978

Kinsey A, Pomeroy W, Martin C: Sexual Behavior in the Human Male. Philadelphia, PA, WB Saunders, 1948

Kinsey AC, Pomeroy WB, Martin CE, et al: Sexual Behavior in the Human Female. Philadelphia, PA, WB Saunders, 1953

Kiser LJ, Ackerman BJ, Brown E, et al: Post-traumatic stress disorder in young children: a reaction to purported sexual abuse. J Am Acad Child Adolesc Psychiatry 27:645–649, 1988

Kluft R: Childhood Antecedents of Multiple Personality. Washington, DC, American Psychiatric Press, 1985

Knittle B, Tuana S: Group therapy as primary treatment for adolescent victims of intrafamilial sexual abuse. Clinical Social Work Journal 8:237–242, 1980

Landis J: Experiences of 500 children with adult sexual deviation. Psychiatric Q (Supplement) 30:91–109, 1956

Lewis M., Sarrell P: Some psychological aspects of seduction, incest and rape in childhood. J Am Acad Child Psychiatry 8:606–619, 1969

Livingston R: Sexually and physically abused children. J Am Acad Child Adolesc Psychiatry 27:413–415, 1987

Lukianowicz N: Incest. Br J Psychiatry 120:301–313, 1972

Lustig N, Dresser J, Spelman S, et al: Incest. Arch Gen Psychiatry 14:31–40, 1966

MacVicar K: Psychotherapy of sexually abused girls. J Am Acad Child Psychiatry 18:342–353, 1979

McLeer SW, Deblinger E, Atkins M, et al: Post-trauamtic stress disorder in sexually abused children. J Am Acad Child Adolesc Psychiatry 27:650–654, 1988

Meiselman L: Incest: A Psychological Study of Causes and Effects With Treatment Recommendations. San Francisco, CA, Jossey-Bass, 1978

Mrazek P, Lynch M, Bentovim A: Recognition of child abuse in the United Kingdom, in Sexually Abused Children and Their Families. Edited by Mrazek P, Kempe H. New York, Pergamon, 1981

Nakashima I, Zakins G: Incest: review and clinical experience. Pediatrics 60:696–701, 1977

Oppenheimer R, Howells K, Palmer L, et al: Adverse sexual experiences in childhood and clinical eating disorders: a preliminary description. J Psychosom Res 19:157–161, 1985

Putnam F: The psychophysiologic investigation of multiple personality disorder. Psychiatr Clin North Am 7:31–40, 1984

Reich JW, Gutierres SE: Escape/aggression incidence in sexually abused juvenile delinquents. Criminal Justice and Behavior 6:239–219, 1979

Revised Report from the National Task Force on Juvenile Sex Offending, 1993, of the National Adolescent Perpetrator Network (recommendations). Juvenile and Family Court Journal 44:25, 1993

Rosenfeld A, Bailey R, Seigel B, et al: Determining incestuous contact between parent and child: frequency of children touching parent's genitals in a nonclinical population. J Am Acad Child Psychiatry 25:481–484, 1986

Russell DE: The incidence and prevalence of intrafamilial and extrafamilial sexual abuse of female children. Child Abuse Negl 7:133–146, 1983

Sgroi S: Handbook of Clinical Intervention in Child Sexual Abuse. Lexington, MA, Lexington Books, 1982

Sgroi SM, Blick LC, Porter FS: A conceptual framework for child sexual abuse, in Handbook of Clinical Intervention in Child Sexual Abuse. Edited by Sgory SM. Lexington, MA, Lexington Books, 1982

Singer JB, Flavell JH: Development of knowledge about communication in children: evaluation of explicitly ambiguous messages. Child Dev 52:1211–1215, 1981

Sloan P, Karpinski F: Effects of incest on participants. Am J Orthopsychiatry 12:666–673, 1942

Sloan G, Leighner P: Is there a relationship between sexual abuse or incest and eating disorders? Can J Psychiatry 31:656–660, 1986

Terr L: Chowchilla revisited: the effects of psychic trauma four years after a school bus kidnapping. Am J Psychiatry 140:543–550, 1983

Terr L: Remembered images and trauma: a psychology of the supernatural. Psychoanal Study Child 40:493–533, 1985

Thoennes N, Tjaden TJ: The extent, nature and validity of sexual abuse allegations in child custody/visitation disputes. Child Abuse Negl 14:151–163, 1990

Tong LK, Oates K, McDowell M: Personality development following sexual abuse. Child Abuse Negl 11:371–383, 1987

Tsai M, Wagner N: Incest and molestation: problems of childhood sexuality. Medical Times (Special Section):16–22, 1978

U.S. Department of Health and Human Services: Child Maltreatment 1993: Reports from the States to the National Center on Child Abuse and Neglect. Washington, DC, U.S. Government Printing Office, 1995, p 2-6

U.S. Department of Health and Human Services, National Center on Child Abuse and Neglect: Study Findings: National Study of Incidence and Severity of Child Abuse and Neglect. Washington, DC, U.S. Government Printing Office, 1988

Weinberg K: Incest Behavior. New York, Citadel Press, 1955

White S, Strom G, Santili G, et al: Interviewing young sexual abuse victims with anatomically correct dolls. Child Abuse Negl 10:519–530, 1986

Wyatt GE: The sexual abuse of Afro-American and white American women in childhood. Child Abuse Negl 9:507–519, 1985

Yates A: Children eroticized by incest. Am J Psychiatry 139:482–485, 1982

Yates A, Musty T: Preschool children's erroneous allegations of sexual molestation. Am J Psychiatry 145:989–992, 1988

Yorukoglu A, Kemph J: Children not severely damaged by incest with a parent. J Am Acad Child Psychiatry 5:111–124, 1966

# CHAPTER 4

## Treatment and Prevention of Child Sexual Abuse

*Christine B. L. Adams, M.D.*

## Treatment

Intervention or treatment in child sexual abuse can begin at the moment a child first tells someone about the abuse. Yet most often, in spite of burgeoning knowledge and formal treatment programs, most children do not receive treatment either for being abused or for abusing others; or, if they do, it is not of long duration (Adams-Tucker 1984). Remediation of a psychiatric nature can be given to the abused child, the person who abused the child, and other adults close to the child. Such treatment ideally begins as crisis help, soon after a child's disclosure, and continues on to long-term therapy. Many and varied forms of treatment have evolved for all the people involved in child sexual abuse cases.

In this chapter's discussion of treatment, I first look at treatments geared toward aiding the abused child and his or her supportive adult(s)—most often the mother. Second, I enumerate treatment modalities available for people who commit sexual abuse. Third, I examine treatment programs that offer multiple modalities to abused children, adults who abuse children, and their families, most often in one physical location. Finally, I discuss consultation with other professionals who are or may become involved with the child, family, and abuser.

**105**

# ▌ Treatment of Abused Children and Their Supportive Adults

## Crisis Help

Crisis help following the child's disclosure consists of providing consciousness raising to help the child realize that the person who abused him or her is the one at fault; that the child owns his or her own body and has the right to say "no" to abusers; that although the child may have been brainwashed by the person who committed the abuse, that is not the same as complicity in the abuse; and that adults should protect children and not exploit them (Adams-Tucker and Adams 1984).

Another function of crisis help is to support the child through residential rearrangements that often occur, especially in incestuous abuse. A child may leave home to enter a hospital or foster care, or the person who committed the abuse may leave home, which provides even more support to the child. The child may feel tremendous guilt at these changes, and this guilt may be buttressed by family and professionals who blame the child for "breaking up the family." The most helpful course of action for the sexually abused child is to quickly determine which adult(s) can best provide emotional nurturance and to strengthen the relationship between that person and the child (Adams-Tucker and Adams 1984).

## Diagnostic Evaluation

Additionally, some psychiatric assessment, diagnosis, and treatment planning needs to be done for the child and his or her supportive adult following the first 4 to 6 weeks after disclosure and as the crisis subsides somewhat. At this point, many children are diagnosed as having DSM-IV (American Psychiatric Association 1994) PTSD, accompanied by symptoms of reexperiencing the sexual abuse in a traumatic, intrusive manner. The often overused diagnosis of adjustment disorder is inappropriate because sexual abuse is not a stressor that falls within the range of common experience. Additionally, heretofore unrecognized problems in development, behavior, and personality style of the abused child may be documented and diagnosed for the first time, coincident with the sexual abuse and not resulting from it.

## Adjunctive Treatments

Several treatment modalities are used that fall between crisis therapy sessions and long-term individual therapy for abused children. These modalities are best seen as extensions of individual psychotherapy. They are family group therapy, conjoint supportive adult-child therapy, individual therapy for the supportive adult, peer group therapy, group therapy for the abused child and the supportive adult, self-help groups, environmental alterations, and pharmacotherapy.

**Family group therapy.**    First pioneered in the treatment of sexual abuse by Henry Giarretto, this therapy treated the family group in which incest had occurred; treatment took place after individual and dyadic therapies for different family members had been performed (Giarretto et al. 1978). The group consisted of the perpetrator (most often the father), the mother, and the abused child. The approach was to view the family as a pathological system that created and maintained the perpetrator's incestuous sexual behaviors with the child. The goal was to "fix" the family by using the same theoretical systems approach for treatment that was used for dynamic understanding of the family. Family reunification was sought through a process of reorienting family interrelationships among the members.

Two problems may arise with this treatment modality. For one, the abusing person's overt sexual activity with the child might stop, but there may be no real intrapsychic change, and therefore his or her emotionally exploitative manner may continue to affect the child. The second problem is that the child may derive no therapeutic benefit from just the palliative alteration of not being sexually abused by her or his parent. The child's needs and turmoil may not be considered, because family group therapy usually subtly shifts to focus on the problems in the marital dyad.

Treatment of the family as a group in instances of intrafamilial sexual abuse usually takes place when the parent who abused the child continues to reside in the original family with the child or children he or she abused. At best, this modality and the concomitant family living arrangement foster hypervigilance in the child and other nonabusing adult to undesired sexual advances from the perpetrator.

Alternatively, another form of family group therapy is that composed of at least one supportive adult and the child(ren) under the adult's care. It does not include the molester in either intrafamilial or extrafamilial abuse. Such adults who can give support to the child may include grandparents, stepparents, foster parents, or neighbors. Most often such groups are composed of mothers and children if intrafamilial abuse has taken place and of both parents (or caregivers) and child if extrafamilial abuse has occurred (Roesler et al. 1993).

**Conjoint supportive adult-child therapy.**   Whether the sexual abuse is intrafamilial or extrafamilial, conjoint work between the child and a supportive adult is of tremendous benefit, perhaps all the more so when incest has occurred. Parent and child often are making adjustments to a new household arrangement (if the parent who abused the child has left home) in which most often the mother assumes a new role as the sole head of the household. She must help her child cope with the realities of court appearances (if criminal charges are brought against the person who committed the abuse). She herself must cope with symptomatic behaviors that have cropped up in the child since being abused (and since disclosure of the abuse). The mother must also cope with a host of changes in her relationship with the child that must be instituted to ensure the child's emotional protection by a trustworthy parent. Such conjoint therapy sessions can be held with the same or different therapists involved in treating the child and adult. What matters is that sessions are held regularly and that they allow the adult and child to work together on common issues.

**Individual therapy for the supportive adult.**   This type of therapy is most often necessary in incest cases. Many and varied issues confront a parent (usually the mother) in such a situation, and because she will become the bulwark of emotional support for the abused child, it is important that she have her own sessions to work through her grief, self-blame, guilt, and anger at her child's abuse. In extrafamilial abuse, each parent may need individual sessions to help clarify how the child was abused. Parents often must deal with overwhelming emotions evoked because of their own past histories of sexual abuse. Parents usually need to achieve a better understanding of their own emotional makeup to answer the perennial question, "How did this happen?"

**Peer group therapy.**   Group therapy that extends individual therapeutic work has been employed for abused children and for supportive adult(s). Many formats and goals exist for such groups. Parents' groups may serve a cathartic and educational function. Groups for abused children have evolved with the rationale that children should acquire a positive self-image in the context of developing peer group relationships (Berliner and Ernst 1984). Such groups may be brief and behavioral, seeking to teach sex education and abuse issues (Damon and Waterman 1986). Some groups have preplanned formats and fixed-length sessions, focusing on topics such as dealing with strangers, good and bad touching, molesters, keeping secrets, and the family (Berliner and Ernst 1984; Nelki and Watters 1989; Vizard 1987). Other group therapies are long term and psychodynamic; they do not have a preplanned format but instead focus on what children bring to each session (Steward et al. 1986).

Psychotherapeutic work in groups helps abused children to break their isolation and to stop feeling different, because all the group members have been sexually abused. Coeducational groups work well for younger children but preadolescents and adolescents prefer same-sex groups. Cotherapists, one of each sex, work best for all age groups and allow each child to work through transference distortions, most often ones in which the male therapist is identified with the person who abused the child.

**Group therapy for the abused child and the supportive adult.** Yet another type of group therapy is composed of supportive adults and abused children. This type of group is used most often for families in which a father has committed incest and is usually made up of mothers and daughters. These groups can be unified, composed of mother-daughter units that meet together after each session. In this way the group therapy functions as an extension of conjoint mother-child therapy and also follows a self-help format. Mothers and daughters can explore the broad, stigmatizing issues of child sexual abuse and can also discuss more mundane issues, such as what to tell a child's school about the abuse and when, what to tell siblings about the incest, how to deal with an abused teenager's dating, and how to negotiate the legal aspects of criminal or civil litigation regarding the abuse. Mother-child groups can also be set up to work in parallel—mothers meeting separately from the children, yet both groups having the same agenda (Nelki and Watters 1989).

**Self-help groups.**   Groups such as Parents United, Adults Molested as Children, and Sons and Daughters United—whose members either have an abused child or were abused as children themselves—provide enormous support to abused children and their families. Such groups work most effectively if a mental health professional is involved in running or supervising the group so that referral of group participants for psychiatric care will be done in a timely way. In some locales self-help groups provide the majority of nonprofessional aid to sexually abused persons by helping with finances, jobs, transportation, legal concerns, and babysitting (Giarretto 1981).

**Environmental alterations.**    Families in which a child has been sexually abused require practical support for daily tasks, for understanding what has happened to them and their child, and for working through the trauma of abuse. All of these changes can be and are aided by a network of family members, neighbors, welfare and child protective services (CPS) workers, attorneys, clergy, and psychiatric professionals.

**Pharmacotherapy.**    Because symptoms of anxiety—sometimes including fully developed PTSD—are the most common emotional sequelae for the abused child, many pediatricians and family practitioners prescribe medications to reduce anxiety and enhance the child's sleep. The antihistamines hydroxyzine (Atarax or Vistaril) or diphenhydramine (Benadryl) are prescribed most often. However, the best approach for the child may be candor, not medication. The physician should urge the abused child and the family to talk about all facets of the sexual abuse and thus begin the healing process by breaking the taboo on silence about the whole topic.

## *Individual Long-Term Psychotherapy*

Few children victimized sexually are permitted the opportunity to embark on long-term individual psychotherapy, although such abuse, particularly incestuous abuse, is regarded as creating a "developmental failure" in emotional growth (Gaddini 1983). Another notion is that preexisting emotionally conditioned pathology acts in concert with sexual abuse experiences in childhood to worsen later emotional difficulties. Such difficulties take place in two forms: 1) repeated sexual victimization and choice of exploitative relationships, or 2) choice of relationships in which one becomes the exploiter and sexual abuser of others.

**Goals.**  Some laudable goals for this lengthier psychotherapeutic process are for the child to

➤ Gain some self-understanding as someone who has been involved in sexual activity with a parent, adult, or older child, as well as gain some self-understanding as a whole person
➤ Appreciate how symptoms or problems arose in connection with and apart from the sexual abuse via gains in insight, in reality testing, and in a stronger ego
➤ First understand, then eradicate, any difficulties perceived by him or her as troublesome
➤ Inoculate himself or herself against future repetitions of past behaviors and conflicts perceived by the child as unwanted and undesirable

Such goals or changes encompass both intrapsychic and interpersonal levels. Most often, long-term therapy seeks to repair, through a deconditioning process, the well-taught omnipotent child's low self-esteem and help the child understand his or her self-devaluation, isolation, and self-blame. Thus, therapy aims to move the child from functioning in an overly strong, omnipotent role, which acquiesces to sexual abuse, to being less strong and saying "no" to future abuse and abusive relationships.[1]

For other sexually abused children, the problem may be that they identify with exploiters and sexual aggressors. These children have been impotently conditioned early in life to behave as if and to believe that they must gratify their impulses regardless of the effect on others. Such impotent youngsters need help in understanding their emotionally conditioned penchant for exploiting and devaluing others—especially sexually, if they have experienced sexual abuse. Their therapy seeks to alter their functioning from a too weak, irresponsible, and impulsive role to one that helps them become stronger, learning more autonomy, self-

---

[1] Omnipotence is an unconscious, conditioned role (behavior and thought pattern) acquired early in a child's life. Such a role makes the child feel and believe that he or she operates from a role of strength, allowing whatever another person wants; in sexual abuse, this would be allowing another's sexual contact (Adams 1994). The less strong role is one in which the child feels and believes that he or she cannot acquiesce to a sexual abuser. Untreated, the omnipotent children, in later childhood and in adulthood, enter repetitively into relationships in which they are exploited by others.

control, and responsible behavior toward others so they will not victimize others in future relationships. If untreated, these youngsters form relationships, in later childhood and in adulthood, that exploit and abuse others sexually and otherwise.

The discussion that follows is directed toward treatment of the children most often seen by clinicians and toward those experiencing the most subjective distress—omnipotent children. For such children, there are a number of issues that arise in the course of psychotherapy.

**Power imbalance.**   Within the framework of the sexually abused child seeking help through therapy and the therapist being the provider of that help lurks the possibility that the child will transfer onto the therapist the assumption of an exploitative role. The child will erroneously perceive a power imbalance, wherein he or she is to be exploited by an adult. The problem is that the child trusts too much. Much time in treatment must be devoted to undoing and avoiding replication of the child's prior vulnerability at the hands of a too-trusted adult. In therapy he or she can begin to know that adults are bigger and more powerful, but that this imbalance can be drawn on for support, nurturance, and empathetic guidance. It does not result in the child's coercion and betrayal by all adults. In therapy the child can learn which adults can be trusted and which cannot.

Abused children, accustomed as they are to exploitation by overly trusted adults, avidly scan their therapists for clues about how to please them. Therapists must be aware of this and avoid falling into this role reversal or pattern that reenacts the abusive relationship in which the child tried to take care of the sexual impulses of the abuser. The therapist must convey that therapeutic time and interaction are not exploitative and, likewise, that real-life relationships need not be based on exploitation.

**Anger at abuser.**   At some point in every therapy, the omnipotent child begins to voice anger with the person who abused him. When this happens early on, it bodes well for the child. The more severely coerced and brainwashed child denies this anger and instead accepts the abusive person's projections that the sexual experience was "good for her" or took place because he was "special." Getting angry with the abusive person is an indication that the child accepts the reality of the sexual abuse because she can see more appropriately that she was not at fault but rather was acted upon by an exploitative adult.

**Man-hating and fear of men.** Many abused children, especially girls, will bring up their phobia of all males in conjunction with voicing anger toward and fear of the man who abused them. Even very young girls make the association of knowing that their pan-heterophobia originated with their sexual molestation by a male. They will say, "I know all men are not like my daddy, but I still get very scared any time a man gets near me or even if I have to talk to one."

Fear of men and man-hating often go hand in hand. Teenage girls especially may ventilate hatred of men in general and forswear dating, marriage, and all future sexual activity with men. Many of these children grow up to adopt celibacy or homosexuality in a compulsive style. The point is these young women should be allowed time to ventilate and to understand their hateful and enraged feelings toward the men who abused them as a normal prelude to healing their emotional wounds. When that is done they do not compulsively assume any particular adult life-style, be it prostitution, misogynist heterosexuality (with overvaluation of men), man-hating homosexuality, drug addiction, or sexual abuse of their offspring, to mention a few.

**Does this mean I'm gay?** Most often boys who have experienced homosexual abuse from older boys or men worry about and question their sexual orientation as a result of the abuse and wonder if they will be homosexual as adults. This quandary about their sexual object choice arises out of self-devaluation and perhaps the child's acceptance of the abusing person's projections of his own homosexual proclivities. It arises from the child's omnipotent role, feeling he will be unable to choose for himself his own sexual orientation later in life, but that instead he must accommodate to a homosexual orientation because of sexual abuse by a man.

**Who should leave home?** In recently disclosed incest cases that came to the attention of a children's protective agency, the issues arose of who the family is and who should leave their usual home. All too often, if anyone is designated to leave, it is the child—with a move to a temporary shelter, foster care, or the home of a relative. Abused children of all ages are usually very frightened at the prospect of moving to new surroundings, particularly away from their mothers. The principal exceptions to this tendency are older teenagers who, although anxious at the prospect, do feel they are capable of living on their own and often choose to move into group home living arrangements. At best, the spotlight on who leaves home centers on the abused child and the abusing father. Children who in some way recognize their own fears and their father's culpability want him to leave. On the other hand, those who accept the projections of their father-aggressors activate regrets and culpability in themselves and want their fathers to stay with them at home. The therapist should work through these distortions in therapy and help children become reoriented to living in a family with adults who will protect rather than exploit.

**Whose fault is it?**  During lengthy therapy, sexually abused children will attempt to sort out who is to blame for their abuse. Most children in the omnipotent role blame themselves first. After all, this is what an abusive relationship confirms to them: they are to blame; the person who abused them is blameless. In addition to self-blame, a child may also blame another adult who failed to protect him or her. This may be reasonable blame of a mother or father, for example, if that parent actually witnessed the sexual molestation and failed to protect the child. The child's blame of the parent may also be unreasonable, however, as in sexual abuse at a preschool about which the parents knew nothing. In the latter example, the child would need to work through in therapy her expectation of her mother's (or father's) omniscient and omnipotent role as parent. The therapist should gather the facts about which person or persons actually participated in molesting the girl or boy and then aid the youngster in working through distorted thinking about blame for the abuse so that the child has a reality-based understanding that the person who committed the abuse is the culpable one. The therapist can help abused children to understand that they are not the culprits and that other adults are not to blame if they do not know that the child is being abused.

**Fear of retaliation and recurrence.**  Abused children faced with the prospect of being reunited with their incestuous fathers or with returning to school, day care, or a setting where the abuse occurred and where the abuser may be show fearfulness about recurrence of the molestation. The child's worry of recurrent sexual abuse crops up even when the child and her incestuous father have each had a long-term therapy experience, as well as when they have participated jointly in family therapy for a considerable period of time. Concomitantly, these children fear reprisals, some retaliation from the person who abused them for breaking the secret and telling about the incest. This fearfulness is often realistic and not unfounded, even when fathers have "apologized" and "taken responsibility for the incest"; even when extrafamilial abusers are home on bond from jail and awaiting trial, or after their criminal prosecution and incarceration. These children appear to know their incestuous fathers' deceptive tactics and incorrigibility better than therapists who push for reuniting these fathers and children. If the therapist decides to push strongly for reunion, the child should be helped to acknowledge his or her fear and discomfort about the abuser and to use it as a barometer of the need to distance himself or herself from the abuser and to learn how to say "no" to his unwanted behaviors.

Part of successful therapy is helping the omnipotent child to identify his or her own feelings of fear, anxiety, and mistrust when in the presence of people who might be emotionally, physically, or sexually exploitative. The child needs to learn to trust his or her own feelings and reactions to others. After all, the abuse occurred because the child trusted too much in an adult who betrayed him or her. Even very young children can learn to use their emotional reactions to adults as a gauge of whom they can and cannot trust for support and nurturance.

**Sexualized talk and behavior.**   Sexualization as a coping style is prevalent among sexually abused children. After all, they have been typecast or programmed on some adult's template of sexual gratification. Their sexualized behavior or talk is most often the result of abusive experiences rather than the cause of the abuse.

The children may talk "sexy," use gutter language, mimic intercourse on the office floor with dolls, invite the male therapist to be fellated by them, ask to see the therapist's genitals, masturbate in front of the therapist, and so on. These behaviors represent a variety of coping maneuvers: identification with the adult sexual aggressor (exploiting the therapist), conversion of passive to active (seducing the therapist before he or she seduces the child), role reversal (pleasing the therapist by inviting exploitation of himself or herself and recapitulating the omnipotent role of victim).

Within the therapy, however, it is paramount to aid the child in understanding what the sexualized behavior means. After that, we can help the child learn that dichotomizing into exploiter versus exploited or aggressor versus victim is not the level on which human relationships need be based. That is to say, the child can be helped to gain an understanding that neither adults nor children need be victims or sexual oppressors. The same holds true for the child patient and therapist in the therapeutic transaction. The therapist must neither exploit the child in therapy nor allow the child to exploit the therapist, sexually or otherwise. The control over this rests squarely with the therapist.

**Looking into the future for delayed consequences.**  At a point near the end of therapy, abused children begin to take stock of what they have accomplished and of what their therapy has yielded for them. At this point, they should be encouraged to look ahead and anticipate what issues, concerns, worries, or problems might arise as they get older and become young women and men. Their concerns are anticipated astutely in many instances:

➤ *7-year-old girl:*  "I might get real scared again and think about what he did when I grow up and get married."
➤ *10-year-old girl:*  "I guess when I start having boyfriends in a few years, I'll think about it a lot."
➤ *11-year-old girl:*  "When I get my period for the first time—because that's what makes you old enough to have babies—I'll think about having babies and get all nervous 'cause I'll think about sex and what my dad did."
➤ *13-year-old boy:*  "Next summer at camp when we all share a cabin and shower and dress with the counselors, I'll probably feel nervous and remember what my neighbor did to me."
➤ *15-year-old girl:*  "I think a problem might come up when I get a boyfriend and we have sex. It will remind me a lot of the abuse . . . and if I have a little girl, I'll worry about somebody making her have sex."

In sum, these children anticipate future problems in same-sex and opposite-sex relationships, in marriages, and in sexual functioning; and they worry about abuse occurring in the next generation. These are exactly the problems that we see in adults who were sexually abused as children.

As therapy terminates, it is important to urge these youngsters to keep in touch and to plan for follow-up appointments whenever they feel the need. The goal of psychiatric treatment is to assist each child in becoming a happy and competent adult—an adult who can continue to probe and understand the ramifications bequeathed to him or her by a history of being sexually abused.

## ▌ Treatment of People Who Commit Sexual Abuse

The sexual abuse of children is so widespread and each abusive person exploits so many children that there is tremendous concern in the psychiatric community about how to stop sexual exploitation of children. The dilemma is whether to incarcerate abusive persons without any form of treatment, treat them without incarcerating them, or do both—that is, incarcerate them and provide treatment while in prison. Robert Prentky and Ann Burgess (1990) performed a cost-benefit analysis of treating incarcerated abusive persons compared to not treating them (Prentky and Burgess 1990). They found lower recidivism rates (repeated legal charges for sexual offenses) for incarcerated and treated abusive persons than for incarcerated and untreated abusive persons. Because of these differences in recidivism rates, it is also more expensive to treat each subsequent victim of an untreated incarcerated sexually abusive person than to treat each victim of an incarcerated sexually abusive person who has received treatment. Prentky and Burgess's data suggest that offenders should be treated for the sake of the people who might be abused.

If treatment of sexually exploitative people is efficacious, then what treatment modalities work best? Individual psychotherapy is difficult, if not impossible, because people who commit sexual abuse are unmotivated to seek intrapsychic or behavioral changes. The sexual abuse of children signifies a deeply entrenched and conditioned personality pathology (Barnard et al. 1989). Sexually abusive people find their pathological actions very gratifying, and they often believe they have done nothing wrong in pleasing themselves. Sexually abusive behavior is also chronic, most often beginning in adolescence. The use of projection by such persons is so entrenched and their superegos are so nonexistent that they never feel culpable, nor do they even experience sufficient anxiety or other dysphoric symptomatology to engage in individual therapy. Also, sexually abusive people often have substance abuse disorders, which, to their way of thinking, can be "blamed" for their sexually abusive involvement with children (Barnard et al. 1989).

Abel et al. (1980) have found that penile plethysmography can be used to break through some persons' denial and projections about the abuse they committed. This technique will then induce them to be more amenable to undertaking treatment. Their premise is "the penis does not lie." The person is shown slides or videos, or hears audiotapes, with sexually arousing content while a strain gauge is attached to his penis. Penile erections or tumescences are recorded in concert with the audio or video sexual stimuli. They demonstrate sexual arousal at deviant sexual content involving sex and children.

Behavior modification treatments have been conducted by Abel et al. (1985); these treatments show more promise than individual psychotherapy. The goals of these behavior modification techniques are for sexually abusive persons to learn some control over their deviant patterns of sexual arousal, thereby preventing future sexually abusive behavior with children. The two techniques most often used are masturbatory satiation and covert sensitization. The technique of masturbatory satiation requires the abusive person to masturbate after having experienced an orgasm, all the while trying to create his fantasies of sexually molesting a child. The desired result is to alter something that is very sexually stimulating (the fantasies) into something more boring (decreased sexual arousal paired with the fantasies). Covert sensitization pairs the abusive person's early sexual arousal and sex-abuse fantasies with self-imposed thoughts of aversive consequences such as incarceration.

In addition, broad-based group therapy work for adult and adolescent offenders (Smets and Cebula 1987) that provides education in sexual matters, social skills, and propriety in adult relationships has been found to be a beneficial part of treatment because the abusive person's poor fund of knowledge and immaturity in many areas are noteworthy (Becker et al. 1978; Lang et al. 1988). Further, antiandrogenic medication, medroxyprogesterone acetate, has been used in treatment and found to be efficacious in diminishing sexual drive (Berlin and Meinecke 1981) and rates of reoffending(Meyer et al. 1992).

## Comprehensive Sexual Abuse Treatment Programs

Keller et al. (1989) surveyed 553 sexual abuse treatment programs within the United States to discern their characteristics as to affiliation, clients served, and treatments or services provided. They found that over 70% of the programs were affiliated with larger private or public agencies providing mental health and social services. Further, almost 90% of the programs focused on adults and children who had been abused as recipients of their treatment services. Types of therapy offered most often were individual and family oriented. Most programs placed stringent exclusion criteria on persons who had committed abuse and wound up treating only the least disturbed persons. Additionally, less than one-quarter of the programs performed any follow-up on their cases and, if they did so, it was for a brief period of time—an average of less than 11 months. Keller and colleagues concluded that they could not assess which program models work best and therefore which programs should be replicated in the future.

Cohn and Daro (1987) studied 89 demonstration treatment programs evolved for treating all forms of child abuse. They concluded that treatments dispensed within such programs are not successful in that reabuse of children by the same people is highly likely. However, they did note lower rates of recidivism among people who committed incestuous abuse when compared with people who committed nonsexual child abuse. They concluded that secondary and tertiary prevention, such as attempting treatment after abuse has occurred, is not as efficacious as once thought and that more emphasis should be placed on primary prevention strategies and techniques.

## ▮ Consultation With Other Professionals

The general or child psychiatrist often is called upon for expertise and input by a myriad of other professionals in cases of sexual abuse. The psychiatrist is in a position to offer a lot during such consultation because of his or her thorough training in medicine and because of his or her knowledge of child development, of psychopathology, of diagnosis, and of how to treat a variety of conditions. All too often when the psychiatrist should be called upon or included in collaboration on cases, he or she is not. As a result, there are times when the psychiatrist must provide input and advocacy for a sexually abused youngster over the objections of and in spite of devaluations by other professionals.

### Schools

Treatment of individual sexual abuse cases may warrant the psychiatrist's consultation with professionals in a child's school—teachers, guidance counselor, or principal. Case-oriented consultation may focus, for example, on a child's symptomatology of heightened anxiety with overactivity and masturbation in class. Through hands-on contact such as a school visit, the psychiatrist gleans information about the child when at school and about the school's expectations of and behavior with the child. Then the psychiatrist is able to discern what the actual problems are and what solutions to recommend.

In addition to targeting specific problematical behaviors in the child, consultation often is provided at the request of parents who ask, "What should I tell the school about the sexual abuse?" The psychiatrist can then plan with the child and parents what, if anything, to communicate to the school and can arrange for a consultation time with school personnel and the family.

Consultation with schools that is not case focused is most often done on an instructional basis. The psychiatrist may be asked by a school's parent-teacher association to teach students or their parents about intra-and extrafamilial sexual abuse as part of a prevention program. Or the psychiatrist may be asked to instruct teachers about sexually abused children outside their school setting as part of their continuing education.

### Pediatricians, Family Practitioners, and Emergency Room Physicians

Most often when the psychiatrist is called upon to consult with other physicians or elicits such consultation, it is case centered and seeks medical information relating to the physical examination of a molested child. The psychiatrist may supply information to the emergency room examining physician, for example, as to the types of sexual abuse the child has talked about so the examining physician knows where to focus his or her physical examination of the child. Or, alternatively, the family practitioner may consult a child psychiatrist regarding diagnosis and treatment of a child with intense anxiety or other emotional or behavioral symptomatology following sexual abuse. Yet another type of collaboration occurs when a sexually abused child under psychiatric treatment has another medical condition, such as diabetes mellitus, anorexia, anal fistulae, or sexually transmitted diseases. The psychiatrist consults the other physician concerning treatment of these other medical conditions. Medical colleagues also teach one another on formal and informal bases about psychiatric conditions resulting from sexual abuse, the forensic physical examination, and so on.

## Child Protective Services

Often the most resistance to collaboration with psychiatrists in cases of sexually abused children comes from state investigative agencies, such as CPS, who perform the initial investigation of cases reported to them because of mandated state laws. CPS workers may lack substantial training in pathological family dynamics, yet their goal often is to investigate an allegation of a child's sexual abuse within a family systems perspective and to reunite an abused child with the parent who abused him or her, if possible. They may opt for such reunification when a treating psychiatrist would not do so. Existing psychopathology in families and in individual children may be unjustly minimized by workers not trained in these areas.

One research study found that CPS underidentified actual cases of sexual abuse and referred few youngsters for psychiatric care (Adams-Tucker 1984). Many true cases were termed invalid by CPS workers because the person who committed the abuse did not admit to the abuse or because children exhibited the "sexual abuse accommodation syndrome" (Summit 1983) and retracted their earlier abuse allegations. Most cases were closed within a few months, often because the abuser had left home, the assumption being that the abuser's absence makes a child safe from repeated sexual abuse (Adams-Tucker 1984).

## Attorneys, Judges, and the Legal System

For psychiatrists, probably the most frequent collaboration in sexual abuse cases is with the legal system. Forensic consultation is also, no doubt, the most time consuming and thwarting for the psychiatrist. Because the sexual abuse of a child is illegal in all states, such cases enter the legal arena to protect the child (dependency actions), to punish the person who committed the abuse (criminal litigation), and/or to sue the culpable parties for a monetary award (civil litigation). Additionally, custody and visitation determinations in which sexual abuse is alleged also warrant legal consultation by the psychiatrist.

Collaboration may take place with attorneys to help them prepare a civil or criminal action against a person accused of sexual abuse. In such a situation, the psychiatrist is a consultant but not a witness in the litigation. He or she consults with the attorney to plan strategy and may read reports and documents from evaluations carried out by other mental health experts.

In contrast to the above, consultation with the legal system may be more focused around the case of a sexually abused child whom the psychiatrist has evaluated or treated. In such an instance, the psychiatrist testifies, giving an expert opinion about what the child is suffering emotionally, the pros and cons regarding whether abuse has occurred, and suggestions for the type and duration of psychiatric treatment.

Another form of consultation the psychiatrist offers to the legal process is that of testifying as an expert witness who has not examined the child involved in the case. Such testimony provides expertise in the area of child sexual abuse and serves to educate the court (judge and jury) about the topic of sexually abused children: epidemiology, true and false allegations, recanting, symptomatology in child victims, forms of emotional distress suffered by adults abused as children, available treatments, and so on. This topic expertise often is requested in both civil and criminal proceedings.

The overwhelming frustration for the psychiatrist in working with the legal system is the expectation that the court will listen to the psychiatrist and take seriously his or her suggestions about what would most benefit the child. Yet, this may not occur. Legal colleagues, with little understanding of the psychopathology of sexually abusive persons, may seek custody for or award custody to a sexually abusive parent and may deny visitation to a supportive parent. Attorneys and judges are educated about legal principles, whereas mental health professionals are educated about intrapsychic processes, human relationships, and psychopathology. Collaboration between mental health and legal professionals enhances support for the person who was abused and assists in effective adjudication and rehabilitation planning for the person who committed the abuse.

It is best to be aware that attorneys and judges may unconsciously expect the psychiatric expert witness to be omnipotent. The court system may desire unequivocal and absolute statements from the psychiatrist expert that sexual abuse has definitely occurred or not occurred. The psychiatrist can almost never render such a statement unless he or she actually witnessed the abuse. Legal professionals also expect the psychiatrist to predict with certainty what a specific child will experience emotionally as an adult and how long treatment should last. The psychiatrist should strive to make the court aware that he or she offers professional opinions and not absolute fact.

Another point for the psychiatrist to keep in mind is the need to be an advocate for the child rather than a part of the adversarial process. The adversarial court process most often neglects the child anyway. For example, in a custody dispute involving an allegation of intrafamilial child sexual abuse, a judge may approve a mother's motion for the psychiatrist to evaluate her child and herself, but omit the father from the evaluation order. The psychiatrist knows that to properly evaluate an allegation of sexual abuse from a forensic perspective, especially if the abuse was intrafamilial and is being alleged in the context of a custody dispute, the child and both the parents need to be seen. The psychiatrist should convey to the court that everyone involved needs to be evaluated and that both time and money are wasted if the court orders only the mother and child to be evaluated.

# Prevention

In this discussion of prevention, I give overviews of rationales for prevention, programmatic contents and locales, and some opinions of sexually abusive persons on the prevention of abuse.

Three types of prevention of suffering and morbidity typically are considered within systems of health care: primary, secondary, and tertiary. Primary prevention seeks to increase awareness of a disease or condition such as sexual abuse in childhood, before the condition occurs—that is, before a child is sexually abused. Secondary prevention can be defined as finding cases of sexual abuse soon after the abuse takes place and instituting rapid treatment so that more chronic and severe morbidity are prevented. Tertiary prevention aims to intervene via psychiatric treatment and other means to diminish suffering in sexually abused children and in adults sexually abused as children who already suffer from extensive psychiatric illness.

## ▌ Rationales

Within the arena of child sexual abuse, many prevention programs have arisen within the past decade. These programs in part aim to do consciousness raising with children of all ages and with adults to increase awareness that children are sexually abused. There are at least seven rationales for preventive approaches:

1. Many young children are potential targets of sexual abuse (Trudell and Whatley 1988).

2. Adults abused as youngsters report that with hindsight they might have avoided such abuse had they been given information about sexual abuse as children (Conte et al.1989; Wurtele 1987).
3. It may be easier to prevent abuse among large numbers of children than to treat them because so few disclose their abuse (Wurtele 1987) and because treatment is expensive and its effectiveness considered dubious (Budin and Johnson 1989).
4. Children aren't taught about intrafamilial sexual abuse at home (Brassard et al. 1983).
5. Schools are a good locale for teaching prevention because of their long-term contact with children and their parents (Brassard et al. 1983).
6. Some abused children become sexual abusers themselves (Dimock 1988).
7. Primary prevention programs unintentionally yet beneficially augment secondary and tertiary prevention because many heretofore silent sexsully abused children disclose their abuse following such programs (Trudell and Whatley 1988).

## ▌ Program Content

The contents or aims of prevention programs are to provide children with factual knowledge and skills that will enable them to deter sexual abuse should they be approached by an adult or older child. They are given data about potential offenders—both family members and strangers; about their being the "boss" of their own bodies; about responsibility for sexual abuse resting with perpetrators and not with children; about trusting their own feelings, especially about touching by others; about "good" and "bad" touches; about self-assertion, saying "no" when they don't like or want touches or hugs; and about telling an adult they do trust if they have fended off or experienced sexual abuse (Budin and Johnson 1989; Conte 1987; Trudell and Whatley 1988).

## ▌ Locales

Locales for prevention programs are most often elementary schools, but high schools, preschools, and day care centers also have programs or less "packaged" formats. In addition to these programs, many children and their parents do educate themselves at home with instructional materials such as videos, pamphlets, coloring books, comic books, television specials, and news reports (Wurtele 1993).

Day care programs strive to educate staff, parents, and children—educating the adults so they in turn can provide an atmosphere conducive to teaching about sexual abuse to the children (Spungen 1989). Parents and staff are taught in workshops separate from children. Professionals outside the day care center may be called in to provide expertise to the adults. Then the staff and parents in turn teach the youngsters using role playing, songs, artistic work, discussion, and books.

School-based prevention programs usually rely on several formats—pamphlets, coloring books, theatrical presentations, lectures, and films (Plummer 1986; Trudell and Whatley 1988; Wurtele 1987). Both teachers and professionals from the community teach prevention to the children while at school.

Parental involvement in such programs is warranted because of the sensitivity toward teaching other people's children about sexual matters (Brassard et al. 1983). One manner of accomplishing this is to provide parents, through the parent-teacher association (PTA), with facts concerning definitions, signs of sexual abuse, and where to seek help for a child and family who have experienced abuse. Often, Parents United and Sons and Daughters United can be invited to lecture to parents. Another way of involving parents is to supply parents and children with similar information given in separate sessions. Separate programs for youngsters can be taught by PTA members, teachers, or community professionals. For elementary-school-age children this often will mean a hands-on approach with role playing, whereas for adolescents the approach more appropriately may be discussion of issues with a focus on nonexploitative interactions in relationships and the choices to be made with sexual encounters (Brassard et al. 1983).

Of course, the ideal goal for prevention programs is to prevent the first potential episode of sexual abuse of a child. That is, when a child is approached to be sexually abused, he or she deters abuse by some type of preventive behavior: getting away, self-protection, or immediately telling a trusted adult. Most programs attempt to prevent abuse solely by altering the child's knowledge base (supplying new information) in the hope that this will result in preventive behavioral strategies. However, teaching new knowledge to children is not synonymous with preventing sexual abuse, because the teaching in such prevention programs may not alter a child's behavior (Pelcovitz et al. 1992; Poche et al. 1981).

One unusual attempt at prevention involves actual on-the-spot training for youngsters. An attempt is made by a "surrogate" stranger to lure children away from their school (Fryer et al. 1987). The results show that children do learn from the instruction in the prevention program and can alter their behaviors following such instruction. However, one critique of such a behaviorally oriented prevention program is that children may be desensitized to actual strangers by the use of simulated strangers in a teaching program (Conte 1987).

There are other criticisms of school-based prevention programs for children that are subtle but perhaps major in consequence. Because these programs address what children can do to prevent sexual abuse, they may inadvertently make children feel and believe the onus lies with them to prevent abuse. The perpetrator's behavior is not altered by these programs and the fallacy may be fostered that altering children's behavior to ward off sexual abuse simply solves a very complex problem (Trudell and Whatley 1988).

Such programs can also create problems for the teachers who must present the didactic content of the programs. Prepackaged curricula are developed by others yet delivered to teachers for them to teach. They do not utilize the teachers' skills. Such curricula may be brief in nature and not allow for adequate assimilation time for students and teachers alike. In addition, prevention curricula with a nonsexual focus can impart to youngsters the notion that sexuality in sexual abuse is a forbidden topic—the opposite idea from what the prevention package wants to convey. Yet these watered-down curricula, which speak of "private parts" as being "inside bathing suits" rather than using correct anatomical terminology, may be more palatable to teachers who may not be accustomed to lecturing about sexuality (Trudell and Whatley 1988).

Other problems for teachers are how to handle the sequelae of their teachings: what to do if a child discloses abuse to them; when to report to CPS; how to handle a child's or family's distress following disclosure of abuse when teachers are not usually able to provide intensive support to individual youngsters (Trudell and Whatley 1988).

## ▌ What Sexually Abusive Persons Say

Yet another approach for preventing child sexual abuse links prevention concepts or programs to sexually abusive persons' preferences in the characteristics of the children they abuse. People who have committed sexual abuse suggest teaching children much of the same information that is included in prevention curricula: 1) tell a trusted adult if you have been abused, 2) say "no" to potential offenders, 3) understand that you are the "boss" of your own body, and 4) don't get into strangers' cars (Budin and Johnson 1989). People who commit sexual abuse look for lonely, troubled children who are unaccompanied and in public places. They resonate best with friendly, trusting children who talk with them and who are willing to become comfortable with the abusive person. The abusive person then gradually desensitizes the child to touch and sexual behaviors, at the same time insuring their physical isolation with the child (Conte et al. 1989).

Offenders also have suggestions for ways parents can aid in preventing sexual abuse of their children, which may be very telling about the origin of childhood sexual abuse in general. They suggest that parents be attentive to their child's emotional state and involved in their child's life; that parents maintain dialogue with their child, especially about sexual abuse; and that they provide good supervision for their child (Budin and Johnson 1989). The overwhelming idea of sexually abusive persons, both in intrafamilial and extrafamilial settings, is that a loved child, meaning an emotionally supported child, is less likely to be abused (Budin and Johnson 1989). When this advice is considered along with the finding from the surrogate stranger prevention program described by Fryer et al. (1987)—that children who deter abuse have higher self-esteem than those who are lured by strangers—the question is raised, does children's higher self-esteem act efficaciously in preventing sexual abuse? And, if so, abuse prevention and the teaching of self-esteem both begin very early in a child's life with reasonable parental emotional support. In this manner, preventing abuse may be learned as a corollary to a child's learning to value himself or herself and to say "no" to abusive devaluations from adults and other children.

---

# Legal Commentary

## ▌ Issues Related to Victims, Other Family Members, and Offenders

Over the past decade, the criminal laws that define child sexual abuse offenses have been substantially revised. New laws on sexual conduct and contact with children have replaced many old laws on statutory rape, age of consent, and child molestation. There are now, in many states and in the United States Code, separate laws and penalties for a wide range of prohibited sexual acts involving children. Many of these laws establish a multilevel structure of offenses, with graduated penalties based on the age of the person abused and the relationship between the person who was abused and the person who committed the abuse, as well as on the severity of the offensive sexual contact.

All states have special laws directed at protecting children from sexual abuse by family members or others in a position of authority over a child. However, there is still a lack of uniformity among the states with respect to certain specifics. For example, the upper age limit for what constitutes a protected child under different laws ranges anywhere from preteen to the age of majority. In addition, statutes exist in most states that specifically prohibit the crime of incest. Usually, however, incest may be charged only if penetration can be proven, because most states require evidence of sexual intercourse to convict someone for this offense. Thus, prosecution for having sexual contact short of penile penetration with a child, even when there has been oral or anal sodomy, could not occur under the incest laws in many states.

There are different trends in the reform of incest laws in the United States. Many incest statutes have moved toward greater protection of the minor child. For example, at least half the states have expanded the scope of their incest laws to include offenses committed by stepparents and adoptive parents. However, even when charges are filed for incestuous sexual intercourse with a child, the incest statutes rarely are used alone; rather, they are invoked in conjunction with other criminal child sexual offense provisions.

There are many other statutes that deal with the problem of sexual abuse. These include family violence and "sexual psychopath" or sexually dangerous offender laws. Family violence statutes are relevant to sexual abuse cases even though they were primarily designed to address spouse abuse. Provisions in these laws, as they appear in many states, can be applied to cases of child sexual abuse. For example, in many states through the use of these statutes, the alleged sexual abuser can be ordered to vacate the marital home; to stop the abuse or not have contact with the abused child; to engage in counseling; or to pay support, restitution, or attorney's fees. Sexual psychopath or sexually dangerous offender statutes allow for the commitment—

often for longer periods than specified in criminal sentences—of seriously ill and dangerous sex offenders to mental health facilities instead of jailing them for particular sex crimes.

Laws dealing with child sexual exploitation have been enacted in all states. In 1978, Congress broadened the definition of sexual abuse in the federal Child Abuse Prevention and Treatment Act (42 U.S.C. Sec. 5101) to include "sexual exploitation." This required states to make their laws consistent with the federal Act in order to be eligible for federal assistance. Further, several times between 1984 and 1992, Congress amended the federal Protection of Children Against Sexual Exploitation Act of 1977 (18 U.S.C. Sec. 2251 et seq). This law addresses the sexual exploitation of children through their use in interstate prostitution activities, the production of pornography, and their transportation across state lines for the purposes of committing unlawful sexual acts.

The amendments to the Sexual Exploitation Act have increased the penalties for offenses and changed the law's definition to permit prosecution of individuals who either possess or trade child pornography materials, who use the U.S. mails or computer networks to exchange information related to child pornography and prostitution, or who sell child pornography or commercially benefit from the use of children in prostitution. The law also now provides children who have been abused with a civil cause of action in federal court for the damages caused by their abusers.

Over the past decade, the use of the judicial system (both the juvenile court and criminal court) for cases of sexual abuse increased significantly. However, many authorities have asserted that traditional methods of legal intervention can cause severe trauma to the sexually abused child and family. In the past, it was not uncommon for such harmful procedures to include multiple, detailed, and insensitive interrogations of the child by law enforcement, medical, and social service professionals; forced gynecological examinations of the child to obtain medical evidence; requiring, without exception, the child's testimony and cross-examination in open court and in the presence of the offender; and the use of polygraph tests to assess the child's veracity.

Based on a 2-year project that examined legal issues related to child sexual abuse cases, the American Bar Association developed a set of guidelines for improving legal intervention in intrafamilial child sexual abuse cases. Its recommendations included promoting innovative and interdisciplinary procedures, coordinating civil and criminal court proceedings involving the same child, establishing a range of judicial intervention procedures designed to reduce trauma to the child, providing a system advocate for the sexually abused child (such as a guardian ad litem), implementing procedures to prevent duplicative interviews with the child, instituting a specialized "vertical prosecution" approach in district attorney offices, avoiding the need for a child to testify in open court whenever possible, providing specialized training to professionals who deal with intrafamilial child sexual abuse cases, amending state legislation to improve existing child sexual abuse laws, and using specialized procedures for the handling of juvenile sex offenders (Bulkley 1982).

During the last 5 years, many communities, and some entire states, have significantly altered investigative techniques, evidence rules, and trial procedures to minimize the trauma of legal intervention on the child and family and to improve outcomes in prosecution. Many of these effective innovations do not require any statutory change. Examples include limiting the number of interviews; enhancing the child's communication skills through the use of dolls, artwork, and simplified vocabulary; modifying the physical environment of the courtroom; and preparing and sensitizing children for their experiences in the courtroom. In addition, some states have enacted special laws (generally upheld by the courts) intended to ease the child's anxiety throughout the criminal justice process. Such legislation includes the following reforms:

➤ Laws permitting child witnesses to have a supportive person present during court proceedings to sit with them while they testify, explain the proceedings, assist the family and child, and advise the court and prosecutor

➤ Laws permitting closing of the courtroom during the testimony of an abused child based on special findings by the judge, in individual cases, that the child would be injured if the courtroom were kept open

➤ Laws directing law enforcement, social service agencies, and prosecutors to conduct joint (or at least coordinated) investigations in child sexual abuse cases whenever possible, using trained interviewers

➤ Laws expediting the adjudication process by giving precedence in trial scheduling to sexual offense cases or to cases in which the abused person is a minor

➤ Laws creating special exceptions to the legal hearsay rule, so that a child's out-of-court statement concerning the abuse is admissible if the court finds sufficient indicia of its reliability and the child either testifies or is held to be unavailable as a witness

➤ Laws and court rules changing witness competency rules by moving away from mandatory child witness competency criteria or any formal distinguishing differences between child and adult witnesses

➤ Laws permitting the use of videotaped testimony of children, if either the defendant is present during the videotaping or a judge finds that testifying in open court would be traumatic to the child, or both

➤ Laws permitting the use of children's testimony via closed circuit television

➤ Laws, or court decisions, permitting the use of mental health expert testimony to aid the judge and jury in understanding issues related to child sexual abuse

The most controversial of these reforms have been the use of videotaped and closed circuit testimony and the admission of mental health expert testimony. In the matter of closed circuit testimony, the U.S. Supreme Court in the case of *Maryland v. Craig* (1990) ruled that state laws permitting the use of closed circuit television testimony at a criminal trial—on a case-by-case basis—do not violate the constitutional rights of the accused.

One area in which the response to reported child sexual abuse has presented communities with great challenges involves the alleged abuse of children in out-of-home care settings. Cases in which large numbers of children were allegedly molested in individual day care, preschool, or other similar programs have garnered much media and public attention. A few of these cases involved allegations that more than one person in the program had committed sexual abuse, but most involved only one accused individual.

Cases in which children are allegedly abused in schools, residential facilities, or other licensed programs present unique investigative challenges because of the multitude of government agencies that have responsibility for the children and the program. A planned, coordinated response to reports of child sexual abuse in out-of-home care, including how therapists will be used, is essential.

Both children and adults have problems, as well as strengths, re-

lated to their serving as witnesses. Although some jurors may regard
children as less credible in general than adults, research suggests that
children are not necessarily less reliable witnesses (Whitcomb et al.
1994). Children may even remember details that some adults would
overlook in their testimony. In recent years, the number of criminal
child sex abuse prosecutions involving very young alleged child victims
has increased. Because of the legal reforms and innovative, child-
sensitive practices described above, it has become more common to
find criminal prosecutions involving children under 6 years upon
whose disclosures and testimony the sex abuse trial will be based.

There is a widening interest among researchers on the capacities
of very young children to accurately perceive, interpret, report without exaggeration, and ultimately give reliable testimony related to
traumatic events that may have happened to them. Researchers and
practitioners also want to gain a better understanding of whether the
memory recognition of extremely young children may fade apprecia-
bly over time, to the extent that it might adversely affect the accuracy
of their delayed reports of child sexual abuse.

It is known that young children spontaneously recall less information than do older children, so that they may leave out important details in their recounting of events without directed or "leading"
questions. Young children may also, because they can get confused by
questioners and have difficulty in freely remembering peripheral details of an event, appear to give inconsistent accounts in successive
interviews. Extremely young children may be susceptible to social
pressures to say what they think an adult interviewing them wants to
hear.

Long after the interviews, the issue of what the child actually said
to the interviewer and what interviewer questions prompted which responses may become a pivotal concern at trial. Therefore, clinicians
should keep as precise a written record as possible of the facts sur-
rounding the interview: who asked the questions, what the questions
were, and how the child responded to each question. Some child advocates recommend audiotaping or videotaping all interviews so that
they can be properly preserved; others are opposed to this because a
recording of the interview may later be used to invade the child's privacy and to improperly discredit the child's revelations of abuse. The
decision whether to routinely record interviews with a possibly abused
child should be made only with knowledgeable legal consultation.

Researchers, joined by prosecutors, defense attorneys, and child advocates, want to know to what extent—if any—preschool- and school-age children are suggestible by overly zealous or inept interviewers. Can very young nonabused children resist making or agreeing to erroneous statements that something wrong happened to them when it did not?

## ▌ Guidance for Mental Health Professionals and Practitioners

In child sexual abuse cases, most jurisdictions require immediate reporting by the CPS agency to the police or prosecutor, and vice versa. Some state reporting laws do not limit reportable sexual abuse to that caused only by a parent or person responsible for the child's care. Many states now require immediate reporting of any suspected sexual assault of a child committed by any person, regardless of the relationship to the child of the person committing the abuse. Clinicians must be aware of the scope of their child sexual abuse reporting responsibilities under state law.

The use of mental health expert witnesses in juvenile and criminal court child sexual abuse cases has become increasingly common. These cases are often characterized by limited evidence, because there are usually no eyewitnesses (except the child) and often no physical or medical indications of the abuse. Courts disagree about whether expert testimony—providing opinions as to whether a certain child has been abused—should be admissible to prove or disprove that a child has in fact been sexually abused. Courts generally have rejected expert testimony regarding the truthfulness or credibility of a child alleged to have been abused.

Many of the ways that experts are being employed in child sexual abuse trials are controversial. Some judges and attorneys are anxious to use mental health expert testimony to aid the jury in determining the credibility or veracity of the child, but this has generally not been legally permitted, given the great prejudicial effect of such testimony and its usurpation of the role of the jury as the "trier of fact." Testimony about child witness credibility—on whether children as a rule are truthful, whether they can be easily coached to lie, or how suggestible they are to interviews that may lead them to testify about things that never happened—can lead to an improper "trial by the experts" (intensified by differences of opinion in the field) rather than a trial based on evidence. This same criticism applies to cases in which ex-

pert testimony might be sought to determine the "typical" characteristics of persons who abuse children, or "profiles" of persons who
abuse children. These types of testimony will generally not be permitted.

Mental health professionals are more likely to be permitted by the
court to testify concerning the general behavioral characteristics of
"normal" children and the common behaviors exhibited by children
who have been sexually abused (the latter has been dubbed the "child
sexual abuse syndrome" or the "child sexual abuse accommodation
syndrome"). Because the average person may possess misconceptions
or myths about the behaviors or symptoms of a child who has been
abused, expert opinion is sometimes used to assist the court by explaining that a child's seemingly paradoxical behavior (such as a delay
in reporting or a retraction) is not inconsistent with sexual abuse.

Most courts will allow such testimony only after the veracity of
the child's testimony has been challenged by the defense on cross-
examination, and when such testimony is designed to rebut defense
assertions that a child fantasized his or her claims of abuse or to explain the child's recantation or inconsistencies in his or her testimony.

(See Appendix H for legal resources.)

# References

Abel GG, Becker JV, Skinner LJ: Aggressive behavior and sex. Psy-
    chiatr Clin North Am 3:133–155, 1980
Abel GG, Mittelman M, Becker JV: Sex offenders: results of assessment
    and recommendations for treatment, in Clinical Criminology: Cur-
    rent Concepts. Edited by Ben-Aron H, Hucker S, Webster C.
    Toronto, Ontario, M & M Graphics, 1985
Adams CBL: Examining questionable child sex abuse allegations in
    their environmental and psychodynamic contexts. J Child Sexual
    Abuse 3:21–36, 1994
Adams-Tucker C: The unmet psychiatric needs of sexually abused
    youths: referrals from a child protection agency and clinical evalu-
    ations. J Am Acad Child Psychiatry 23:659–667, 1984
Adams-Tucker C, Adams PL: Treatment of sexually abused children, in
    Victims of Sexual Aggression: Treatment of Children, Women and
    Men. Edited by Stuart IR, Greer JG. New York, Van Nostrand Rein-
    hold, 1984, pp 57–74

American Psychiatric Association: Diagnostic and Statistical Manual of Mental Disorders, 4th Edition. Washington, DC, American Psychiatric Association, 1994

Barnard GW, Fuller AK, Robbins L, et al: The Child Molester. New York, Brunner/Mazel, 1989

Becker JV, Abel GG, Blanchard EB, et al: Evaluating social skills of sexual aggressiveness. Criminal Justice and Behavior 5:357–368, 1978

Berlin FS, Meinecke C: Treatment of sex offenders with antiandrogenic medication: conceptualization, review of treatment modalities, and preliminary findings. Am J Psychiatry 138:601–607, 1981

Berliner L, Ernst E: Group work with preadolescent sexual assault victims, in Victims of Sexual Aggression: Treatment of Children, Women and Men. Edited by Stuart IR, Greer JG. New York, Van Nostrand Reinhold, 1984, pp 105–124

Brassard MR, Tyler AH, Kehle TJ: School programs to prevent intrafamilial child sexual abuse. Child Abuse Negl 7:241–245, 1983

Budin LE, Johnson CF: Sex abuse prevention programs: offenders' attitudes about their efficacy. Child Abuse Negl 13:77–87, 1989

Bulkley J: Recommendations for Improving Legal Intervention in Intrafamil Child Sexual Abuse Cases. Washington, DC, American Bar Association Center on Children and the Law, 1982

Cohn AH, Daro D: Is treatment too late: what ten years of evaluative research tell us. Child Abuse Negl 11:433–442, 1987

Conte JR: Ethical issues in evaluation of prevention programs. Child Abuse Negl 11:171–172, 1987

Conte JR, Wolf S, Smith T: What sexual offenders tell us about prevention strategies. Child Abuse Negl 13:293–301, 1989

Damon L, Waterman J: Parallel group treatment of children and their mothers, in Sexual Abuse of Young Children. Edited by MacFarlane K, Waterman J. New York, Guilford, 1986, 224–298

Dimock PT: Adult males sexually abused as children: characteristics and implications for treatment. Journal of Interpersonal Violence 3:203–221, 1988

Fryer GE, Kraizer SK, Miyoshi T: Measuring actual reduction of risk to child abuse: a new approach. Child Abuse Negl 11:173–179, 1987

Gaddini R: Incest as a developmental failure. Child Abuse Negl 7:357–358, 1983

Giarretto H: A comprehensive child sexual abuse treatment program, in Sexually Abused Children and Their Families. Edited by Mrazek PB, Kempe CH. New York, Pergamon, 1981, 179–198

Giarretto H, Giarretto A, Sgroi SM: Coordinated community treatment of incest, in Sexual Assault of Children and Adolescents. Edited by Burgess AW, Groth AN, Holmstrom LL, et al. Lexington, MA, DC Heath, 1978, pp 231–240

Keller RA, Cicchinelli LF, Gardner DM: Characteristics of child sexual abuse treatment programs. Child Abuse Negl 13:361–368, 1989

Lang RA, Pugh GM, Langevin R: Treatment of incest and pedophilic offenders: a pilot study. Behavioral Science and the Law 6:239–255, 1988

Maryland v Craig, 110 S. Ct. 3157, 1990

Meyer WJ, Cole C, Emory E: Depo-Provera treatment for sex offending behavior: an evaluation of outcome. Bull Am Acad Psychiatry Law 20:249–259, 1992

Nelki JS, Watters J: A group for sexually abused young children: unravelling the web. Child Abuse Negl 13:369–377, 1989

Pelcovitz D, Adler NA, Kaplan S, et al: The failure of a school-bsed child sexual abuse prevention program. J Am Acad Child Adolesc Psychiatry 31:887–892, 1992

Plummer CA: Prevention education perspective, in The Educator's Guide to Preventing Child Sexual Abuse. Edited by Nelson M, Clark K. Santa Cruz, CA, Network Publications, 1986

Poche C, Brouer R, Swearington M: Teaching self-protection to children. J Appl Behav Anal 14:159–176, 1981

Prentky R, Burgess AW: Rehabilitation of child molesters: a cost-benefit analysis. Am J Orthopsychiatry 60:108–117, 1990

Roesler T, Savin D, Grosz C: Family therapy of extra-familial sexual abuse. Am Acad Child Adolesc Psychiatry 32:967–970, 1993

Smets AC, Cebula CM: A group treatment program for adolescent sex offenders: five steps toward resolution. Child Abuse Negl 11:247–254, 1987

Spungen C: Child personal safety: model program for prevention of child sexual abuse. Social Work 34:127–131, 1989

Steward M, Farquar LC, Dicharry DC, et al: Group therapy: a treatment of choice for young victims of child abuse. Int J Group Psychother 36:261–277, 1986

Summit RC: The child sexual abuse accommodation syndrome. Child Abuse Negl 7:177–193, 1983

Trudell B, Whatley MH: School sexual abuse prevention: unintended consequences and dilemmas. Child Abuse Negl 12:103–113, 1988

Vizard E: Self-esteem and personal safety: comments on secondary prevention group work with young sexually abused children. Association for Child Psychology and Psychiatry Newsletter 9:16–22, 1987

Whitcomb D, Runyan DK, Toth PA, et al: The Child Victim as a Witness: Research Report. Washington, DC, Office of Juvenile Justice and Delinquency Prevention, 1994

Wurtele SK: School-based sexual abuse prevention programs: a review. Child Abuse Negl 11:483–495, 1987

Wurtele SK: The role of maintaining telephone contact with parents during the teaching of a personal safety program. J Child Sex Abuse 2:65–82, 1993

# Chapter 5

# Domestic Violence

*Mary Lystad, Ph.D.*
*Matilda Rice, M.D.*
*Sandra J. Kaplan, M.D.*

## Overview

## ▍ Definition

*Domestic violence,* sometimes referred to as *partner abuse, spousal assault,* or *spouse abuse,* is defined in this chapter as violence between adults who are intimates, regardless of their marital status, living arrangements, or sexual orientations. In this chapter the term *domestic violence* is used to refer to partner or spousal abuse or assault. Such violence includes minor aggressive acts of throwing, shoving, and slapping; as well as major aggressive acts of beatings, forced sex, threats with a deadly weapon, and homicide (Straus and Gelles 1986). This book's introduction noted that females more often than males are targets of domestic violence, sexual abuse, elder abuse, and adolescent physical abuse (Earls et al. 1991).

## ▍ Historical Perspective

Domestic violence, in which women were the most likely to be injured, has a long-standing history. For thousands of years, being a target of spousal assault was considered a woman's lot. Wives who were not beaten were considered lucky, and women were taught how to behave in order to avoid being beaten (Walker 1986).

139

The long tradition of domestic violence has blended with religious beliefs and legal rights holding men responsible for the deeds of their wives and children, and making it their duty to discipline those who were viewed as disobedient (Walker 1986). The "rule of thumb" expression comes from an old common-law statute that imposed a limitation on men's disciplinary authority over "their" women by enjoining husbands from hitting wives with a stick wider than their thumbs. Given the long traditions that legitimized male supremacy, it is not surprising that family violence has been closely linked with discrimination against women.

The substantial achievements of women in obtaining social justice and equality over the last decade have prompted analyses of women's relationships both inside and outside the home. Women's groups have brought domestic violence to the attention of lawmakers, professional service workers, and the general public. They have identified spousal assault and rape as forms of family violence and have identified as destructive myths the traditional beliefs that a "man's home is his castle" and that a man's female partner is his property, both of which have been licenses for criminal assault.

Studies of domestic violence document its existence in all social classes and ethnic and racial groups in this country (Straus et al. 1980; Straus and Gelles 1986). Both men and women are targets of domestic violence; however, women are injured more often than men during spousal assault (American Medical Association 1992).

People who commit acts of violence toward their domestic partners are often those who were themselves beaten or who witnessed violence against their mothers as children. There is also an intergenerational cycle of abuse: persons who were abused as children often abuse their own children and/or intimate partners (Steinmetz et al. 1986). In addition, many adults who commit family sexual assaults have a history of having been assaulted as children.

# ▌ Prevalence

Until recently, there were no formal statistics on domestic violence cases known to the police or to social service agencies (Lerman 1981). As an academic topic of research, domestic violence is barely 20 years old. There have been numerous articles in the mass media during the last decade on the "epidemic" of domestic violence. This attention probably reflects a growing awareness and recognitionof this long-standing social problem.

Nonfatal spousal or partner assault has been reported to occur in the United States in one out of six homes each year with two million females a year severely injured by their male partners (Straus and Gelles 1986). It has been found that severe husband-to-wife violence occurs in about 30/1,000 married couples (Straus and Gelles 1986), and that assaulted partners are at high risk for repeated injury from spousal assault (U.S. Department of Justice 1991). During 1992, 3.9 million women were physically abused by their partners (Commonwealth Fund 1993). Between 1976 and 1985 there were 16,595 deaths from partner abuse. More than half of the women who die as a result of homicide are killed by partners or ex-partners (Browne and Williams 1989; Zahn 1989). Spousal homicides are responsible for 8.8% of homicides in the United States with white wives 1.3 times more likely to be killed than white husbands and with black husbands 1.3 times more likely to be killed than black wives. As already mentioned, females have been found to be injured more often than males during spousal or partner assaults (American Medical Association 1992).

Unmarried women during dating or cohabitation (Makepeace 1983; Roscoe and Benaske 1985) and separated or divorced women have been reported to be at even greater risk of severe injury by their current or, in the cases of separated or divorced women, their estranged partners, than remarried women (Ellis 1989; Gaquin 1978).

Marital rape was reported by 14% of San Francisco women who had ever been married (Russell 1980). It has also been reported that marital rape may occur antecedent to marital homicide (Browne 1987).

In 1975–1976, Straus et al. (1980) conducted the first national survey of family violence, using a probability sample of 2,143 currently married or cohabiting persons. A random half of the respondents were women and the other half men. Face-to-face interviews lasted approximately 1 hour. The completion rate of the entire sample was 65%. In 1985, Straus and Gelles (1986) did a national resurvey of family violence. Partner abuse data were based on 3,520 households containing a currently married or cohabiting couple. The response rate, calculated as a proportion of eligibles, was 84% (Straus and Gelles 1986). Because of interview time limitations, the term *abuse* was restricted to physical abuse. Psychological abuse and sexual abuse were not included.

The findings are in the form of three indices—husband-to-wife, and couple. These indices differentiate between minor violence (pushing, slapping, and throwing things) and severe violence (kicking, biting, and punching). All but one of the six comparisons show that the rate of violence was lower in 1985 than in 1975, although none of the changes were statistically significant. The fact that the 1985 interviews were by telephone and the 1975 interviews were in person may account for the apparent decline in violence reported in 1985.

### Husband-to-Wife Violence

The overall rate of violence by husbands declined from 121/1,000 couples to 113/1,000 couples over the 10-year period. Thus, the husband-to-wife violence rate declined by 6.6%. The rate of severe violence by husbands according to Straus' measure of "wife beating" declined from 38/1,000 couples to 30/1,000 couples in 1985. In addition, a decrease of 9/1,000 in the rate of wife beating is worth noting because it represents a large number of couples. Specifically, if the 1975 rate for husband-to-wife severe violence had remained in effect, the application of this rate to the 54 million couples in the United States in 1985 would have resulted in an estimate of at least 2,052,000 severely assaulted wives each year. However, if there has been a 27% decrease in the rate, that translates to 1,620,000 beaten wives, which is 432,000 fewer than would have been the case if the 1975 rate had prevailed. That would have been an extremely important reduction. On the other hand, as Straus and Gelles (1986) point out, the 1985 estimate of 1.6 million beaten wives is not an indicator of domestic tranquillity.

### Wife-to-Husband Violence

Although the trend for husband-to-wife violence is encouraging, the situation for wife-to-husband violence is at best mixed. As already mentioned, both men and women are targets of assault during domestic violence. However, women are more likely than men to become victims of both fatal (Mercy and Saltzman 1989) and nonfatal spousal assault and are more likely than men to be injured during such assault (Gelles and Straus 1988). It is estimated that 95% of the intimate partners who are severely assaulted are women (Schecter 1982). Acts of physical aggression between intimate partners have been reported to occur in 1 in 6 American homes (Straus and Gelles 1988; Gelles and Straus 1990). The overall violence rate actually increased slightly between 1975 and 1985 from 116/1,000 couples to 121/1,000 couples

(Straus and Gelles 1986). The rate for severe violence against a husband decreased during this same time period, but only slightly: from 46/1,000 couples to 44/1,000 couples. Neither of these changes is statistically significant.

In addition to the trends, the violence rates reveal an important finding about violence in American families: in marked contrast to the behavior of women outside the family, within the family women are often as violent as men. However, this equivalence in rate does not take severity of injury into account. This highly controversial finding of female assaultive behavior in the 1975 study is confirmed by the 1985 study and also by findings on other samples and by other investigators. Although the two national surveys and other studies cited by Straus and Gelles (1986) leave little doubt about the high frequency of wife-to-husband violence, the meaning of such violence needs to be understood. As pointed out by Straus (1977), Straus and Gelles (1986), and Straus et al. (1980), the greater average size and strength of men and their greater aggressiveness mean that the same act (for example, a punch) is likely to vary considerably in the amount of pain or injury inflicted depending on whether it is delivered by a woman or a man. Even more important, a great deal of violence by women against their husbands is committed in retaliation or self-defense.

## Couple Violence

Couple violence refers to the data on combined violence by husbands and wives or by male and female cohabiting partners. In 1975 a violent act occurred in 160/1,000 families, and the 1985 rate was almost as high—158/1,000 families. Similarly, only a small decrease in the rate of severe assaults on an intimate partner—from 61/1,000 couples to 58/1,000 couples—occurred over the 10-year span.

Straus and Gelles (1986) write that the lower rates of severe violence in the 1985 study could have been produced by a number of factors, including 1) differences in the methodology used in the two surveys, 2) a greater reluctance on the part of the respondents to report violence, or 3) a decrease in the amount of child abuse and wife beating. It is unlikely that the decrease is due to differences in the methods used in the two surveys because the increased anonymity afforded by the telephone survey would tend to increase rather than decrease the 1985 rate. Most likely, these researchers say, the findings represent a combination of changed attitudes and norms along with changes in overt behavior. This interpretation is based on a number of changes in American society that took place during or immediately before the decade of this study, including changes in the family, the economy, the social acceptability of family violence, the alternatives available to women, the social control processes, and the availability of treatment and prevention services.

## ▌ Domestic Violence in Homosexual Relationships

Domestic violence has been recognized to be a problem not only between heterosexual partners, but also between homosexual partners. Lie and Gentlewarrior (1991) found that among 1,099 lesbians surveyed, more than half reported having been abused by a female lover. The most commonly indicated type of abuse was combined physical and psychological abuse. Lobel (1986) and Renzetti (1988) also reported on domestic violence between lesbian partners, and Letellier (1994) reported on male homosexual partner abuse.

## ▌ Sexual Assault and Domestic Violence

Although the Gelles and Straus studies did not address sexual assault as spousal assault, other research does address this form of family violence. Marital rape appears to be quite prevalent. Finkelhor and Yllo (1983) report that 36% of 304 battered women in 10 shelters had been raped by their husband or cohabiting partner; a similar rate among battered women was found by Giles-Sims (1983). Of a sample of 119 battered women in California, 37% had experienced marital rape (Pagelow 1980); and 14% of a sample of 930 women reported an unwanted sexual experience with a husband or an ex-husband (Russell 1982). Although forced sex in marriage is probably the most frequent type of sexual assault, women who have been sexually assaulted by their husbands or partners often avoid defining themselves as raped (Gelles 1979).

## ▌ Association of Child Abuse with Domestic Violence

In reviewing the clinical literature, Nadelson and Sauzier (1986) found that wife beating is often accompanied by physical and/or sexual abuse of the children. Gayford (1975), in a study of battered wives, reported that 37% of the women and 54% of the men who had been abused beat their own children. Hilberman (1980), in a study of battered women, identified physical and/or sexual abuse of children in a third of the families studied. Emotional neglect of children, parental alcoholism, and frequent separations of parents from children were occurrences in these families. Children in these violent homes were witnesses as well as targets of abuse.

## ▌ Family Background and Domestic Violence

Hilberman (1980) also reported that suicides and homicides were frequent occurrences among the family members and neighborhood acquaintances she studied. Most of the women had left their family of origin at early ages to escape from violent and sexually abusive fathers. They tended to marry in their teenage years; many of them were pregnant at the time of marriage or already had children. These women viewed pregnancy as a way to leave their family of origin. Further, most battered women in this study reported an increase in their husband's violence during pregnancy. This violence often led to miscarriages and premature births.

Women raised as children in violent homes were found to have an increased risk of being assaulted by their partners. In addition, women raised in violent families as children were found to have an increased risk of inflicting partner assault (American Medical Association 1992).

## Risk Factors for Domestic Violence

Although domestic violence occurs in all socioeconomic classes, socioeconomic disadvantage does increase risk. In spousal assault, an important risk factor, regardless of social status, is power imbalance, with the highest prevalence rates in male-dominated dyads and the lowest prevalence in egalitarian spousal dyads (Straus and Gelles 1990). However, Babcock et al. (1993) found that among domestically violent couples, husbands who had less power were physically abusive toward their wives. This may indicate that violence is a compensatory behavior that results from the husband's lack of power in other areas of the marriage.

Earls et al. (1992) have also hypothesized that in addition to sex role socialization, which may legitimize the use of violence by males toward females, other risk factors for assault among partners and other intimates in dyads may be cultural norms and the privacy of family interactions coupled with an absence of societal restraints (Fagan and Wexler 1987; Shield et al. 1988). Women between the ages of 17 and 28 have also been found to have increased risk of assault by their partners (American Medical Association 1992). In addition, social isolation has been reported in child-abusive families; given the approximately 50% overlap in families with either spousal abuse or child abuse, a lack of acculturation to a nonassaulting community may be a factor (Salzinger et al. 1986).

## ▌ Substance Abuse, Depression, and Domestic Violence

Substance abuse and depression are both risk factors for, and probably effects of, domestic violence. Hotaling and Sugarman (1986) reported that alcohol use was associated with child abuse and husband-to-wife violence. Campbell and Gibbs (1986), Hotaling and Sugarman (1986), and Ladoucer and Temple (1985) showed that alcohol was related respectively to sexual assault and to adolescent violence in social settings. Illicit drug use, particularly powdered and crack cocaine, has also been associated with increases in severe interpersonal violence between adults, and in neglect and abuse of children in these families (Campbell and Gibbs 1986). Slade et al. (1991) examined the relationship between domestic violence and the intake of alcohol and other drugs. Findings showed that alcohol was revealed in 85% of the cases and cocaine was found in 30% of the cases. A combination of both was found in 20% of the cases.

Kaplan et al. (1988) found that major depressive episodes in assaulted partners often antedated the onset of spousal assault, thereby rendering the assaulted partner vulnerable.

## Emotional and Behavioral Symptoms and Disorders and Domestic Violence

### ▌ Assaulted Partners

Nadelson and Sauzier (1986) surveyed studies of the impact of abuse. They cited Hilberman and Munson's (1977–1978) description of a response pattern among 60 battered women that is similar to that of the rape-trauma syndrome. Hilberman and Munson wrote of constant terror plus the presence of severe agitation and anxiety with fears of imminent doom. These women were unable to relax or sleep and experienced violent nightmares. During the daytime they were passive and lacked energy. They experienced a sense of hopelessness, helplessness, and despair, and often saw themselves as deserving of abuse and as powerless to change their lives.

Frequent somatic symptoms were reported—such as headaches, asthma, gastrointestinal symptoms, and chronic pain. More than half of these women had prior psychiatric histories, with depression being the most frequent diagnosis. They had often sought medical help and many had been treated for drug overdoses and suicide attempts. Although they had multiple medical contacts over many years, they did not talk with their physicians about the abuse. The tendency of assaulted partners not to tell and of physicians not to ask has been frequently reported (Dewsbury 1975; Hilberman and Munson 1977–1978).

Stark and Flitcraft (1981) and McLeer and Anwar (1989) have reported the tendency of physicians not to diagnose domestic violence in emergency rooms. McLeer and Anwar (1989) reported increased rates of domestic violence diagnoses following emergency room personnel training.

Kaplan et al. (1988), in a study of 20 women who had been assaulted by their husbands and of 24 control-group women who had not been assaulted, found that a significantly higher percentage of abused partners were diagnosed, using the Schedule for Affective Disorders and Schizophrenia, Lifetime Version (SADS-L), as having a depressive disorder or a labile personality (characterized by affective lability). The onset of a psychiatric disorder usually antedated the abuse, suggesting, as previously mentioned, that these women's affective disorders made them vulnerable to being assaulted by their husbands.

Depression, suicidal behavior, and psychoses of assaulted partners have been reported by Gayford (1975), Hilberman and Munson (1977–1978), Hughes (1988), Myers et al. (1985), and Pfeffer (1985). Cascardi and O'Leary (1992) found that among a group of battered women, as the frequency and severity of the physically aggressive acts increased, depressive symptoms increased and self-esteem decreased.

AIDS infection risk associated with domestic violence has not been specifically studied. However, because alcohol abuse has been reported to be a risk factor for HIV (human immunodeficiency virus) infection (Stall et al. 1986) and alcohol abuse has been associated with domestic violence (Hotaling and Sugarman 1986), it would be reasonable to anticipate increased risk of HIV infection in violent families.

## ▋ Assaulting Partners

Studies have shown behavioral and emotional symptoms and disorders associated with violent partners as well as with the partner who is assaulted. Walker (1984) noted that the best predictors of future violence are a history of exposure to violent behavior: witnessing, receiving, and committing violent acts in the childhood home; committing violent acts toward pets, inanimate objects, or other people; having previous criminal records; having spent a longer time in the military; and a history of violent behavior toward women.

Certain psychosocial characteristics suggest higher risk potential for domestic violence perpetration. Straus et al. (1980) found that batterers tend to be less educated and from lower socioeconomic classes than their abused partners. Men who are more traditional than women in their attitudes toward women's roles are more likely to be batterers. These men measure a woman's feelings for them by how well she meets their sex-role expectations.

Certain personality traits as well as various psychological and cognitive characteristics suggest a higher risk potential for the violent partner. Else et al. (1993) found that men who commit domestic violence have poor problem-solving skills, certain hostility traits, borderline antisocial personality traits, and histories of abuse as children. These factors may predispose them to violent behavior.

Hilberman (1980) reported that such men are in need of a great amount of nurturance and are very possessive of a woman's time. Hilberman, as well as Gayford (1975), Gelles (1974), and Scott (1974), reported extreme jealousy in a large percentage of violent marriages. These husbands made active efforts to keep their wives isolated, and if the women left the house for any reason, they were often accused of infidelity, and were then assaulted. Women as well as men use violence during spousal assault (Straus and Gelles 1986). The association between substance abuse and domestic violence has been discussed earlier in this chapter.

## ▋ Child Witnesses

A number of studies describe a high incidence of somatic, psychological, and behavioral dysfunctions in the children of battered women. Salzin-

ger et al. (1992) found that children showed general behavioral disturbances as a result of experiencing different constellations of family
violence.

Somatic dysfunctions reported in the children of battered women
include headaches, abdominal complaints, asthma, and peptic ulcers
(Nadelson and Sauzier 1986).

Behavioral problems reported among young children include stut-
tering, school phobias, enuresis, and insomnia. Insomnia has often
been reported to be accompanied by intense fear, screaming, and resistance to going to bed at night. Many of these children have been
found to have impaired concentration and difficulty with schoolwork.
Ragg and Webb (1992) reported that when a preschool child has witnessed partner abuse, the risk of negative effects on the emotional
development and the adaptive behavior of the child is increased.

Disruptive behaviors have been described among older children.
Such behaviors in boys include stealing, temper tantrums, truancy, and
fighting with siblings and schoolmates. Somatic symptoms have been
described as more characteristic of girls (Hershorn and Rosenbaum
1985; Hilberman 1980). The higher numbers of behavior problems
among these children have usually been accompanied by reports of lower
social competence ratings (Jaffe et al. 1986; Wolfe et al. 1985). Wolfe et
al. also noted that the children's psychosocial adjustment worsened as
their mother's depression and anxiety worsened. Jaffe et al. (1990)
stated that, in addition to age and sex, stage of development and role in
the family are important factors in children's responses to partner abuse.

A number of researchers have pointed out that partner abuse and
child abuse often occur together in the family (Giles-Sims 1985;
Jouriles et al. 1987). Abuse of parents by children also may occur
(Kratcoski 1985). Davis and Carlson (1987) write that children who
both witness partner abuse and experience abuse appear more seriously affected than those who just witness the behavior. Malmquist
(1985) pointed out that attendant problems must be addressed from
both medical and legal perspectives in order to protect the child from
further harm in the home and in the courts.

## Dynamics of Domestic Violence

In the past, domestic violence was viewed by providers of mental
health care as a situation existing when a woman with masochistic

tendencies unconsciously or consciously encouraged abuse by her husband. This view also assumed that women stayed in battering relationships in order to suffer (Snell et al. 1964).

The witnessing of parental partner abuse during childhood and having experienced child abuse (Straus 1977) have both been reported to be associated with experiencing or committing domestic violence oneself. The witnessing (Straus et al. 1980) or experiencing of interpersonal violence during childhood may lead to the belief that violence is a legitimate way to resolve interpersonal conflict. In addition, this exposure to violence may enable the learning of specific aggressive behaviors from parents who are behavior role models. The witnessing or experiencing of family violence against a woman also promotes impairment of self and a devaluation of women by both girls and boys in a family. Child witnesses identify their mothers and women in general as accepting of violence. They may expect violence to be part of marriage (Dutton and Painter 1981).

Walker (1979) applied "learned helplessness" (Seligman's term [1975]) as a theory of the mechanism by which people who experience domestic violence become entrapped in abusive relationships. This theory proposes that assaulted partners expect battering as part of their intimate relationships. It also proposes that assaulted partners blame themselves for the violence, and that they have impaired self-esteem because they feel unable to control the violence in their intimate relationships.

Traumatic bonding has been presented as another theory to explain the domestic violence process; it postulates that assaulted partners form strong emotional attachments under conditions of intermittent positive and negative reinforcement. Positive feelings and attitudes for the violent partner then form in the assaulted partner (Dutton and Painter 1981). A cycle of dependency is created, during which a power imbalance occurs. The assaulted partner experiences both enhanced self-esteem, through identification with and overvaluing of the violent partner, and impaired self-esteem, through feelings of disempowerment (Dutton and Painter 1981).

## Role of Mental Health Professionals

The role of the psychiatrist and other mental health professionals is multifaceted and depends on many factors. One factor involves the place of the intervention—a hospital inpatient unit, an emergency room, a clinic, an office, or a court setting. Another factor involves the time of the intervention—in the acute period immediately after the violence has occurred, in an intermediate period of apparent peaceful coexistence, in the chronic period, or during a separation period. The psychiatrist's work with assaulted partners usually begins during a separation period. Batterers do not usually accept psychiatric intervention unless treatment is court ordered.

Help cannot begin until a diagnosis of family violence is established. The clinician then needs to network with social services, police, domestic violence advocacy groups, and the legal system in order to plan a therapeutic intervention. On many occasions networking also involves other physicians who may be working with the family, such as the family physician, the pediatrician, the obstetrician, and the emergency room physician. The treatment plan formulated first needs to consider how to ensure the assaulted partner's protection both from further assault and from suicide risk—particularly during the acute period. The cessation of the battering is the immediate concern, but the long-term therapeutic goal is to facilitate the assaulted partner's independence by treating assault-related psychological symptoms.

Admission of an assaulted partner to a hospital is often therapeutic, particularly for treatment of severe physical injury and high suicide risk. The person assaulted is usually physically and emotionally exhausted, and hospitalization can hasten the healing process. It also provides a safe temporary refuge and a chance to establish new and vital therapeutic alliances. The assaulted partner then has time to think and to decide on a course of action. Before discharge from an inpatient service or an emergency room, the assaulted partner should be given the telephone numbers of and appointments with the local helping agencies dealing with domestic violence. To ensure protection, it is highly desirable to set up interviews with an advocacy agency before discharging the assaulted partner from medical services.

Private physicians and outpatient clinics see smaller numbers of assaulted partners in the acute phase. Women often visit their doctors for somatic concerns, yet never confide in them about ongoing domestic violence. Assaulted partners often consider it less of a risk to see doctors for physical complaints than for psychological concerns related to domestic violence.

Some battered women are identified by health care providers during their pregnancies. At this time the violence often escalates, and is expressed by repeated blows to the woman's protruding abdomen (Saltzman 1990).

Battered women rarely consult with mental health professionals before they have endured long periods of violence. They then often do so only after they have exhausted many physicians and many possible diagnoses. These women often report that they did not disclose battering incidents to mental health professionals. This may be explained by the failure of many nonpsychiatric physicians, as well as psychiatrists and other mental health professionals, to suspect abuse or to make routine inquiries about family violence (Stark and Flitcraft 1981). In order to provide effective treatment and to prevent further spousal assault, domestic violence needs to be suspected in the absence of direct complaints, and it must be asked about tactfully yet persistently (McLeer and Anwar 1989).

## Assessment

### ▌ Physical Signs and History

Those suspected of being targets of domestic violence require physical examinations for accurate diagnosis and treatment planning. The physical injury pattern and history associated with domestic violence typically includes one or a combination of the following:

1. *Location of injuries.*   Injuries are often located on the face, head, neck, chest, breasts, abdomen, or genital areas, often with bilateral distribution.
2. *Types of injuries.*   Common types of injuries are contusions, lacerations, abrasions, ecchymosis, stab wounds, burns, human bites, fractures (particularly of the nose and orbits and spiral wrist fractures), and multiple injuries in various stages of healing. In addition to these types of injuries, there are often explanations by those injured that fail to account for the type or pattern of injuries sustained.
3. *Complaints.*   There may be complaints of pain in the absence of tissue injury, complaints of sexual assault, multiple injuries in various stages of healing, and again, explanations by those injured that fail to account for the type or pattern of injuries sustained.

4. *Injuries during pregnancy.* There may be vaginal bleeding, threatened abortion, or spontaneous abortion, in addition to the types of injuries, complaints, and explanations listed above for all patients.
5. *Previous emergency room visits for trauma.*

It is helpful for the clinician to be familiar with symptoms resulting from domestic violence and to separate the symptoms from primary psychiatric symptoms. It is also important for the psychiatrist to know patterns of behavior often associated with domestic violence, frequently referred to as the cycle of battering.

### Sample Interview

Interviews specifically to discover domestic violence are helpful during clinical assessment. McLeer and Anwar (1989) have prepared a sample interview for diagnosis of domestic violence, which can be used by clinicians during case assessment.

**Clinician-patient interview.** The first part of the interview consists of 30 questions for the clinician to ask the woman:

1. How were you hurt?
2. Has this happened before?
3. When did it first happen?
4. How badly have you been hurt in the past?
5. Was a weapon involved? Is there a weapon in the house?
6. If so, what kind?
7. Who lives in the home?
8. What are the children's ages?
9. Are the children in danger?
10. Have they been hit or hurt by him?
11. How badly have they been hurt?
12. Have you ever told anyone about this before? If so, who?
12. What have you done in the past to protect yourself?
14. What have you done in the past to get help?
15. Have you ever called the police?
16. If yes, when, and what did they say or do?
17. Did you report this incident to the police? If not, why not?
18. If yes, what precinct?

19. What did they say?
20. Have you ever obtained a protective order?
21. Have you ever tried to press charges this time or before?
22. Does your boyfriend/husband have a criminal record?
23. Has he beaten up or hurt other people?
24. Has he threatened to kill you?
25. Has he tried to kill you?
26. What did he do?
27. Are you afraid to go home?
28. Where can you go?
29. Have you ever called Women Against Abuse, Women in Crisis, etc.?
30. If yes, do you have a contact there? Who?

**Questions for the clinician to answer.**   The second part of the interview consists of 10 questions the clinician answers separately after having spoken with the woman.

1. Is the woman able to function at home and at work?
2. What efforts has she made in the past to cope with battering?
3. Whom has she contacted?
4. How often?
5. What has been the response?
6. Has her behavior or mental status changed?
7. Is she more aware of the danger or harm, or less?
8. Is she reaching out, or is she withdrawing?
9. Does she seem in a fog or emotionally dulled?
10. Does she seem to feel hopeless, as if nothing she does will help her to extricate herself from the situation?

**Behavior and emotional status assessment by the clinician.**   In addition to interviewing the battered woman and determining the answers to the questions above, the clinician should assess her behavior and emotional status. The type of symptomatology that has been observed in abused women includes the emotional reactions described below:

1. *Agitation.*   Agitation and anxiety, bordering on panic or including panic, are often present, together with a chronic apprehension of imminent doom. Abused women often have anticipatory terror that causes them to stay vigilant and makes them unable

to relax or sleep. Nightmares are often present with themes of violence and danger (Hilberman 1980).

2. *Immobilization.* The woman's response to the violence committed by an explosive partner is often profound terror. Symonds (1978) conceptualizes this fear as a form of traumatic psychological infantilism, or frozen fright, similar to the acute psychological response to rape and other violent crimes.

3. *Learned helplessness.* When people experience trauma that they cannot control, motivation for controlling later trauma often wanes. They become helpless (Seligman 1975).

4. *Hopelessness.* Battered women often believe that they can never escape the batterer's domination. This expectation of powerlessness and inability to control their own destiny, whether or not it is real, prevents any effective action. Most such women anticipate their own defeat and do not seek or accept assistance because they do not believe that it will be effective (Walker 1977–1978).

5. *Dependence.* Walker (1977–1978) describes the mental paralysis that besets battered partners and states further that compelling psychological factors often bind the woman and the man together in a symbiotic relationship: both of them are frightened that they cannot survive alone.

6. *Obsessive thinking.* Abused persons develop strange mechanisms of self-protection; major parts of their lives are spent thinking of ways to please their partners in order to avoid violence. Battered women often lose their ability to plan ahead because they do not feel themselves to be in control of their lives. They can plan only for short periods of time in direct connection with the violence. As a consequence, they lose their problem-solving skills and are inadequately prepared for independence.

7. *Pathological transference.* According to Ochberg (1980), battered partners develop the same type of transference to the batterer that develops between hostage and hostage takers in a terrorism situation. The transference includes positive feelings toward the captor and negative feelings toward the authorities responsible for rescue. This pathological transference is based on terror, infantile dependence, and gratitude; it may, in fact, be a survival effort. This phenomenon has also been described as a "traumatic bonding" similar to captor-hostage relationships (Ochberg 1980). Loneliness, isolation, shame, guilt, and negative self-image also contribute to the severity of the syndrome.

Therapeutic interventions for battered partners are facilitated by correctly diagnosing symptoms that result from battering and following up with an effective treatment plan involving identification and clarification of the stressor event(s) of domestic violence. Battering is a series of physical attacks on an intimate or family member, repeated in a habitual pattern; as pointed out above, domestic violence may be considered analogous to a hostage situation. Battered partners have negative perceptions of themselves and their pasts, presents, and futures. They are often afraid of change and develop adaptive defense mechanisms that offer immediate protection for minimal survival and self-preservation. They may rationalize the violence as normal and justified. They often become compliant and submissive and will go to any length to avoid the violence. They are in a no-win situation: if they are passive, they may invite the abuse and be unable to protect themselves, and if they are aggressive, they may be seen as provoking the abuse.

It is important to note that the personalities of battered partners may have been changed by the experience of abuse itself. The relationship of the battered person to the batterer is often dependent and symbiotic. The battered person may consider death to be an acceptable alternative and the only way to stop the abuse. The clinician assessing someone who has been beaten, and perhaps suggesting separation from the batterer for the battered person's protection, must be alert to any signs of suicide.

## Treatment for the Battered Partner

Modalities of treatment for the battered partner include

- Crisis intervention
- Psychotherapy (individual and group)
- Couple therapy
- Family therapy
- Parenting therapy
- Substance abuse treatment
- Consideration of medication for incapacitating depression or other psychiatric disorders that may be associated with the domestic violence and that may lead to an inability to take action to protect oneself

# ▌ Crisis Intervention

Crisis intervention techniques are very appropriate after an acute battering incident, especially before Phase 3 of the cycle, the repentant batterer (see the following section, "The Cycle of Battering Behavior"). After an acute incident, the battered partner is often concerned enough with her lack of control of becoming a target of partner assault to want to change her behavior. A goal in crisis intervention is to teach battered partners how to resolve possible future crises by applying conflict resolution techniques. To maintain a wedge of useful intervention, denial and minimalization must be counteracted. Battered partners are helped by recognizing themselves as battered and by having their batterers exposed as violent and uncontrollable.

# ▌ Psychotherapy

The mental health professions generally emphasize the value of keeping families intact. However, in dealing with domestic violence, at least a temporary separation, or "time out," should be encouraged. The major difficulty in achieving time out is that although battered partners want the therapist to stop the batterer from abusing them they fear any separation from the batterer.

Techniques of psychotherapy vary, but the goals remain the same. It is important to clarify the ambivalent feelings of the battered partner, which center around issues of love and hate, anger, passivity, depression and anxiety, symbiotic relationships and independence, omnipotence and impotence. A combination of behavioral and insight-oriented psychotherapies has proved most effective.

## *Individual Psychotherapy*

The battered person (usually a woman) who comes to a psychiatrist and already has admitted her critical situation is trying to cope with her feelings of guilt, anxiety, and anger. The psychiatrist can help her express these feelings by having her recount every detail of the battering incidents, emphasizing that she was powerless over the violence. Mastery of her anger by techniques of cognitive therapy and behavior modification can be an important part of the therapy.

Behavioral alternatives to violence, such as time out between the battering adults, should be recommended. It is important that angry pairs avoid each other's physical presence. Anger-control sessions and self-control skills, as well as assertive behavior, should be part of therapy. The couple should be urged to use a set time to solve disputes, a time other than the height of a conflict.

Present alternatives and future goal planning should also be explored in individual therapy. Goals of the therapy should always include strengthening the battered person's independence and self-esteem. Career goals also need to be explored. Action-oriented approaches are useful and, as therapy progresses, adjunctive therapies can be recommended: assertiveness training, vocational counseling, self-help groups, self-awareness education, couple groups, and marital therapy. Role playing is also a helpful technique in teaching the patient how to stop an argument and how to negotiate a conflict; the therapist should help the patient build up her confidence, so as to avoid constant compromise.

Battered partners have to be reassured at all times that they are not at fault and that abuse is a crime. It is helpful to encourage the battered person to recount details of battering incidents. This helps in the process of reality testing. The psychiatrist or other mental health professional can then discuss the battering with the person who has been battered and help her or him interpret behavior and motivational factors involved in the violence. It is helpful to discuss the social context in which domestic violence against women occurs: sexual stereotypes, false beliefs about men's rights in battering, and the social stigma faced by the battered.

It is often helpful for the clinician to refer the patient to hot lines, support groups, safe houses, legal assistance programs, and public assistance, as necessary. The therapist can then help by supporting the patient's choices and by following up to learn the results.

The decision to use tranquilizers and antidepressants is a pragmatic one. Obviously, tranquilizers may be beneficial for anxiety, insomnia, and agitation, but there is a risk of sedation that could impair the battered partner's alertness and readiness to react quickly to danger. The use of antidepressants has proved beneficial to some, but the psychiatrist must recognize that the patient may react to such benefit by minimizing the real and dangerous spousal nightmare as merely a derivative of a treatable depression in herself.

## Group Psychotherapy

Group work has some benefits over individual therapy, particularly in the great sense of support it generally provides for battered women who are usually socially isolated and thus rarely meet other battered women. Effective group therapy is often action oriented, with a focus on changing behaviors. Members often derive a sense of strength from the group, which helps them overcome the immobilization that their terror brings.

Group psychotherapy conducted by a professional leader who is active, available, and involved with all aspects of the patients' lives is seen as most beneficial. A combination of individual and group psychotherapy is often successful.

## Couple Therapy

Couple therapy offers an opportunity both for primary prevention of domestic violence and for intervention (provided safety for the battered person is ensured) following the onset of domestic violence. Regarding prevention, because Steinmetz (1977b) found that male-dominated marital relationships were more frequently associated with domestic violence than were other types of power relationships between couples, it follows that focusing on power balance may prevent spousal assault. An evaluation to determine safety and appropriateness of couple therapy once domestic violence has begun has been suggested by Rosenbaum and O'Leary (1986).

## Parenting Therapy

Because child witnessing of domestic violence is associated with emotional and behavioral sequelae in children, parenting therapies are an important component of the rehabilitation of all members of families with children (Grusznski et al. 1988). Davies (1991) describes a treatment approach appropriate for male toddlers. This intervention helps the parent and child overcome the traumatic experience of witnessing domestic violence through the mother-child bond. Ragg and Webb (1992) present a group method for working with preschool children growing up in violent families. The method consists of safety, clinical, and preventive programming for children of this age group. These groups can help preschoolers deal with their anxieties.

Another option is to combine the different modalities of treatment. Kirschner and Kirschner (1992) used a case study of partner abuse to demonstrate a comprehensive therapy approach. This approach integrates individual, couple, and family therapy.

## Treatment of Violent Partners

Browne (1984) described the importance of arrest and other law enforcement efforts in beginning rehabilitation of violent partners. Saunders and Hanusa (1984) described behavioral treatments that deal with battering partners' problems with anger control and also substance abuse treatments as indicated.

### ▌ The Cycle of Battering Behavior

An assessment of the interpersonal stages of domestic violence is an important part of treatment for violent partners. Walker (1984) described a sequence of interactional events that lead to domestic violence. Although described in terms of battered women, this model is also pertinent for battered men.

#### *Phase 1*

Minor battering incidents occur. The battered partner usually attempts to calm the batterer, using techniques that have been successful in the past. The battered partner believes that she is doing everything to prevent his anger from escalating. However, the batterer interprets his partner's behavior as an acceptance of the abuse and does not bother to control himself. The battered partner is powerless to prevent the behavior from recurring and her psychological humiliation increases.

#### *Phase 2*

The batterer's rage is out of control. Severe injuries occur. The battered partner often senses the incontestability of this phase, cannot tolerate her terror and anxiety, and knows that Phase 3—calm—will follow. Therefore, she provokes the batterer into exploding, "to get it over with." Police are usually called in this phase, but most partners report that acute battering increases after the police leave. Only the batterer can end Phase 2, which may last hours or days.

At the end of this phase, women are relieved that it is over and grateful that it was not worse. They usually do not seek medical care, partly to deny the seriousness of their injuries, and partly to appease the batterer.

## Phase 3

The batterer behaves in a charming and loving manner. He begs for forgiveness and promises never to batter again. The battered woman either believes or wants to believe that he is sincere. She is reinforced for staying in the relationship. The battered woman fantasizes that this is the "good man," the man she married, the man she loved. At this time it is usually very difficult for her to decide to leave him. It is in this phase that the family is usually referred for mental health intervention.

## ▌ Treatment of Family Members in Domestic Violence

### ➤ Case Example

Mrs. C, a 30-year-old Caucasian, was a married, pregnant college graduate who was a homemaker and the mother of a 4-year-old daughter and a 1-year-old son. She presented at the emergency room of a community hospital affiliated with a medical school. Physical examination revealed a lip laceration and bruises on the left cheek and above the left eye, mouth, and nose.

Mrs. C was examined by the emergency room physician, treated for her injuries, and evaluated with a protocol for domestic violence assessment. While completing a specific history for source of injury, Mrs. C disclosed that her husband Mr. C, who was physically abused as a child, beat her often when he drank more than two glasses of Scotch. These beatings had occurred at least once a week for the past 5 years of Mrs. C's 6-year marriage. The beatings began during her first pregnancy.

Mrs. C reported to emergency room personnel that she loved Mr. C and that she was hesitant to speak with the police. She reported that for the past 2 months Mr. C had also begun to hit their 4-year-old daughter Pam when she cried and clung to Mrs. C during Mr. C's beatings of Mrs. C.

A psychiatric consultation was obtained in the emergency room. Mrs. C gave a history of sustained depressed mood, early morning awakening, and thoughts of worthlessness, helplessness, and hopelessness since the beatings had begun 5 years before. She reported that she never saw friends and usually stayed in her house. She also stated that 4 months ago she had attempted to kill herself by ingesting 20 Advil and a 6-pack of beer and was surprised that she had not died. She also reported appetite loss during the previous 4 months and weight loss of 20 pounds without dieting.

Mental status examination revealed a thin, disheveled woman who appeared older than her stated age. Mood was depressed. Psychomotor retardation was noted. There were no hallucinations or delusions. Mrs. C denied any suicidal or homicidal ideation or plan. She expressed fear for her safety and for that of her children. Thoughts revealed low self-esteem and self-blame regarding partner abuse.

## ➤ DSM-IV Diagnosis
### (American Psychiatric Association 1994)

Axis I:     Dysthymic disorder with major depressive episode
Axis II:    None
Axis III:   None
Axis IV:    Severe—partner abuse and child abuse
Axis V:     50

## ➤ Treatment Plan

1.  The Coalition for Domestic Violence, located in the same community as the treating hospital, met Mrs. C in the emergency room and made arrangements for Mrs. C and her children to enter a shelter for abused women. Consultation in child and general psychiatry, internal medicine, and pediatrics is routinely provided for the residents of this shelter by the hospital containing the emergency room.

2.  Legal advocacy referral, which included an Order of Protection process, were initiated for her and her children in the emergency room of the hospital.

3.  A child abuse report was made in the emergency room to the Department of Social Services, naming Mrs. C's husband as a perpetrator of physical child abuse.

4.  Mrs. C accepted a referral to the department of psychiatry of the same hospital for individual and group outpatient psychiatric treatment.

5.  Antidepressant medication was prescribed for her in addition to the psychotherapy, and was continued for six months.

6. Mrs. C's husband was referred by the county probation department for treatment for substance abuse and spousal and child assaultive behavior.

7. After successful alcohol detoxification, regular attendance at Alcoholics Anonymous (AA) meetings, and compliance with partner abuse group therapy, Mr. C began to have brief visits with Mrs. C and his children. Marital and family therapy were also initiated at this time.

### ➤ *Follow-Up*

Mr. C and Mrs. C complied with the above treatment plan for 2 years. At the time of this report, Mr. C was continuing in AA. Mrs. C was no longer depressed, and she and her children had been able to leave the shelter and return to her home and her husband. The family was intact.

## Community Prevention and Intervention by Psychiatrists and Other Mental Health Professionals

The mental health professional is able to play a major role in community prevention and intervention strategies for battered partners and their families (Lystad 1986). It is critical that the professional know the community resources available to the battered partner, to the battering partner, and to the children in the family, and that he or she network with health, social service, and criminal justice providers of care. It is also critical that support be provided for education and training of psychiatrists and other health and mental health specialists in the emotional sequelae of partner abuse.

The mental health professional is not expected, or able, to address all the facets of this social problem. He or she cannot fully address the economic needs of the battered partner, who usually has little job experience, and so may suffer further assault in terms of economic deprivation if her partner declines support. Neither is the mental health professional able to fully address the child care needs of the battered partner, who may become a single parent and the sole support of her children at the same time. But knowledge of available community resources enables the psychiatrist to maximize support for all the family members.

# ▮ Recommendations of the Workshop on Violence and Public Health

In the fall of 1985, the Surgeon General of the United States, C. Everett Koop, sponsored an Invitational Workshop on Violence and Public Health (U.S. Department of Health and Human Services 1986). Partner abuse was among the topics for which recommendations for evaluation, treatment, and prevention were made. These recommendations are set forth here because they are a significant part of the psychiatrist's role.

## *Evaluation and Treatment*

In the areas of evaluation and treatment, recommendations were made for education, research, and services.

In the area of professional education, it was recommended that

➤ Information on interpersonal violence, including partner abuse, be part of the basic education and training curriculum, as well as postgraduate and continuing education, for all health professionals and faculty
➤ Certification, licensing, coordination, and board examinations include questions on interpersonal violence and partner abuse so that health professionals and faculty have at least minimal knowledge of these phenomena
➤ Identification of abused and abusive partners and knowledge of appropriate intervention strategies be part of standards of practice and recommended standards of care for the health disciplines

In the area of research, it was recommended that areas of clinical exploration include

➤ Longitudinal studies of abused partners
➤ Evaluation of models of intervention and prevention in domestic violence
➤ Studies of the relationship between an abusive partner's intake of alcohol and drugs and the frequency, severity, and lethality of his abusiveness
➤ Studies of the ways in which personal and environmental factors interact and escalate domestic violence
➤ Studies of the ways in which psychological assessment tools may

be adapted to measure the psychological impact and posttraumatic stress disorder (PTSD) associated with partner abuse

➤ Studies of the relationship between stress-related disorders and partner abuse

➤ Studies of the long-term effects on health care and social service providers who work in the area of domestic violence

➤ Studies of the long-term impact on children who witness partner (parent) abuse

In the area of services, it was recommended that the first priority for intervention in domestic violence be to provide shelters, safe homes, and other protective environments for abused partners and their children. Domestic violence services include

➤ Innovative treatments that address the specific economic, social, and cultural needs of vulnerable populations

➤ Intervention strategies that hold abusive partners accountable for their violent behavior

➤ Protocols for partner abuse identification and intervention that can be developed and used by health care professionals in emergency rooms, trauma centers, primary care sites, mental health centers, psychiatric hospitals, and physicians' offices

➤ Examination of all existing and proposed topologies to eliminate blaming the abused partner

➤ Secondary treatment sites primarily concerned with alcohol and drug abuse, suicide prevention, rape and sexual assault, emergency psychiatric problems, child abuse, and problems of homelessness

Finally, it was recommended that new programs in education, treatment, and counseling be developed to help stop abusive men from committing further acts of violence.

## Prevention

The workshop participants also made three major recommendations for partner abuse prevention in the areas of education, research, and services:

1. *Education.* National leaders in health care should declare their opposition to partner abuse and develop and distribute appropri-

ate educational materials to the public. It has been found that medical education often does not include a domestic violence focus (Centers for Disease Control 1989).

2. *Research.* Research and demonstration projects should be designed for the prevention of partner abuse; the different dynamics and consequences of abuse for men and for women—and the service implications of these differences— should be identified.

3. *Services.* Health and social service personnel should uniformly define partner abuse as any assault or threat of assault by a social partner, regardless of gender or marital status and regardless of whether or not the partners are present or former cohabitants.

The CDC (1989) have pointed out the importance of targeting high risk populations in order to prevent further violence. Because assaulted partners are at risk for repeated assault, the necessity for therapeutic interventions is apparent. These interventions should include mental health and substance abuse assessments as well as treatments for abused partners, abusive partners, and child witnesses of partner abuse.

Research is needed to further understand etiology and efficacy of interventions. Training for health care providers in assessment and management is also needed. This training must include the development and use of systematic protocols and curricula for health care providers. And finally, public education targeted at youth in elementary and secondary schools that teaches nonviolent conflict resolution was recommended (U.S. Department of Health and Human Services 1986).

---

## Legal Commentary

### ▌ Issues Related to Victims, Other Family Members, and Offenders

Although the term *partner abuse* has at times been used throughout this chapter, legal analysis of the underlying issues more commonly uses the terms *spouse abuse, domestic violence,* or *family violence.* Many of the cases reported to law enforcement agencies concerning the infliction of injury by one adult on another in the home do not, of course, involve legally married persons. Although legal and judicial reforms of recent years have been driven by horrific stories of wife beating and the inadequate governmental response thereto, the scope of the problem of violence in the home is far wider than that. The terms *partner abuse* and *domestic violence* are used herein. These terms are intended to encompass 1) the battering of unmarried as well as married people by their adult cohabitors and past cohabitors, 2) the subjection to violence by another person presently or recently living in the home, whether a blood relation or not (although this would include abuse of an elderly parent and that topic is covered separately elsewhere), and 3) abuse committed by both adult partners of the same sex as well as different sexes.

The appropriate legal response to partner abuse has been studied and debated for many years. Initially, few laws were specifically directed at protection of individuals from abuse by their partners. Indeed, the outrageous "Rule of Thumb," which permitted a husband to beat his wife with a rod no thicker than his thumb, was enacted in nineteenth-century England as a liberal reform to provide some legal protection to women who traditionally had been considered the property of their husbands and could be beaten at whim. U.S. law and public policy during the past several decades has reflected an increasing consciousness of the scope and severity of this major social problem.

Unlike intrafamilial child abuse and elder abuse, where the primary effective legal responses may be focused on civil judicial protective actions, cases of partner abuse are likely to be adequately and fully addressed only within the criminal justice system. Most legal reform has therefore been aimed at improving the criminal justice process, instituting policies that reflect the serious criminal nature of partner abuse. The goal has been to eliminate the disdainful regard by some members of the criminal justice community (e.g., police, prosecutors, and judges) for the handling of domestic violence, so as to overcome the traditional avoidance and mishandling of these cases. Laws and policies have thus been sought to ensure both that abused partners are protected and that their abusive partners will be handled just as aggressively as if they were strangers.

State legislative reforms have focused on improving the entire community response to domestic violence. New laws and policies have been enacted that 1) define the boundaries of proper police arrest practices (including the concept of mandatory arrest of abusive partners), 2) mandate data collection and reporting, 3) require professional education and training, 4) provide various forms of special assistance to abused partners, 5) authorize the use of civil court orders for protection of abused partners, and 6) increase the penalties for abusing a partner. Some of these law reforms will be found in special state domestic violence legislation, and others will be found throughout the state's statutes.

Assault and battery are crimes, generally categorized as misdemeanors, in every state. However, there is substantial documentation that law enforcement officers have traditionally handled domestic violence complaints as noncriminal disputes in which the parties merely need "calming down" or referrals. This problem has been aggravated by the traditional legal principle that police are prohibited from making misdemeanor arrests without having a warrant, unless the offense was committed in an officer's presence. Over the past 20 years, many states have changed their laws in this area, giving police warrantless arrest powers when they have probable cause to believe that a misdemeanor has been committed, or that a previously granted civil protection or restraining order has been violated.

Many states have enacted mandatory arrest laws, even covering misdemeanor cases of partner abuse, following research that has established the efficacy of arrest as the most appropriate police response to domestic violence cases. These laws have resulted in police more aggressively responding to domestic disturbance calls, more carefully determining the facts of the case so that a proper decision can be made as to whether there is "probable cause" to conclude that partner abuse has occurred, and making more arrests of alleged abusive partners. Experts who have studied the impact of new mandatory arrest policies have found that mandatory arrest is effective in preventing further domestic violence.

Another means of police intervention in these cases is to ensure that the alleged abusive partner cannot simply be released immediately after being taken into custody. Some law enforcement policies permit overnight incarceration or an enforced cooling-off period for those arrested for abusing their partners. Additionally, some states permit pretrial detention for alleged abusive partners deemed to be dangerous. This may include situations where the abuser has violated the terms of an earlier pretrial release or an earlier protection order. In every case in which judges permit the release of an alleged abusive partner, it is advisable for them to condition the release upon the alleged abusive partner having no contact with the abused partner and upon other special requirements that will protect the abused partner and other family members. Furthermore, the abused partner should be notified of any pending release of the abusive partner so that adequate provisions can be made for her safety. Finally, it is important for the court to have the imposed conditions of release monitored.

Two of the most significant reforms of state criminal laws related to domestic violence concern the abrogation of the spousal exemption for marital rape and the creation of special criminal sanctions for acts of partner abuse. Under traditional legal principles, the crime of marital rape did not exist, because partners were presumed to consent to conjugal relations even if they were not living together. Many states, especially if the parties have been living apart or are unmarried cohabitors, have abolished the marital exemptions to sexual assault laws. In the absence of legislative reform on this issue, appellate courts are showing an increased willingness to reject the applicability of the exemption.

In order to give legislative recognition of the seriousness of domestic violence, many states have separated out in their penal codes violent family crimes from offenses committed by strangers. These special statutes also may have sanctions that are specifically geared toward the batterer, such as increasing the degree of the offense or the permissible punishment for repeat offenders. Some state laws give criminal judges broad authority to issue protection orders similar to those available in civil courts. Judicial actions that have become commonplace in partner abuse cases are diversion agreements (avoiding the incarceration of, or establishment of a criminal record for, the batterer) predicated upon a cessation of assaultive behavior or upon the abusive partner's getting treatment, deferred (delaying with a view to potential dismissal of) prosecution, or the reduction of charges based on no further violence and on participation in treatment.

Often these compromises have been thought to be inappropriate, given the severity of the abuse and the dangerousness of the person who has committed the abuse. All actions by criminal court judges in partner abuse cases must ensure that the abusive partner not only is held accountable for his actions, but that he is also ordered to be involved in activities specifically designed to reduce future partner abuse, that he be evaluated for substance abuse, and that—if evidence of substance abuse is found—treatment be required, monitored, and successfully completed.

Traditionally, abused partners have experienced great frustration in seeking, obtaining, and enforcing civil "protection from abuse" or "restraining" orders. As criminal law reforms have progressed, so have concomitant improvements in civil judicial proceedings related to partner abuse. The broader powers of civil courts provide the opportunity for remedies of abuse that might be unavailable in a criminal court. Judges can use their power to issue civil court orders to evict abusive partners from shared residences (in some cases, even if solely owned or leased by the abusive partner—especially if the abused partner is married to the person abusing her or if he has a legal duty to support her children). Judges can also order abusive partners to stay away from the abused partner and other family members. They can order counseling for abusers, order the payment of child support, make child custody awards or restrict visitation, require restitution to the abused partner, and compel the abusive partner to pay the abused partner's legal fees.

Under revised state laws that have evolved over the past 20 years, judges can issue emergency domestic violence protective orders ex parte—that is, with only the complaining partner present at the hearing. Violation of such an order (or any civil protective order) is punishable either as contempt of court, or, in some states, as a separate criminal offense. An emergency protective order usually is valid only for a limited time or until a full hearing with both parties present can be held.

Today most states have civil protection-from-abuse laws specifically targeted at partner abuse situations. However, these laws vary widely in terms of who may petition the court for protection (e.g., current or ex-spouses, present or former cohabitors), the courts that are empowered to issue protective orders, and the types of abusive behavior that can be enjoined. Filing and processing procedures also vary (e.g., some courts make it simpler than others for an abused woman to institute action, including waiving filing fees). Laws vary in terms of the proof necessary to substantiate an abuse allegation, the period during which court orders apply, and the ways in which these orders can be enforced. In the few states that do not have special domestic violence civil protection order laws, abused partners who are married, separated, or divorced can still obtain a hearing through traditional domestic relations court proceedings.

Civil protection orders have been criticized for not being immediately helpful to the abused partners, who find themselves continually harassed, stalked, and even reabused by their partners. They are, some partners have stated, merely "pieces of paper" that police and the abusive partner have felt free to ignore. However, some courts have held that the protective order creates a special relationship between the police and the abused partner. The police therefore may be more likely to feel that they owe an abused partner a special duty of care, because they know that they may be held civilly or criminally liable for failing to enforce a protective order. The leading case on this topic is the federal court decision of *Thurman v. City of Torrington* (1984). Increasingly, federal civil rights claims are being used by attorneys on behalf of battered women against government agencies that fail to respond adequately to abuse complaints, or that fail to enforce court orders of protection.

Some state civil protection laws still have limited enforcement authority, but they are increasingly containing special enforcement provisions that, for example, give the police specific power to arrest the abusive partner if they have probable cause to believe that a protection order has been violated. Even more effective are laws that make violation of the order a separate criminal offense (with judges in many states now able to sentence violators of these orders to jail). However, in 1993 the U.S. Supreme Court held in the case of *U.S. v. Foster* (1993) that a criminal contempt prosecution for a violation of an order of protection could bar later criminal prosecution for the same underlying action. One other problem with protection orders is that they may be, and too often are, inappropriately imposed on both parties, thus negating the clearly unlawful behavior of the batterer.

Another trend in civil laws related to domestic violence is the growing number of states that make the occurrence of abuse prior to divorce or marital separation, or where there has been a prior civil protection order issued, a specific criterion to be considered by the court in making any child custody and visitation orders. Some of these laws further provide that the court 1) develop safety plans designed to protect the child and mother from further harm, particularly in any visitation situations, 2) refrain from using the abused parent's departure from the home against her, and 3) presume that a person committing domestic violence not be given sole custody of a child, or that a joint custody order would not be in the child's best interests. Increasingly, trial and appellate courts are considering partner abuse a key factor in both child custody and child visitation (access) decisions. In 1990, Congress passed legislation, sponsored by Representative

Constance Morella (R-MD), which expressed the "Sense of the Congress" that evidence of partner abuse should create a statutory presumption that it is detrimental to the child to be placed in the custody of an abusive parent (H.R. Con. Res. 172, 101st Cong., 2nd Sess., 1990), and a number of states have adopted such presumptions.

## ▌ Guidance for Mental Health Professionals and Practitioners

It is critical for all mental health professionals and practitioners to know that almost every state has a crime victim compensation program created by statute. Under these laws, abused partners are entitled to receive reimbursement for mental health counseling, as well as for medical costs and lost wages. States annually spend millions of dollars on compensation to abused partners specifically for mental health services.

State programs complying with the federal Victims of Crime Act (42 U.S.C. Sec. 10601 et seq.) receive federal financial support for their compensation programs. Each state sets a maximum dollar benefit for compensation paid to individual abused partners. Generally, any medical insurance (including Medicaid) coverage available to the abused partner must be used before government crime victim compensation programs will cover treatment costs.

Crime compensation programs are operated either by independent government agencies or by worker's compensation systems, attorney general offices, criminal justice agencies, or the courts. To be eligible for government compensation, a person must be 1) the target of a violent crime as defined in the statute, and 2) must report the crime to law enforcement, usually within 72 hours, and file a claim, typically within 1 year of the crime.

Harm or injury to oneself resulting from domestic violence (as well as child physical and sexual abuse, and elder abuse) is generally compensatable, although surprisingly few people who have been assaulted by their partners ever seek the compensation that is available to them. The Victims of Crime Act prohibits states receiving federal support for their compensation programs from denying coverage because of a familial relationship between the person who was abused and the person who committed the abuse.

Most programs either waive or extend the reporting and filing requirements for children, partners, or elderly people who have been abused. In addition, family members of abused children, partners, or elderly people may themselves be entitled to compensation to cover the costs of mental health treatment. For abuse that has occurred over an extended period of time, the time limit for reporting and filing begins at the conclusion of the abuse. To help ensure that children who have been abused receive compensation when needed, some programs have modified their reporting requirement to within 1 year after the abused child reaches the age of majority.

The Victims of Crime Act also provides financial support for state crime victim services programs. These services include programs providing counseling, therapy, and group treatment to people who have been abused or assaulted and their families. In recent years, there has been a special focus on the state level to expand these services to abused partners, as well as to children and elderly people who have been abused.

Another subject that mental health professionals and practitioners need to better understand is expert testimony on the *battered woman syndrome*. Such testimony is now generally accepted within the scientific community and has been receiving an increasingly favorable response from the courts, especially in custody and visitation-related cases (including cases in which a battered woman has been required to flee from a batterer and seek a safe haven elsewhere). This testimony is also typically offered as part of a self-defense theory by an abused partner who has been criminally charged with an act of violence against the abusive partner and needs to convince the jury that she truly believed she had to use violent force to protect herself. The syndrome may also be used offensively by a prosecutor to help explain an abused woman's behavior related to the offense.

Appellate court decisions have been split on the issue of the admissibility of battered woman syndrome testimony in criminal proceedings. Recently there has been increased media attention to the fact that legislators, state governors, and pardon and parole authorities have been reconsidering the sentences and convictions of battered women who killed or severely injured their abusive partners, on the basis of the application of the battered woman syndrome theory.

Privacy and confidentiality concerns related to domestic violence are also evolving rapidly. It is extremely important for those professionals working with abused partners to understand their state's laws concerning the privileged nature of communications made to them by battered women. Given the "duty to warn" principle enunciated in the case discussed in Chapter 1, *Tarasoff v. Regents of the University of California (1974)*, a special relationship may exist between the abused partner and her therapist that may warrant disclosure to law enforcement or child protective authorities. It is possible that the *Tarasoff* doctrine will in future years be further interpreted and extended by the courts to apply to those who work in battered-women's shelters, as well as to others who work with abused and abusive partners. The duty to warn may apply when: 1) a battered woman is about to return to her partner and there is reason to suspect that she, her children, or both she and her children may be placed in great danger, 2) the woman threatens to kill or maim her husband or partner, or 3) the woman is at risk for suicide, but provisions have not been made to protect her from harming herself or others.

States are increasingly enacting special laws to protect the confidentiality of communications made between battered women and domestic violence mental health counselors. These laws may prohibit a counselor from testifying in court proceedings or from disclosing records related to the contacts between the woman and her counselor. The location (i.e., temporary residence) of a battered woman may also be legally privileged information.

Specially designed treatment programs for batterers are becoming more common, and their use as referral programs by civil and criminal courts is more widespread. Because batterers generally refuse voluntary treatment, successful participation of batterers in court-ordered counseling in lieu of a sentence of incarceration may provide a powerful incentive for abusive partners to enter and remain in such programs. Because the long-term behavior patterns or substance abuse addiction problems of some batterers may render them poor candidates for such programs, some courts will refer abusive partners for a special assessment as to their appropriateness for a program prior to making any treatment-related order.

Finally, mental health professionals should be aware that, although court-ordered mediation in family conflict cases has become widespread, partner abuse advocates, domestic relations lawyers, and family court judges increasingly are considering the use of mediation inappropriate when there is clear evidence that partner abuse has occurred (especially when it has been serious, of relatively recent occurrence, or both). In particular, because mental health professionals and practitioners may be involved in mediating family disputes, they should be careful to avoid participating in the development of mediated "agreements not to batter," which offer virtually no protection and which imply that the victim is somehow at fault for her battering. Also, the power imbalance between batterers and battered women renders the voluntary nature of mediation meaningless.

(See Appendix H for legal resources.)

## References

American Medical Association: Diagnostic and Treatment Guidelines on Domestic Violence. Chicago, IL, American Medical Association, 1992

American Psychiatric Association: Diagnostic and Statistical Manual of Mental Disorders, 4th Edition. Washington, DC, American Psychiatric Association, 1994

Babcock JC, Waltz J, Jacobson NS, et al: Power and violence: the relation between communication patterns, power discrepancies, and domestic violence. Special section: couples and couple therapy. J Consult Clin Psychol 61:40–50, 1993

Browne A: Making peace at home: models for ending family violence. Paper presented at the annual meeting of the American Psychological Association, Toronto, Ontario, August 1984

Browne A: When Battered Women Kill. New York, Macmillan/Free Press, 1987

Browne A, Williams KR: Exploring the effects of resource availability and the likelihood of female-perpetrated homicides. Law and Society Review 23:75–94, 1989

Campbell A, Gibbs J (eds): Violent Transactions. New York, Basil Blackwell, 1986

Cascardi M, O'Leary KD: Depressive symptomatology, self esteem, and self blame in battered women. Journal of Family Violence 7:249–259, 1992

Centers for Disease Control: Education about adult domestic violence in United States and Canadian medical schools. MMWR 38:17–19, 1987–1988, 1989

Commonwealth Fund: First Comprehensive National Health Survey of American Women. New York, The Commonwealth Fund, 1993

Davies D: Intervention with male toddlers who have witnessed parental violence. Special Issue (family violence). Families in Society 72:515–524, 1991

Davis L, Carlson B: Observation of spouse abuse: what happens to the children? Journal of Interpersonal Violence 2:278–291, 1987

Dewsbury A: Family violence as seen in general practice. Review of Social Health Journal 95:290–294, 1975

Dutton D, Painter SL: Traumatic bonding: the development of emotional attachments in battered women and other relationships of intermittent abuse. Victimology: An International Journal 6:139–155, 1981

Earls F, Slaby RG, Spirito A, et al: Draft of a position paper. Presented at the Panel on Violence Prevention at the Third National Injury Control Conference, Denver, CO, April 1991

Earls G, Slaby RG, Spirito A, et al: Prevention of violence and injuries due to violence. Position papers from the Third National Injury Control Conference, U.S. Department of Health and Human Services, Public Health Service, Centers for Disease Control. Washington, DC, Government Printing Office, 1992

Ellis D: Male abuse of a married or cohabitating female partner: application of sociologic theory to research findings. Violence Victims 4:235–255, 1989

Else L, Wonderlich SA, Beatty WW, et al: Personality characteristics of men who physically abuse women. Hosp Community Psychiatry 44:54–58, 1993

Fagan J, Wexler S: Crime at home and in the streets: the relationship between family and stranger violence. Violence Victims 2:5–23, 1987

Finkelhor D, Yllo K: Rape in marriage: a sociological view, in The Dark Side of Families. Edited by Finkelhor D, Gelles R, Hotaling G, et al. Beverly Hills, CA, Sage, 1983

Gaquin DA: Spouse abuse: data from the National Crime Survey. Victimology: An International Journal 2:632–643, 1978

Gayford J: Wife battering: a preliminary survey of 100 cases. BMJ 1: 195–197, 1975

Gelles R: The Violent Home. Beverly Hills, CA, Sage, 1974

Gelles R: Family Violence. Beverly Hills, CA, Sage, 1979

Gelles RJ, Straus MA: Intimate Violence: The Definitive Study of the Causes and Consequences of Abuse in the American Family. New York, Simon & Schuster, 1988

Giles-Sims J: Wife Beating: A Systems Theory Approach. New York, Guilford, 1983

Giles-Sims J: Family relations. Journal of Applied Family and Child Studies 34:205–210, 1985

Grusznski RJ, Brink JC, Edleson JL: Support and education groups for children of battered women. Child Welfare 67:431–444, 1988

Hershorn M, Rosenbaum A: Children of marital violence: a closer look at the unintended victims. Am J Orthopsychiatry 55:260–266, 1985

Hilberman E: Overview: the "wife-beater's wife" reconsidered. Am J Psychiatry 137:1336–1347, 1980

Hilberman E, Munson M: Sixty battered women. Victimology: An International Journal 2:460–471, 1977–1978

Hotaling GT, Sugarman DB: An analysis of risk makers in husband to wife violence: the current state of knowledge. Victims and Violence 1:101–124, 1986

Hughes H: Psychological and behavioral correlates of family violence in child witnesses and victims. Am J Orthopsychiatry 58:77–90, 1988

Jaffe P, Wolfe D, Wilson S: Children of Battered Women. Newbury Park, CA, Sage, 1990

Jaffe P, Wolfe D, Wilson S, et al: Family violence and child adjustment: a comparative analysis of girls'and boys' behavior symptoms. Am J Psychiatry 143:74–77, 1986

Jouriles E, Barling J, O'Leary K: Predicting child behavior problems in maritally violent families. Journal of Abnormal and Social Psychology 15:165–173, 1987

Kaplan S, Pelcovitz D, Salzinger S, et al: Psychopathology of nonviolent women in violent families, in The Child in His Family. Edited by Anthony EJ, Chiland C. New York, Wiley, 1988

Kirschner DA, Kirschner S: Comprehensive family therapy in the treatment of spouse abuse. Special issue: Psychotherapy in independent practice: current issues for clinicians. Psychotherapy in Private Practice 10:67–76, 1992

Kratcoski P: Youth violence directed towards significant others. Journal of Adolescence 8:145–157, 1985

Ladoucer P, Temple M: Substance abuse among rapists. Crime and Delinquency 31:269–294, 1985

Lerman L: Prosecution of Spouse Abuse: Innovations in Criminal Justice Response. Washington, DC, Center for Women Policy Studies, 1981

Letellier P: Identifying and treating battered gay men. San Francisco Med 67:16–19, 1994

Lie G, Gentlewarrior S: Intimate violence in lesbian relationships: discussion of survey findings and practice implications. Journal of Social Service Research 15:41–59, 1991

Lobel K: Naming the Violence: Speaking Out About Lesbian Battering, 2nd Edition (National Coalition Against Domestic Violence publication). Seattle, WA, Seal Press, 1986

Lystad M: Interdisciplinary perspectives on family violence: an overview, in Violence in the Home: Interdisciplinary Perspectives. Edited by Lystad M. New York, Brunner/Mazel, 1986

Makepeace JM: Life events, stress, and courtship violence. Journal of Applied Family and Child Studies 32:101–109, 1983

Malmquist C: Children who witness violence: tortuous aspects. Bull Am Acad Psychiatry Law 13:221–231, 1985

McLeer SV, Anwar R: The role of the emergency room physician in the prevention of domestic violence. Annals of Emergency Medicine 16:1155–1161, 1987

Mercy JA, Saltzman LE: Fatal violence among spouses in the United States, 1976–85. Am J Public Health 79:595–599, 1989

Myers K, Burkey P, McCauley E: Suicidal behavior by hospitalized preadolescent children on a psychiatric unit. J Am Acad Child Psychiatry 24:474–480, 1985

Nadelson C, Sauzier M: Intervention programs for individual victims and their families, in Violence in the Home: Interdisciplinary Perspectives. Edited by Lystad M. New York, Brunner/Mazel, 1986

Ochberg F: Victims of terrorism. J Clin Psychiatry 41:73–74, 1980

Pagelow MD: Does the Law Help Battered Wives? Some Research Notes. Madison, WI, Law and Society Association, 1980

Pfeffer C: Self-destructive behavior in children and adolescents. Psychiatr Clin North Am 8:215–226, 1985

President's Commission on Mental Health, Report of the Subpanel on Women's Mental Health, Volume 3 (Appendix). Washington, DC, U.S. Government Printing Office, 1978

Ragg DM, Webb C: Group treatment for the preschool child witness of spouse abuse. Journal of Child and Youth Care 7:1–19, 1992

Renzetti CM: Violence in lesbian relationships: a preliminary analysis of causal factors. Journal of Interpersonal Violence 3:381–399, 1988

Roscoe B, Benaske N: Courtship violence experienced by abused wives: similarities in patterns of abuse. Journal of Applied Family and Child Studies 34:419–424, 1985

Rosenbaum A, O'Leary KD: Treatment of marital violence, in Clinical Handbook of Marital Therapy. Edited by Jacobson NS, Gurman AS. New York, Guilford, 1986, pp 385–406

Russell D: The prevalence and impact of marital rape in San Francisco. Paper presented at the annual meeting of the American Sociological Association, 1980

Russell DEH: The prevalence and incidence of forcible rape and attempted rape of females. Victimology: An International Journal 7:81–93, 1982

Saltzman L: Battering during pregnancy: a role for physicians. Atlanta Medicine 64: 1990

Salzinger S, Samit C, Krieger R, et al: A controlled study of the life events of mothers of maltreated children in suburban families. J Am Acad Child Psychiatry 25:419–426, 1986

Salzinger S, Feldman RS, Hammer M, et al: Constellations of family violence and their differential effects on children's behavioral disturbance. Child and Family Behavior Therapy 12:23–41, 1992

Saunders DG, Hanusa DR: Cognitive-behavioral treatment of abusive husbands: the short term effects of group therapy. Paper presented at the Second National Conference for Family Violence Researchers, Durham, NH, August 1984

Schecter S: Women and Male Violence. Boston, MA, South End, 1982

Scott P: Battered wives. Br J Psychiatry 125:433–441, 1974

Seligman M: Helplessness: On Depression, Development and Death. San Francisco, CA, W.H. Freeman & Company, 1975

Shield N, McCall GJ, Hannecke RR: Patterns of family and non-family violence: violent husbands and violent men. Violence Victims 3:83–98, 1988

Slade M, Daniel LJ, Hoisler CJ: Application of forensic toxicology to the problem of domestic violence. J Forensic Sci 36:708–713, 1991

Snell JE, Rosenwald J, Robey A: The wife-beater's wife. Arch Gen Psychiatry 11:107–112, 1964

Stall R, McCusick L, Wiley J, et al: Alcohol and drug use behavior during sexual activity and compliance with safe sex guidelines for AIDS: the AIDS behavioral research project. Health Education Quarterly 13:359–371, 1986

Stark ED, Flitcraft A: Wife abuse in the medical setting: an introduction for health personnel, monograph #7. Washington, DC, Office of Domestic Violence, 1981

Steinmetz S: Wifebeating-husbandbeating—a comparison of the use of physical violence between spouses to resolve marital fights, in Women: A Psychosociological Study of Domestic Violence. Edited by Ray MM. New York, Van Nostrand Reinhold, 1977b

Steinmetz S et al: The violent family, in Violence in the Home: Interdisciplinary Perspectives. Edited by Lystad M. New York, Brunner/Mazel, 1986

Straus M: Wife-beating: how common, and why? Victimology: An International Journal 2:443–458, 1977

Straus M, Gelles R: Societal change and change in family violence from 1975 to 1985 as revealed by two national surveys. Journal of Marriage and the Family 48:465–479, 1986

Straus MA, Gelles RJ: Physical Violence in American Families: Risk Factors and Adaptations to Violence in 8,145 Families. New Brunswick, NJ, Transaction Publishers, 1990

Straus M, Gelles R, Steinmetz S: Behind Closed Doors: Violence in the American Family. Garden City, NY, Doubleday/Anchor Press, 1980

Symonds M: The psychodynamics of violence-prone marriages. Am J Psychiatry 38:213–222, 1978

Tarasoff v Regents of the University of California, 118 Cal Rptr 129, 529 P2d 553 (1974)

U.S. v Foster, 113 S., Ct. 2849 (1993)

U.S. Department of Health and Human Services: Surgeon General's Workshop on Violence and Public Health: A Report. Washington, DC, U.S. Government Printing Office, 1986

U.S. Department of Justice: Female Victims of Violent Crime (No NCJ-126826). Washington, DC, U.S. Department of Justice, 1991

Walker L: The Battered Woman. New York, Harper & Row, 1979

Walker L: The Battered Woman Syndrome. New York, Springer, 1984

Walker L: Battered women and learned helplessness. Victimology: An International Journal 2:525–534, 1977–1978

Walker L: Psychological causes of family violence, in Violence in the Home: Interdisciplinary Perspectives. Edited by Lystad M. New York, Brunner/Mazel, 1986

Wolfe D, Jaffe P, Wilson S, et al: Children of battered women: the relation of child behavior to family violence and maternal stress. J Consult Clin Psychol 53:657–665, 1985

Zahn MA: Homicide in the 20th century: trends, types and causes, in Violence in America. Vol. 1: History of Violence. Edited by Gurr TR. Newbury Park, CA, Sage, 1989

# CHAPTER 6

## Elder Maltreatment

*Marion Zucker Goldstein, M.D.*

---

### Issues in Studying Maltreatment of Elderly Persons

Vague definitions, lack of random sample surveys, lack of case comparison studies, and reliance on individual professional reports have made the epidemiology of elder abuse, neglect, and exploitation a subject of much speculation over the past two decades. It is the most recent type of maltreatment to come to public attention. With increasing awareness of what was once termed a hidden problem, the consensus now is that well over one million older Americans are physically, financially and emotionally abused by persons they live with in other than institutional settings (Subcommittee on Health and Long-Term Care 1990). In this chapter, the focus is on the abuse that occurs in family settings, not in institutional settings. We must be aware that this leaves out the relatively large number of elderly women who live alone or in institutional settings.

In addition to the need for clarification of definitions, the following issues need to be considered in studies of prevalence of elder maltreatment, abuse, neglect, and exploitation. First, although the group of elderly individuals living with adult children has been of special interest to researchers, only 10% of persons age 65 and older reside with their adult children. Second, whereas older persons who live with others are at higher risk for abuse, those living alone are more likely to be objects of neglect (H. O'Malley, H. Segars, R. Perez, V. Mitchell,

**181**

and G. Krumppel, "Elder Abuse in Massachusetts: A Survey of Professionals and Paraprofessionals," unpublished manuscript, Legal Research and Services for the Elderly, Boston, 1979; Wolf et al. 1984, 1986). Third, considerably more elderly women than elderly men live alone, because more elderly men have a living spouse and because a higher proportion of widowed men than women live with their children. Therefore, studies of spouse abuse in the elderly population include a disproportionately larger number of men than women as abusers. Finally, interviews with abusers revealed that abusers were more willing to admit to abuse than were those abused (Finkelhor and Pillemer 1984; Straus and Gelles 1986). Those abused often fear placement in unfamiliar surroundings and greater abandonment than they have already been subjected to, and they are often fearful even for their lives.

Although a systematic assessment of care needed by elderly persons is essential, it must be remembered that the need to establish a trusting relationship with their caregivers, as well as an assessment of the limitations and stresses experienced by these caregivers, is equally essential. Speaking only of "victims" and "abusers" does not do justice to the situation. Interviews with victims are more likely to be limited by the incapacities of elderly persons and often need to be supplemented with collateral information. Elderly persons with severe physical or mental impairments may be at particular risk for abuse, neglect, and exploitation. It is well known that community resources for impaired elderly persons and their caregivers are extremely limited in many communities. As a nation and as a society, we are only in the process of preparing for the graying of America, although it is already upon us. In this process, we are learning to deal with crisis—to respond only to "screams of anguish," not to the first whimper of distress (Norman 1982, p. 16)—while prevention of the excessive burden and stress of caregiving lags far behind. Hence we use judgmental words, such as *abuse, neglect,* and *exploitation,* and we work at definitions of terms so we can communicate with each other when we speak or write about the maltreatment of a person of advanced years who is unable to protect and care for himself or herself independently.

In this chapter, the focus is specifically on the role of the psychiatrist and other mental health care providers in the assessment, prevention, intervention, and follow-up of elderly individuals and their caregivers as it relates to situations of maltreatment.

Elder abuse, adolescent abuse, child abuse, sexual abuse, and spouse abuse have many of the same risk factors. As mentioned, in elder-abusing families, women are more often the targets of assault. Substance abuse is also often present in all types of violent families. There is often a victim-perpetrator power imbalance, with the victim dependent on the perpetrator as a result of age or illness (Wolf et al. 1984). Depression is frequently present in these families (Carmen et al. 1984), as well as social isolation (Anetzberger 1987; Salzinger et al. 1983), and there is often a lack of empathy and of strategies for nonviolent conflict resolution (Pagelow and Pagelow 1984).

## Epidemiology

A random-sample survey of 2,000 persons in the Boston metropolitan area revealed a prevalence rate of 32/1,000 maltreated elderly persons and an incidence of 26/1,000 (Pillemer and Finkelhor 1988). Nearly three-fifths of the perpetrators were spouses, one-fifth were adult children—among whom were twice as many sons as daughters—and one-fifth were others, such as grandchildren, siblings, and boarders. The rates in this study translate to the maltreatment of about one million elderly people in the United States. The reported incidence rate in Massachusetts during that year, however, was 1.8/1,000, indicating that only 1 case in 14 had come to public attention. The National Center on Elder Abuse and Neglect (1995) estimated that 18,000 elders became victims of elder abuse during 1994. We know from experience that only some of the most extreme cases come to public attention (Subcommittee on Health and Long-Term Care 1990).

In 1978 the Subcommittee on Health and Long-Term Care of the Select Committee on Aging of the U.S. House of Representatives received a letter describing how an 80-year-old paraplegic woman had been sexually abused by her son-in-law, who threatened her with a hammer every time she refused his advances. This letter prompted the committee, under the leadership of the late Senator Claude Pepper (D-FL), to undertake the first congressional examination of elder abuse in the United States (Subcommittee on Health and Long-Term Care 1990). A 1981 report validated this committee's estimate that more than one million elderly Americans are physically, financially, and emotionally abused within family settings.

## History of Recognition of Maltreatment of Elderly Persons and Government Economics

"Granny battering" (Burston 1975) and "the battered old person syndrome" (Butler 1975) were terms coined in the mid-1970s, in Great Britain and the United States respectively, to describe the clinical condition of maltreatment of elderly people. In the United States, states began passing legislation dealing with elder abuse in the early 1970s, and more prominent national attention was drawn to the issue of the battering of parents in the late 1970s. The Pepper committee reviewed the history of domestic violence in America. Committee members learned that congressional assistance to states and state agencies designated to receive complaints about, identify, and treat child abuse had led to improvements in prevention and treatment in this area. States were encouraged by the possibility of financial assistance. Protective service laws regarding elder abuse, with mandatory reporting provisions, increased rapidly during the 1980s. There are now elder abuse laws in all 50 states. Some of these laws require physicians specifically to file a report; other laws use the terms "anyone" or "health care provider." The ethics of these reporting mandates are currently being debated in regard to breach of doctor-patient confidentiality and assessment of ability to consent to reporting or consent to interventions. Terms continue to be redefined to improve clarity. That physical abuse has psychological consequences is often overlooked, and psychological abuse tends to be listed as a separate entity. There is still a wide disparity in opportunities for prevention, assessment of the occurrence of maltreatment, and comprehensive intervention to sustain an optimal quality of life for a dependent elderly individual and a caregiver who is unable to cope without becoming abusive.

Under Chairman E. R. Roybal, the Subcommittee on Health and Long-Term Care of the Select Committee on Aging started major inquiries to determine the adequacy of federal and state efforts on behalf of issues involving elder abuse. This committee concluded that there was an increase of 1%, or 500,000 abuse cases, annually during the 1980s. They also observed that elder abuse was far less likely to be reported than child abuse (1 of 3 child abuse cases, compared with 1 of 8 elder abuse cases), and that the number of unreported cases had been increasing over the past decade. Seventy percent of adult abuse cases reported annually involve persons age 60 and over. In spite of the impressive increase of state reporting statutes and adult protective services laws during the last decade, the relative lack of financial incentives to the states analogous to child abuse funding hampers states in channeling monies into the newly designated social services for the elderly population. On the average, each state spends about $45.00 per child resident for protective services for abused children, but only $3.80 per elderly resident for protective services for abused elderly persons. In addition, although the incidence of elder abuse is increasing annually, the percentage of state budgets allotted for adult protective services declined from 6.6% in 1981 to 4.0% in 1989.

This economic aspect cannot be overlooked when we prepare guidelines for psychiatrists on optimal approaches to an elder abuse situation, once detected. Availability and expertise from members of multidisciplinary teams are needed for appropriate ongoing interventions. Detection and assessment of, and intervention in, a malfunctioning elderly person-caregiver dyad that culminates in maltreatment of an elderly person can only rarely be dealt with effectively by a psychiatrist in an office setting. The balance of the assessment of both the victim and the perpetrator of the abuse must be fine-tuned, and care must be made available for each one in a nonpunitive, therapeutic manner. In instances when blatant, malicious intent and criminal behavior have been determined, punitive measures are appropriate to ensure behavioral changes in the abuse perpetrator and protection of the victim. Financial resources for suitable staffing to implement interventions need to be available. There must be appropriate reimbursement for the time the psychiatrist spends with the elderly persons and their caregivers, and there must be legal, financial, and other community resources.

## Case Histories and Etiologies of Abusive Behaviors

Case histories of elder abuse are remarkably sparse in psychiatric literature (Goldstein and Woods 1993; Woods and Goldstein 1994). More extensive examples can be found in legislative literature and nursing and social work journals (see Bibliography at the end of the chapter). The Subcommittee on Health and Long-Term Care of the Select Committee on Aging (1990) received numerous case examples from state officials who responded to an elder abuse questionnaire in 1989. In addition, the subcommittee issued an invitation to participants at the annual meeting of the National Association of Social Workers to submit summaries of elder abuse cases with which they were familiar. The result was more than 60 case vignettes demonstrating physical abuse and neglect, financial abuse, psychological abuse, self-neglect, sexual abuse, and violation of rights (Subcommittee on Health and Long-Term Care 1990).

The Subcommittee on Health and Long-Term Care (1990) also speculated on the etiology of the behaviors described:

> The abuser may lack community resources to assist him or her in their caregiving role; if mistreated as a child, the abuser may view abuse of the parents as a means of retaliation or revenge; sometimes, after parent and child have been separated emotionally or geographically for lengthy periods, the elderly parent's return is viewed as an intrusion; for certain families violence is the normative response to stress and is a tradition carried from generation to generation; many middle aged family members, finally ready to enjoy time to themselves, are resentful of a frail, dependent elderly parent; increased life expectancy is another factor leading to increased incidences of elderly abuse since the dependency period of old age has been extended; and there are certain environmental conditions which can precipitate stress, which may then lead to abuse or neglectful behavior—quality of housing, unemployment, alcohol and drug abuse and crowded living conditions can by themselves or in combinations with other factors encourage maltreatment of a dependent elderly person. (p. 13)

Review of the case histories reveals that a number of adult children, as a result of mental retardation or other deficits for which they required lifelong parental attention, are now overwhelmed by the dependency of their elderly parent.

In the professional community it is generally felt that sound scientific methodology needs to be applied to find out the true etiologies of elder abuse in order to determine risk factors and interventions.

## Research Status

Case vignettes and exploratory descriptive surveys have become numerous and have convinced the public, professionals, providers of care, and policymakers of the realities of elder abuse (Blunt 1993; Ramsey-Klawsnik 1993; Wolf 1988). Research studies of abused elderly persons (with or without control groups) and of abusive caregivers and nonabusive caregivers (Coyne et al. 1993; Paveza et al. 1992; Pillemer and Finkelhor 1988; Pillemer and Suitor 1992; Saverman et al. 1993) have come to the following conclusions:

1. Violence against elderly people is more likely to occur if men are the caregivers, particularly if the male caregiver has a history of mental health problems and if there is evidence of recent deterioration.
2. The abused or neglected older people themselves are more likely to have emotional and cognitive difficulties and recent deterioration.
3. Although one abused group was similar in physical impairments to a nonabused group, a recent increase in functional dependency was found in the abused group.
4. Unrealistic expectations by caregivers of elderly persons contribute to abuse.
5. Continuation and/or new occurrences of interpersonal problems, with provocative behaviors on the part of elderly persons, contribute to abuse.
6. Changes in living situations, such as having to share a residence for financial reasons, as well as social isolation of the elderly person-caregiver unit, contribute to abuse.
7. Length of time of caregiving and severity of dementia of dependent elderly persons are risk factors for abuse.
8. Depression and stress in caregivers contribute to abuse.

The question of whether there is a higher incidence of parent abuse by children who have been abused by their parents, though a likely hypothesis, has not yet been researched. The fact that a recent change in the physical, mental, or environmental situations of elderly persons and/or the domestic caregiver contributes to abuse alerts us to an area that has a potential for preventive psychiatric interventions.

Terms such as *family violence* and *elder abuse* are ambiguous, at best, and lead to many interpretations. Definitions of terms vary in the legal, clinical, and scientific arenas, and they need to be given careful attention.

# Definitions of Terms

The title of this book begins with the term *family violence,* which makes us think of episodic actions of physical aggression. In practice, nurses report that they encounter continuous neglect of elderly patients that varies in severity but is usually not immediately life threatening (Hudson and Johnson 1986). Because elder abuse laws in many states are based on child abuse laws, clinical practice in cases of maltreatment of elderly persons does not match definitions used by legislators and the legal system. A multidimensional assessment protocol that includes the dependency status of elderly individuals needs to be an integral part of definitions of abuse and neglect as well as of any decision-making process on behalf of an elderly person. The Elder Abuse, Prevention, Identification and Treatment Act (1985), introduced by the late Senator Claude Pepper, defines abuse, exploitation, neglect, and physical harm as follows: "The term *abuse* means the willful infliction of injury, unreasonable confinement, intimidation or cruel punishment with resulting physical harm or pain or mental anguish; or the willful deprivation by a caretaker of goods or services which are necessary to avoid harm, mental anguish or mental illness." The term *exploitation* means "the illegal or improper act or process of a caretaker using the resources of an elder for monetary or personal benefit, profit or gain." The term *neglect* means "the failure to provide . . . the goods or services which are necessary to avoid physical harm, mental anguish or mental illness or the failure of a caregiver to provide such goods or services." The term *physical harm* means "bodily pain, injury, impairment or disease" (Elder Abuse, Prevention, Identification and Treatment Act 1985). This act was modeled after the child abuse act of 1974.

Various assessment instruments have been designed. Clinically, one example of an Elder Assessment Instrument (EAI), developed at Beth Israel Hospital (1986), Boston, covers mandated reporting categories: physical abuse, neglect, mental anguish, and exploitation (Fulmer and Welte 1986). A variety of definitions have been developed for research purposes and tend to precede each study and vary in specificity. For example, in Godkin et al. (1989, p. 211) the reporting category of abuse is classified into physical, psychological, and material abuse. *Physical* is the infliction of physical pain or injury, physical coercion, or confinement against one's will (e.g., being slapped, bruised, sexually molested, cut, burned, physically restrained). *Psychological* is the infliction of mental anguish (e.g., being called names, treated like a child, frightened, humiliated, intimidated, threatened, isolated). *Material* is the illegal or improper exploitation and/or use of funds or other resources (Godkin et al. 1989, p. 211).

The reporting category of neglect is classified into active and passive neglect. *Active* neglect is the refusal or failure to fulfill a caretaking obligation, including a conscious and intentional attempt to inflict physical or emotional distress on an elderly person (e.g., deliberate abandonment or deliberate denial of food or health-related services). *Passive* neglect is the refusal or failure to fulfill a caretaking obligation, in the absence of a conscious and intentional attempt to inflict physical or emotional distress on the elderly person (e.g., abandonment or denial of food or health-related services because of inadequate knowledge, laziness, infirmity, or disputing the value of prescribed services) (Godkin et al. 1989, p. 211). These researchers included being treated like a child under psychological abuse, and they fine-tuned the definition of neglect by not only separating active and passive neglect but also identifying features of the mental status of the caregiver.

The American Medical Association (1985), Department of State Legislation, provided guidelines for physicians in the form of a model bill known as the Elderly Abuse Reporting Act. The model bill reads as follows: "Abuse shall mean an act or omission which results in harm or threatened harm to the health or welfare of an elderly person. Abuse includes intentional infliction of physical or mental injury, sexual abuse or withholding of necessary food, clothing and medical care to treat the physical and mental health needs of an elderly person by one having the care, custody or responsibility of an elderly person." Subsequently the Council on Scientific Affairs of the American Medical Association summarized elderly abuse of the following types: abuse (physical, psychological, sexual), exploitation (financial, material), neglect (active, or physical; passive, or psychological), self-neglect, violation of rights (Council on Scientific Affairs 1987).

A considerably more refined classification for physicians was generated by the Washington State Medical Association (1985). The lists that follow are a combination of clinical manifestations that can be observed in elderly people and behaviors that may be observed in, or asked about, the caregiver.

Manifestations of physical (including sexual) abuse are as follows:

- Bruises
- Welts
- Lacerations
- Punctures
- Fractures
- Evidence of excessive drugging
- Burns
- Signs of physical restraints
- Malnutrition
- Dehydration
- Lack of personal care
- Signs of inadequate heating
- Lack of food and water
- Unclean clothes and bedding
- Lack of needed medication
- Lack of eyeglasses, hearing aids, and false teeth
- Difficulty walking or sitting
- Venereal disease
- Pain or itching
- Bruises or bleeding of external genitalia, vaginal area, or anal area

Manifestations of psychological abuse in the abused person are as follows:

- Resignation
- Fear
- Depression
- Confusion
- Anger
- Ambivalence
- Insomnia

Behaviors indicating psychological abuse by the abuser(s) include the following:

- Threats
- Insults
- Harassment
- Withholding security
- Harsh orders

➤ Refusal on the part of those caring for the elderly person to allow travel, visits by friends or other family members, or attendance at religious observances

Exploitation is considered to be the misuse of a vulnerable adult's income or other financial resources. The exploited elderly person, if capable, is the best source of information, but in most cases money management has been handed over to another person, and as a result there may be some confusion about finances. Information on dealing with financial documents and the elder abuse statutes of each state have evolved into a subspecialty of elder law in the legal profession (Blunt 1993).

Medical abuse is considered to be the withholding or improper administration of medications or necessary medical treatments for a condition or the withholding of aids the person would medically require, such as false teeth, glasses, or a hearing aid. Evidence of such medical abuse may be

➤ Confusion
➤ Disorientation
➤ Memory impairment
➤ Agitation
➤ Lethargy
➤ Self-neglect

Neglectful behaviors that result in deprivation by self or others of care necessary to maintain physical and mental health may be manifested by malnutrition, poor personal hygiene, and any of the indicators above of medical abuse (Washington State Medical Association 1985).

Legislators, researchers, and providers of services in various disciplines have contributed to defining elder maltreatment. As the field of geriatric psychiatry assumes greater prominence as a specialty with an ever broadening knowledge base, and as more general psychiatrists are treating elderly patients, the issues of elder maltreatment are becoming of concern to the psychiatric community. Psychiatrists and psychiatric training programs can have a unique and seminal role in the prevention, detection, assessment, treatment, and advocacy of issues concerning elder maltreatment.

# Role of the Psychiatrist

Psychiatrists, and especially geriatric psychiatrists, as well as other mental health professionals, can make considerable contributions to assessment, prevention, and intervention in conflictual situations in the elderly person-caregiver dyad as well as in gaining access to family and community resources. The fact is that the relationships between elderly people and caregivers often have a past of many years' duration. A variety of patterns of mutual exchange and power balance or imbalance have occurred during this past. Definitions—especially interview techniques and more formal assessment scales—should therefore include elements of the past, as well as changes and the current nature of these relationships. Although legal and medical definitions of elder maltreatment provide guidelines for clinicians, they are—because of their focus on intentionality, concrete outcome, and blame—limiting in nature. A focus on blame and punishment stands in the way of unbiased assessment and optimal treatment. A broader clinical conceptualization than has so far been available to physicians is needed to provide effective guidelines for prevention and intervention.

The evaluation of the elderly patient goes beyond what has traditionally been taught in psychiatric residency training programs and in the training programs of other mental health professionals. Evaluation of the elderly patient (Goldstein 1990) and integration of family assessment (Goldstein 1991) are becoming essential to the psychiatrist's diagnosis and treatment armamentarium. The following are guidelines for special focus on awareness of situations in which maltreatment of elderly people is likely to occur or is taking place.

Psychiatric evaluation of elderly people should be preceded by or—minimally—followed immediately by an extensive and comprehensive physical and neurological examination. A list of the doses and frequencies of all current and recent medications should be available at the time of the psychiatric evaluation. An adequate workup requires the completion of all laboratory tests, X rays, and other imaging techniques indicated by current physical and neurological findings.

The psychiatric evaluation needs to include a comprehensive assessment of cognition, affect and function, organic deficits, and thought content. An evaluation of communication and sensory deficits, mobility impairments, continence, and eating problems gives an overview of the level of care required.

With such a detailed, reality-based assessment, the psychiatrist is prepared to prevent and/or alleviate the emotional abuse that inadvertently occurs when a caregiver has unrealistic expectations of an elderly person. Such expectations can be based on his/her past performance and abilities and on a caregiver's inattention to or denial of actual changes that have occurred. Personal needs of the caregiver that the elderly person can no longer fulfill also contribute to misperceptions of capacity.

The literature referred to previously reveals that abusive situations frequently occur following recent changes that neither the elderly person nor the caregiver has had time to adapt to or understand. It is incumbent on the psychiatrist to use all of his or her interviewing skills to evaluate the elderly patient and the caregiver, both individually and together. A mental status as well as a needs assessment of the elderly patient and of the caregiver(s) must be carried out. Nurses, social workers, and psychologists, who constitute the multidisciplinary team, should be integrally involved in assessment and treatment. A nurse-practitioner or a physician's assistant is a highly desirable member of such a team. Role definition of each member of the team is an ongoing process. The team member's role depends on expertise, skill, initiative, and motivation to render optimal quality and continuity of care. Efforts of team members should complement, not duplicate, each other and should contribute in a well-defined manner to the outcome of services rendered.

Assessment can take place, at least in part, with standardized scales such as the Mini-Mental State examination (Folstein et al. 1975), the Hachinski scale to rule out multi-infarct dementia (Hachinski et al. 1975), and depression scales such as the Geriatric Depression Scale (Yesavage 1986) or the Hamilton Rating Scale for Depression (Hamilton 1960). For functional capacity, a scale such as the Older Americans Resources and Services (OARS) questionnaire (Duke University 1978) or others can be administered as part of the assessment. The CAMDEX (Roth et al. 1986) is a comprehensive instrument taking about 75 minutes that incorporates the information from the caregiver with assessment of dementia and depression.

Psychiatrists need to remain abreast of forensic issues as well as community resources and have knowledge of the state laws on abuse of elderly persons. This knowledge includes the legal base to investigate and gain access to premises, the level of immunity from prosecution for good-faith reporting, and penalties for not reporting. The psychiatrist is the one to assess whether the law diminishes self-determination because it is based on child abuse laws. (See Thobaben and Anderson 1985 for state laws.) The financial and living situations of elderly individuals and their caregivers need to be assessed in order to make reality-based recommendations for interventions. Not only does the psychiatrist need to be aware of the financial situation of a maltreated elderly person and his or her caregiver, but he or she must also know the financial resources in the community for protective services. He or she must also keep abreast of Medicare reimbursements for the complex, comprehensive initial evaluation, as well as for the follow-up needed to implement and supervise recommended interventions. Advocacy for services for maltreated elderly persons and their caregivers must go hand in hand with advocacy for appropriate reimbursement for such services.

It is the psychiatrist who has the medical training to make a medical assessment (e.g., etiology and diagnosis of "confusion") as well as to put information obtained into a developmental perspective. Personal and interpersonal conflicts that originate from lack of adaptation to role reversals (occurring when a provider, nurturing parent, or partner declines into a state of relative dependency) are also within the domain of psychiatric diagnosis and treatment.

Maladaptive feelings, which can lead to maladaptive behaviors such as abuse, neglect, and exploitation, can, it is hoped, be addressed and worked through when elicited in a timely fashion.

## ➤ Case Example

When psychotherapy is needed for the caregiver, who pays the bill? An 87-year-old white widower was referred to the psychiatrist by a neurologist to help the daughter deal with the father's hallucinations and delusions. Nonpharmacological intervention was recommended because of the patient's orthostatic hypotensive episodes. The father was tied in a wheelchair, his head was tilted to one side, and he was bent forward. He drooled on occasion. Responses were coherent but extremely slow, and at times he did not respond at all. During the interview, evidence of hallucinations or delusions was not apparent and could not be elicited. He was unable to participate in the Mini-Mental State Examination. He reported that he ate and slept well. He had been widowed 9 years previously and had worked as an electrician and mail carrier. He was the father of two adult children. He expressed fondness for his daughter.

The daughter, who brought him to the interview, was accompanied by a male aide who looked after the father's personal needs 4 days a week. A married son lived out of town and came to visit several times a year. During the son's occasional visits, the daughter was relieved and handed care of the father over to her brother temporarily. After an assessment of the father, the daughter was seen individually. The HMO with whom the patient had her medical insurance required a referral from the "gatekeeper physician" to a specialist. Because the referral had not been arranged before, this psychiatric interview was not reimbursable. (Modifications of Medicare reimbursement for seeing family with and without the patient have alleviated this problem somewhat, though regional variations persist. Regional Medicare carriers have been known to make their own rules about whether to reimburse for family participation, with or without the patient present or for both situations.)

The 43-year-old single daughter had never moved out of the parental home. She had a bachelor's degree in career planning and a master's degree in personnel and was employed full time. The daughter expressed much fondness for her father. However, she revealed that since the father had begun to hallucinate and had become progressively slower and debilitated, she had become more and more resentful of the burden of his care, to which she had dedicated herself. She had thought of alternatives—such as having the aide come more often, or, as a last resort, nursing home placement—but she had been unable to act on either of these alternatives. She felt her father didn't care for the aide because the aide was talkative and boisterous and her father was quiet and reserved. Therefore, she did not want to employ the aide for more hours. She described her parental home as having been so pleasant that she had never had a desire to move out. She had much conflict about moving her father into a nursing home. She was an attractive person, aware that men were attracted to her, but she could not reciprocate. She recognized many laudatory attributes in her current boyfriend and took the fact that her father was able to remember his name as a sign that the father liked him. She disliked her boyfriend's solicitous approach toward her.

The daughter was getting progressively more resentful of her father's demands and needs. The duration of her father's condition and the intensity of care required aroused feelings of rage that were quite ego-alien to her but nevertheless were mounting in frequency and severity. Psychotherapy was recommended for the daughter, but the referral, which had to be made from the HMO, did not occur.

The psychiatrist faces the resistance not only of the patient—to engage in psychotherapy to resolve some long-standing conflicts and to guide behavior in constructive directions—but also of the primary care physician at an HMO, who might overlook or fail to understand the situation. Although the psychiatrist may recognize his or her role in this situation, the system in which the patient has medical insurance often does not recognize stresses and potential behavioral changes in the elderly person-caregiver dyad.

This example has been chosen to demonstrate how tenderness and caring can turn into anger and rage when the decline goes on for years and years and requires more and more care, and when feelings of the past hinder decisions about the most effective care for both patient and caregiver.

Had there been the opportunity to continue psychiatric interventions in the case discussed here, the following alternatives could have been considered: The growth and development of the daughter-caregiver could have been addressed by psychodynamic psychotherapy. In the course of this process, the daughter might have become able to seek out a nearby nursing home for her father, to share the decision making with her brother, and to assume the responsibilities of caregiving while attending to her own development. This process, with focused, brief psychotherapy, could well have been accomplished in 10–20 sessions. The son could have been contacted for an assessment session while in town, followed by joint appointments as needed to achieve optimal care for the father, as well as to ensure the well-being of his adult children and their significant others and/or families.

## ▋ Consultation-Liaison Service

Identification of the current role of the elderly patient in the family and of the possible multiple roles of the caregiver(s) must precede treatment planning and intervention.

Psychiatrists and other mental health professionals working on consultation-liaison services in general hospitals, where often one-third of the patients are 65 or older, are in a good position to diagnose elder maltreatment and to bring about interventions. Abuse and neglect as "differential diagnoses" need to be kept in mind, especially in patients who are admitted for problems of dehydration, malnutrition, hypothermia, falls, fractures, drug toxicity, fecal impaction, prolonged intervals of illness, and lack of medical treatment. These conditions should increase the psychiatrist's level of suspicion about possible maltreatment.

Medicare reimbursement for length of stay in hospitals varies from region to region, and families must often take their elderly relatives home despite excessive caregiving burdens. Medicare reimbursement is still 50% copay for outpatient care, whereas other outpatient medical care is 20% copay. Seeing the family with and without the patient has a reimbursable code. With the onset of diagnostic-related groups (DRGs), which set regulations for how long a patient may stay for each type of procedure or treatment, the length of stay for medical illness in general hospitals has been greatly curtailed; once a particular condition is attended to in the hospital, the elderly patient is discharged, even if she or he has a multitude of other conditions. These other conditions may be less acute, but are nevertheless at times excessively burdensome for the caretaker to attend to without adequate support.

## Summary

It is for the psychiatrist as well as other mental health professionals to explore past and current behaviors and relationships that may contribute to current maltreatment. It is the psychiatrist who assesses the likelihood that a working alliance can be established and that ongoing psychiatric interventions can contribute to compliance and cooperation with the multifaceted interventions that may be needed. The psychiatrist also has a major role in assessing the patient's competence, level of autonomous functioning, and dependency. The psychiatric team can facilitate exploring the availability of caregiving resources, assess their appropriateness for each individual situation, and enhance receptiveness to interventions.

## Legal Commentary

### ▌ Issues Related to Victims, Other Family Members, and Offenders

To help identify victims of elder abuse, nearly every state has passed laws concerning the reporting of elder abuse incidents. All states and the District of Columbia have adopted elder abuse reporting laws. In most states, there is also legislation creating elder abuse programs. A variety of state agencies are designated to receive and investigate complaints: law enforcement, social service, human service, protection and advocacy (for those with mental health and developmental disabilities problems), and state nursing home ombudsmen (in institutional cases).

In contrast to the central role played by maltreatment reporting in the protection of children, elder abuse reporting laws are viewed by most experts as much less effective in case identification and protection of the elderly than are a range of other responses, including the following:

➤ Expanding the availability of in-home services, respite care, and community-based support services
➤ Reinforcing the public protective agency's response through enhanced staffing and training and clarifying the agency's legal authority to conduct case investigations
➤ Improving interagency coordination (e.g., through elder abuse multidisciplinary teams, in which the participation of mental health and legal services agency personnel is essential)
➤ Raising public and professional awareness of the problem

Physical abuse of an elderly person, in addition to being a reportable condition, is always a crime. In some states there are enhanced penalties for crimes committed against older persons. Some police departments, prosecutors' offices, and crime victim assistance programs have developed special policies and protocols and individual expertise in the handling of crimes related to elder abuse. Although the protective services response to elder abuse has generally taken on the characteristics of the child abuse response system, law enforcement actions or inactions in elder abuse cases have faced problems similar to the early law enforcement responses in domestic violence cases.

One of the interventions for elder abuse that is dependent on the specific state law is to have the court issue an order to restrain the abuser from having contact with the victim. The remedies available under such laws are similar to those available in domestic violence cases. These types of restraints might include the following:

➤ Refraining from contacting the victim in any way
➤ Refraining from abusing a member of the victim's household

➤ Requiring the abuser to move away from and stay out of a shared residence, even if the title of the house or the apartment lease is in the abuser's name
➤ Requiring the abuser to obtain counseling
➤ Requiring the abuser to pay the victim for medical expenses, moving expenses, property damage, court costs, or attorney's fees

The overwhelming majority of reported cases of elder abuse never reach any court, either because prosecutors may not see the maltreatment as a crime or because the victim does not want to pursue legal action. However, in both civil and criminal court actions related to elder abuse, the victim may be required to appear and give testimony. As is true with cases involving young child victims of abuse, it is recognized that the special needs of older witnesses in general should be accommodated by courtroom scheduling and procedures that take their status into consideration.

One of the clearest problems with reliance on reporting laws as the primary public policy response to the problem of elder abuse is that agency resources are insufficient to provide services addressing the problems uncovered through the reporting system. In partial response to this shortcoming, under the 1978 amendments to the federal Older Americans Act (Public Law [P.L.] 95-478), Congress appropriated special funds for elder abuse prevention activities (the first such appropriation was $2.9 million in federal fiscal year 1991). In 1992 the act was further amended to include requirements for states to coordinate state legal advocacy efforts for the elderly population, including those relating to elder abuse (P.L. 102-375, 42 U.S.C. Sec. 3058i).

In addition, a proposal for the reauthorization of this act included a provision for greater funding targeted at state efforts on elder abuse as well as at the creation of a National Aging Resource Center on Elder Abuse. This center is cosponsored by the American Public Welfare Association, the National Association of State Units on Aging, and the University of Delaware. The center publishes a wide variety of materials on state policies and practices relating to elder abuse, offers training assistance, and collects limited statistics on the scope of the problem. Other resources for professionals include a National Committee for the Prevention of Elder Abuse and Neglect; a set of guidelines for elder abuse identification, documentation, and intervention from the American Medical Association (1992); and related work of the National Guardianship Association (which addresses abuse and neglect issues in the context of guardianship proceedings).

It is essential to remember that the response to identified elder abuse may require forcible intervention (i.e., action taken against the abused person's will) by the state, which results in an adult's being moved out of his or her home and into a board-and-care situation or a nursing home. Some laws and policies permit such involuntary removals and relocations without providing the affected adults the same due process of law that would exist in a civil commitment or a guardianship action. At a minimum, written procedural rules and standards for administrative and judicial actions are essential in connection with elder abuse intervention where anyone will be deprived of property or liberty—regardless of the pronouncement that the state is taking protective action.

Some state laws provide for an administrative (nonjudicial) or emergency hearing (before a court or administrative body) prior to the removal of an abuse victim from a living situation. These procedures may include a determination of capacity. In general, however, unless a court proceeding takes place, there is no legal finding regarding capacity. A judicial proceeding to determine partial or full incapacity generally requires a statement by a physician as to the person's ability to function in a decision-making process on issues relevant to the guardianship action. A few states require a judicial decision to place a current ward (person under a legal guardianship) before he or she is placed in a nursing home.

There are different statutory bases, and thus procedures, developed for elder abuse, civil commitment, and guardianship. The legal standards for determining incapacity are different for each of the three types of intervention. As opposed to the formal mechanisms used for guardianship and civil commitment, those used for elder abuse do not have the same legal protections for the older person. It must be noted that cases of elder maltreatment, particularly those involving the victim's finances, may first appear in the context of guardianship proceedings. (Indeed, some believe that financial abuse is a common factor in guardianship actions.) If a court proceeding is brought under civil commitment or guardianship laws, the affected elderly person may have the right to a court-appointed legal counsel. If the case is labeled an elder abuse matter (especially in the informal ways these cases are often handled), there may be no right to an attorney, and no counsel appointed, even though a consequence of the proceeding may be the person's removal from the home and an institutional placement.

It should also be understood that, unlike child abuse and neglect interventions, in which typically a finite set of home-based child welfare or foster care services are accessed, elder abuse cases may require that victims receive a complex set of medical and mental health, legal, and financial management services. Intervening in an older person's life also raises a unique set of ethical issues (e.g., the right to refuse treatment). Additionally, many of these cases have characteristics similar to spouse abuse cases in that a significant proportion (some suggest the largest amount) of elder abuse appears to take place among spouses. The fact that financial exploitation is a commonly reported type of elder abuse also differentiates this from the child abuse model.

Although the generic term *elder abuse* is commonly used (like *child maltreatment*), the single type of elder maltreatment most reported and substantiated is neglect. Just as with the term *child neglect,* the term *elder neglect* is fraught with vagueness—even more so because of the presumed capacity of adults to care for themselves. The most controversial form of reported neglect of older adults is alleged self-neglect, in which adults are considered unable to provide themselves with necessary care to the extent that their well-being is impaired or seriously threatened. As with child neglect intervention, the danger is that individuals with different social and cultural values will seek to impose, through involuntary protective services, paternalistic actions that result in a deprivation of the older person's ability to make his or her own decisions.

In addition to the adult protective laws that provide for government responses to reported abuse of elderly people in their own homes, there is an entirely different set of protections for older Americans who reside in nursing homes and other institutions. Special state and local government agency advocates and ombudsmen for the elderly population are entrusted with responsibilities for responding to reports of institutionally based maltreatment of elderly people. Particular state elder abuse and neglect laws give responsibility to ombudsmen, law enforcement agencies, and other protective service agencies to investigate allegations of institutional abuse.

The 1973 amendments to the federal Older Americans Act added a nursing home ombudsman program whose responsibility it is to investigate reports of abuse in nursing homes. Subsequent amendments have expanded the authority of the ombudsman program to include investigations in board-and-care homes and home care. The types of maltreatment typically reported to ombudsman programs include tying residents to their chairs or beds for long periods, neglect of bedsores, and overprescription of medication, as well as allegations of physical abuse. State Medicaid fraud and abuse units also have responsibility for investigating abuse of elderly persons when it occurs in Medicaid-supported facilities.

## ▮ Guidance for Mental Health Professionals and Practitioners

Elder abuse reporting laws have generally been modeled on child abuse reporting legislation. However, in simply changing the ages of the abused persons, statutory drafters have often forgotten an important concept: that minor children are presumed because of their age to require protection, whereas adults of whatever age are presumed capable of making all necessary decisions about the conduct of their lives. For government to intervene in an elder abuse case, there must be a mechanism for making a prompt and accurate determination of the competence of the alleged abused person. Mental health professionals play a critical role in helping adult protective agencies and courts make an assessment of competence in cases of alleged elder abuse, much as they do in adult guardianship and conservatorship actions.

When elderly persons suspected of being abused appear to be mentally incompetent, an assessment of capacity needs to be made to determine the ability of the older person to participate in decision making. An objection to an intervention proposed for such a person should not be sole grounds for determining incapacity. If the person appears to lack capacity, then a petition for the appointment of a guardian or conservator should be filed with the appropriate court. In many cases, the appointment of only a limited guardian or conservator will be necessary, thus preserving for the adult as many rights as possible. A limited order may be entered to change a place of residence, authorize a medical intervention, or transfer an asset.

When mental health professionals become involved in elder abuse cases, they must remember that, contrary to the procedures in child abuse cases, the alleged abused persons should be accorded the same presumption of mental capacity that would be given any other adult client. They should be given the same rights of response to the alleged abuse as would be given any adult clients seeking professional assistance, without fear of a court proceeding that might have them declared mentally incompetent simply because they choose not to accept assistance offered. Mental health professionals need to be on guard in these cases against making mistakes similar to the all-too-typical governmental protective response in child maltreatment cases: a focus on crisis intervention services, or "rush in and save the victim." Such a response can do more harm than good.

A number of legislative changes would help guide the response to elder abuse reports. The standards for determining whether an intervention is needed to protect an older person need to be reconciled with the standards used for guardianship and civil commitment. In addition, the use of self-neglect as a case-finding mechanism needs to be eliminated from state laws so that unwarranted, intrusive interventions under the guise of elder abuse protection are minimized.

Finally, confidentiality issues are an important aspect of government response to elder abuse. An especially important issue is removing barriers to the effective interagency sharing of relevant case information while generally protecting the privacy of the family involved. Unlike confidentiality in the child abuse arena, where these issues have been studied and debated for decades, confidentiality in elder abuse intervention is still a fledgling issue. Mental health professionals who treat elderly clients, or who find themselves involved in the diagnosis or response planning for cases of elder abuse, will need expert legal consultation on the application of existing privacy and confidentiality laws to these cases.

(See Appendix H for legal resources.)

# References

American Medical Association: Diagnostic and Treatment Guidelines on Elder Abuse and Neglect. Chicago, American Medical Association, 1992

American Medical Association: Model Elderly Abuse Reporting Act. Chicago, American Medical Association, 1985

Anetzberger GJ: The etiology of elder abuse by adult offspring: an exploratory study. Dissertation Abstracts International 47(H8-A):3186, 1987

Beth Israel Hospital, Elder Assessment Team: An elder abuse assessment team in an acute hospital setting. Practice Concepts 26:115–118, 1986

Blunt PA: Financial exploitation of the incapacitated: investigation and remedies. Journal of Elder Abuse and Neglect 5(1):19–32, 1993

Burston GR: Granny battering. BMJ 3:592, 1975

Butler RN: Why Survive? Being Old in America. New York, Harper & Row, 1975

Carmen EH, Rieker PP, Mills T: Victims of violence and psychiatric illness. Am J Psychiatry 141:378–383, 1984

Council on Scientific Affairs of the American Medical Association: Council report: elder abuse and neglect. JAMA 257:966–971, 1987

Coyne AC, Reichman WE, Berbig LJ: The relationship between dementia and elder abuse. Am J Psychiatry 150:643–646, 1993

Duke University: Multidimensional Functional Assessment: The OARS Methodology: A Manual, 2nd Edition. Durham, NC, Center for the Study of Aging and Human Development, 1978

Elder Abuse Prevention, Identification, and Treatment Act of 1985. H.R. 1674, U.S. House of Representatives, 1985

Finkelhor D, Pillemer K: Elder abuse: the relationship to other forms of family violence, in New Directions in Family Violence. Edited by Hotaling G, Finkelhor D, Gelles R, Straus M. Beverly Hills, CA, Sage, 1984

Folstein MF, Folstein SE, McHugh PR: "Mini-Mental State": a practical method for grading the cognitive state of patients for the clinician. j Psychiatr Res 12:189–198, 1975

Fulmer T, Welte T: Elder abuse: screening and intervention. Nurse Practitioner 11:33–38, 1986

Godkin MA, Wolf RS, Pillemer KA: A case comparison analysis of elder abuse and neglect. Int J Aging Hum Dev 28:207–225, 1989

Goldstein MZ: Evaluation of the elderly patient, in Verwoerdts' Clinical Geropsychiatry, 3rd Edition. Edited by Bienenfeld D. Baltimore, MD, Williams & Wilkins, 1990, pp 47–65

Goldstein MZ: Family therapy, in Comprehensive Review Of Geriatric Psychiatry. Edited by Sadavoy J, Lazarus LW, Jarvik LF. Washington, DC, American Psychiatric Press, 1991, pp 513–525

Goldstein, Woods C: Elder abuse, neglect and exploitation. American Association for Geriatric Psychiatry Newsletter 13:8–9, 1993

Hachinski VC, Iliff LD, Zilhka E, et al: Cerebral blood flow in dementia. Arch Neurol 32:632–637, 1975

Hamilton M: A rating scale for depression. j Neurol Neurosurg Psychiatry 23:56–62, 1960

Hudson MJ, Johnson TF: Elder neglect and abuse: a review of the literature. Annual Review of Gerontology and Geriatrics 6:81–134, 1986

National Center on Elder Abuse and Neglect: Understanding the Nature of Elder Abuse in Domestic Settings. Washington, DC, National Center on Elder Abuse and Neglect, 1995

Norman A: Mental Illness in Old Age: Meeting the Challenge. Center for Policy on Aging, 1982

Pagelow MD, Pagelow LW: Family Violence. New York, Praeger, 1984

Paveza GJ, Cohen D, Eisdorfer C, et al: Severe family violence and Alzheimer's disease: prevalence and risk factors. Gerontologist 32:493–497, 1992

Pillemer K, Finkelhor D: The prevalence of elder abuse: a random sample survey. Gerontologist 28:51–57, 1988

Pillemer K, Suitor JJ: Violence and violent feelings: what causes them among family caregivers? J Gerontol 47:S165–172, 1992

Ramsey-Klawsnik H: Interviewing elders for suspected sexual abuse: guidelines and techniques. Journal of Elder Abuse and Neglect 5:5–18, 1993

Roth M, Tym E, Mouvitjoy CQ, et al: CAMDEX: a standardized instrument for the diagnosis of mental disorder in the elderly with special reference to the early detection of dementia. Br J Psychiatry 149:698–709, 1986

Salzinger S, Kaplan S, Artemyeff C: Mother's personal social network and child maltreatment. J Abnorm Psychol 22:253–256, 1983

Saverman BI, Halberg IR, Norberg A, et al: Patterns of abuse of the elderly in their own homes as reported by district nurses. Scandinavian Journal of Primary Health Care 11:111–116, 1993

Straus MA, Gelles RJ: Social change and change in family violence from 1975 to 1985 as revealed in two national surveys. Journal of Marriage and the Family 48:465–479, 1986

Subcommittee on Health and Long-Term Care, Select Committee on Aging, U.S. House of Representatives: Elder Abuse: A Decade of Shame and Inaction. Report by the Chairman. Comm. Pub. No. 101-752. Washington, DC, U.S. Government Printing Office, 1990

Thobaben M, Anderson L: Reporting elder abuse: it's the law. American Journal of Nursing 185:371–374, 1985

Washington State Medical Association: Elder Abuse: Guidelines for Intervention by Physicians and Other Service Providers. Seattle, WA, Washington State Medical Association, 1985

Wolf RS: Elder abuse: ten years later. j Am Geriatr Soc 36:758–762, 1988

Wolf R, Godkin M, Pillemer K: Elder abuse and neglect: report from three model projects. Worcester, MA, University of Massachusetts Medical Center, 1984

Wolf R, Godkin M, Pillemer K: Maltreatment of the elderly: a comparative analysis. Pride Institute Journal of Long Term Home Health Care 5:10–17, 1986

Woods C, Goldstein MZ: Elder abuse, neglect and exploitation. American Association for Geriatric Psychiatry Newsletter 14:6–7, 1994

Yesavage JA: The use of self-rating depression scales in the elderly, in Clinical Memory Assessment of Older Adults. Edited by Poon LW. Washington, DC, American Psychological Association, 1986

# Bibliography

## ▌ Journal Articles and Book Chapters

Beck MC, Phillips LR: The unseen abuse: why financial maltreatment of the elderly goes unrecognized. Journal of Gerontological Nursing 10:26–30, 1987

Beth Israel Hospital, Elder Assessment Team: An elder abuse assessment team in an acute hospital setting. Practice Concepts 26:115–118, 1986

Caulse J: The abusive relationship. New Zealand Nursing Journal 80:16–18, 1987

Cochran C, Petrone S: Elder abuse: the physician's role in identification and prevention. Illinopis Medical Journal 171:241–246, 1987

Daniels RS, Baumhover LA, Clark Daniels, CL: Physician's mandatory reporting of elder abuse. The Gerontologist 29:321–332, 1989

Eastman, M: Granny abuse. Community Outlook, pp 15–16, 1988

Elder Abuse: ethical and practical dilemmas for social work. Health and Social Work 85-94, 1985.

Elder Abuse: The PhYsicians role in Illinois Medical Journal

Fine M: Age of abuse: who cares? The Australian Nurses Journal 15:28–30, 1986

Fulmer T, Cahill VM: Assessing elder abuse: a study. Journal of Gerontological Nursing 10:16–20, 1987

Galbraith MW, Zdorkwoski R: Teaching the investigation of elder abuse. Journal of Gerontological Nursing 10:21–25, 1987

Garrett G: Old age abuse by careers. Professional Nurse 1:304–305, 1986

Gilbert DA: The ethics of mandatory elder abuse reporting statuses. Advances in Nursing Science 9:51–62, 1986

Goldstein MZ: Elder neglect, abuse and exploitation, in Family Violence: Emerging Issues of a National Crisis. Edited by Dickstein L, Nadelson C. Washington, DC, American Psychiatric Press, 1989, pp 101–124

Hickey T, Douglass RL: Neglect and abuse of older family members: professionals' perspectives. Gerontologist 21:171–176, 1981

Hirst SP, Miller J: The abused elderly. Journal of Psychosocial Nursing 24:28–34, 1986

Hirst SP, Miller J: Elder maltreatment: within the family home. Perspectives 12:4–5, 1988

Hudson MJ, Johnson TF: Elder neglect and abuse: A review of the literature. Annual Review of Gerontology and Geriatrics 6:81–134, 1986

Jacobs M: More than a million older Americans abused physically and mentally each year. Perspectives on Aging 19–20, Nov-Dec 1984

Law J: Elder care: houses of horror. Community Outlook 31, 1988

Matlaw JR, Mayer JB: Elder abuse: ethical and practical dilemmas for social work. Health and Social Work 10:85–94, 1985

Mildenberger G, Wessman H: Abuse and neglect of elderly persons by family members. Physical Therapy 66:537–539, 1986

Morley S: Careers: How can we help you? Community Outlook 31:32–37, 1988

Padwell TC: Familial abuse of the elderly: a look at caregiver potential and prevention. Home Healthcare Nurse 4:10–13, 1986

Phillips LR: The list of elder abuse with the family. Public Health Nursing 5:222–229, 1988

Phillips LR, Rempusheski V: A decision-making model for diagnosing and intervening in elder abuse and neglect. Nursing Research 34:134–139, 1985

Phillips LR, Rempusheski V: Caring for the frail elderly at home: toward a theoretical explanation of the dynamics of poor quality family caregiving. Advances in Nursing Science 8:62–84, 1986

Podnieks E: Elder abuse: it's time we did something about it. Canadian Nurse 36–39, Dec 1985

Podnieks E: The victimization of older persons. Canadian Journal of Psychiatric Nursing 28:6–11, 1985

Sayles-Cross S: Profile of familial elder abuse: a selected review of the literature. Journal of Community Health Nursing 5:209–219, 1989

Selkirk D: Family violence: opportunity for change. Axon 9:3–8, 1987

Soule DJ, Bennett JM: Elder abuse in South Dakota, 2: what can be done about it? South Dakota Journal of Medicine 40:5–8, 1987

Steinmetz SK: Elder abuse by family caregivers: processes and intervention strategies. International Journal of Contemporary Family Therapy 10:256–271, 1988

Steur J, Austin E: Family abuse of the elderly. J Am Geriatr Soc 28:372-376, 1980

Thobaben M: Abuse: the shameful secret of elder care at home. RN 52:85–86, 1985

Thobaben M: Elder abuse. Home Health Care Nurse 6:37–38, 1988

# Journals

Journal of Elder Abuse and Neglect. Quarterly. Devoted to the study of the causes, treatment, effects, and prevention of the mistreatment of older people

# Annotated Bibliographies

Johnson T, O'Brien J, Hudson MF: Elder neglect and abuse: an annotated bibliography. Westport, CT, Greenwood, 1985

# CHAPTER 7

## Adult Survivors of Child Abuse and Neglect

*Jean M. Goodwin, M.D., M.P.H.*

In the 1980s it became clear that many adults who sought inpatient, outpatient, or emergency psychiatric treatment had histories of childhood abuse or neglect. Forms of abuse and neglect that have been reported as having occurred during childhood include physical and sexual abuse; emotional, medical, educational, and physical neglect; emotional abuse (such as social isolation, scapegoating, and work exploitation); witnessing family violence; and neglect because of impairment of a parent or other caretaker, sometimes as a result of uncontrolled mental illness or substance abuse. Earlier chapters of this book, on childhood abuse and neglect, give detailed definitions of maltreatment.

## Child Maltreatment as Trauma

Childhood abuse and neglect may be considered a type of oppression that occurs when one group is subjugated by another group with greater power.

Studies of people who have survived traumatic events, such as combat veterans, have provided helpful analogies for work with adults who have experienced childhood abuse and neglect (van der Kolk 1987). Core posttraumatic symptoms reported in combat veterans as well as adult survivors of childhood abuse and neglect include the following (Summit 1973):

209

➤ Flashbacks (reexperiencing perceptions associated with a traumatic episode), which may be misinterpreted as hallucinations
➤ Sleep disturbances with nightmares
➤ High anxiety with easy startle
➤ Reenactments (compelled or automatic behaviors, which may include exact reproductions of complex details of the initial trauma)
➤ Extreme emotional distress
➤ Shattered self-esteem
➤ A tendency to express psychic pain in bodily terms
➤ Multiple symptoms
➤ A tendency on the part of both sufferers and helpers to minimize, deny, and dissociate awareness of the severity of both the initial human-inflicted trauma and the subsequent symptoms

These analogies remain controversial in psychiatry, and some theorists assert that the abuse of children—most of which is inflicted by family members—is fundamentally different from that occurring in combat zones or in concentration camps. However, close examination shows the differences may be quantitative rather than qualitative. Child abuse tends to take place over a long period of time, as do many instances of oppression and war. It is critically important for the abused child to sustain family systems and trusting relationships; supportive group systems are also critical for those in military and concentration camp settings. In all three settings, issues of shame, betrayal, and divided loyalties may become as painful and damaging as the physical harm that was inflicted. In all three categories, one finds evidence for interference with personal development and for the transmission of the hurt to others unless specific interventions are made (Scurfield 1985).

## Historical Perspective

One historical strand of psychiatric and psychoanalytic theory has foreshadowed child maltreatment as a major contributor to adult psychopathology. Early in his career, Freud postulated that hysteria resulted from sexual seductions in childhood. Although he later renounced this hypothesis, some of his clinical work was quite modern, including 1) his use of collateral sources to confirm patients' accounts of maltreatment, 2) his recognition of the abused person's resistance to disclosure, and 3) his tracing of the specific links between symptoms and the initial trauma, including the concept that symptoms represent intrusive repetitions of the event or elaborate restitutive and avoidant fantasies or some combination of the two (Balmary 1979; Goodwin 1989). Despite a greater focus in the twentieth century on tracing the origins of symptoms to intrapsychic conflict, Freudian psychodynamics has retained an emphasis on this genetic or developmental component of psychiatric symptom formation.

Among post-Freudian theorists, both Fairbairn and Winnicott worked with child protection agencies in England (Khan 1975). This experience may have contributed to their view of psychopathology as a complex defensive edifice constructed in childhood to protect the self from an essentially destructive environment. In the United States, Harry Stack Sullivan and Adolf Meyer placed similarly strong emphasis on the interpersonally influenced adaptive function of psychiatric symptoms (Havens 1976). Heinz Kohut postulated that pathological narcissism results from inadequate mirroring of the infantile self and deficient opportunities for the self to idealize and function side by side with the parent figure (Modell 1990).

## Prevalence in Adult Populations

Given the high frequencies of all types of abuse in the general population, even if psychiatric patients had no greater rates of such histories than did the general population, one could expect abuse histories in large percentages of patients. Straus and Gelles (1986), in a study of 1,426 representative households, found that 10.7% of children in these homes experienced severe levels of physical abuse, including being kicked, bitten, hit with a fist, hit with an object, beaten up, and being threatened or injured with a gun or knife. In a sample of 4,695 university students, Berger et al. (1988) found that 12% reported having been injured during childhood by parental discipline. In this study about 1% reported having had bones fractured, and about 1% reported having been locked in or tied up during discipline.

Russell interviewed a general population sample of 930 women in San Francisco in 1978 and found that 152 (16%) described incestuous abuse before 18 years of age. Forty-two (4.5%) described father-daughter or stepfather-stepdaughter incest. These frequencies seem generalizable. Wyatt (1986) interviewed 248 women in Los Angeles in 1985 and found that 72 African-American women (29%) and 82 white women (33%) reported some type of sexual abuse before 18 years of age.

# ▌Adult Psychiatric Populations

Studies of psychiatric patients indicate that histories of childhood maltreatment are even higher in this group than in the general population. In several studies, between 42% and 81% of adult psychiatric patients disclosed histories of physical or sexual abuse when asked directly (Bryer et al. 1987; Carmen et al. 1984; Chu and Dill 1990; Craine et al. 1988; Jacobson 1989; Jacobson and Richardson 1987).

Psychiatric patients with such histories have been found to differ significantly from other psychiatric patients. Van der Kolk et al. (1991) reported that histories of childhood sexual and physical abuse are highly significant predictors of self-cutting and suicide. Bryer et al. (1987) found that psychological distress and symptoms of all types of mental disorders proved to be more severe in a group with a history of childhood maltreatment. Several studies found that self-mutilation and substance abuse were also more frequent in this group (Brown and Anderson 1991; Goodwin et al. 1990; Herman et al. 1989).

Studies of chronically hospitalized patients, mostly diagnosed as schizophrenic, revealed an association between childhood experiences of violence and some of the most florid, disabling psychiatric symptoms. Yesavage (1981) found that schizophrenic patients with histories of childhood maltreatment were significantly more likely to display violence as part of their symptom picture. Beck and Van der Kolk (1987) found, in a small sample ($N = 26$) of chronically hospitalized women, that those reporting childhood incest (46%) had significantly higher frequencies of sexual delusions, affective symptoms, substance abuse, suspected organicity, and major medical problems and spent more time in seclusion than did those without child abuse histories. Childhood rape survivors were more likely than those who had not been raped to have met DSM-III (American Psychiatric Association 1980) diagnostic criteria for a major depressive episode, agoraphobia, obsessive-compulsive disorder, social phobia, or sexual disorder (Saunders et al. 1992).

Craine et al. (1988), working with a larger sample ($N = 105$), found that the significant discriminators differentiating chronically hospitalized women with a history of childhood sexual abuse (51%) from those without abuse histories were 1) the presence of posttraumatic stress disorder (PTSD), 2) sexual problems (compulsive sexual behavior, sadomasochistic fantasies, sexual preoccupation, sexual identity issues, loss of sexual interest, history of rape, homosexuality), 3) chemical dependency, 4) affective symptoms (sleep problems, low energy, feeling slowed down, crying), 5) somatic symptoms (severe reactions to a medical or pelvic exam, gagging response), 6) body mutilation, and 7) school problems.

Several studies have examined correlations between severity of abuse and specific psychiatric symptoms. Saxe et al. (1993) reported that traumatic experiences (physical abuse, sexual abuse, witnessing violence) and disruptions in parental care (neglect, separations, family chaos) played a major role in the development of dissociative symptoms such as amnesia, depersonalization, and identity confusion that can rise to the level of multiple personality disorder (Braun 1986). Chu and Dill (1990) found significant correlations between severity of childhood sexual trauma and dissociative symptoms in adulthood. This association calls into question our very capacity to recognize and study these problems, because it implies that the most severely abused are the least likely to supply an abuse history because of cognitive, behavioral, sensory, and emotional symptoms that block their abilities to be aware of and to relate their histories (Herman and Schatzow 1987). Despite these disclosure difficulties, Herman et al. (1986) found also that overall severity of symptoms in adult survivors of child sexual abuse was correlated with known severity of abuse.

These findings are similar to those of studies of Vietnam veterans: extremity of combat was associated with dissociative symptoms, and it is the best predictor of severity of posttraumatic symptomatology (van der Kolk 1987).

Studies of correlations between symptoms and maltreatment in nonclinical populations give additional data about the kinds of symptoms that may cluster in those with histories of child maltreatment. Briere and Runtz (1988) found suicidality, depression, school problems, dissociation, anxiety, eating problems, conflicts with authority, early sexual behaviors, and somatization to be higher in women college students with histories of child sexual abuse than they were in nonabused college students. Using professional women from various occupations as subjects, Elliott and Briere (1992) found that those women who were molested as children reported more anxiety, depression, dissociation, sexual problems, sleep disturbances, and posttraumatic symptoms than did their nonabused peers. Moreover, adult abuse survivors frequently experienced problems in maintaining positive relationships (Chu 1992a).

## Three Syndromes of Maltreatment Sequelae

In this discussion I organize patterns of symptoms found years after experiences of three levels of increasingly severe childhood maltreatment. All three levels of maltreatment conform to definitions of abuse currently in use by United States child protection agencies. Almost all individuals who suffer these types of physical and sexual assaults would also be defined as maltreated by more psychodynamically derived definitions, such as Alice Miller's "poisonous pedagogy" (1981, 1984) or Leonard Shengold's "soul murder" (1989). However, for purposes of this discussion, the population of adults whose childhood emotional abuse was not complicated by physical assaults has not been included. In the populations considered here, emotional abuse that accompanied physical assaults is best understood as analogous to the suppression tactics that accompany political torture (Stover and Nightingale 1985). These include 1) enforced isolation, 2) interference with free communication, 3) deprivation of opportunity to compete and create, 4) exploitation of work capacity, 5) destruction of property, 5) forced witnessing of violence or participation therein, 6) incarceration, 7) interference with basic functions, including eating, sleeping, shelter, and elimination, and 8) assaults on basic elements of identity and security, such as cherished relationships, family continuity, and the individual's history and future plans. The individuals in the case examples considered here uniformly described their experiences of maltreatment as including moments of certainty that they would be killed, or that the maltreatment would reach a point where survival would not be possible.

Many people who have been abused, even those who have experienced severe violence, have no symptoms. On the other hand, severe symptoms may be seen after single or apparently limited abuse. In general, one can expect all the symptoms present at lower levels of severity to be associated also with the more severe abuse experiences, but this, too, is variable. Treatment is addressed separately in the final section of this chapter. However, some aspects of treatment specific to each case example are presented with the example.

# ▌ Posttraumatic Stress Disorders

Symptoms described in many adult survivors of relatively uncomplicated sexual or physical abuse conform generally to the pattern of PTSD. There is high anxiety, especially around "triggers" for the abuse memories. Certain behaviors, thoughts, and feelings are avoided in order to ward off memories that might be overwhelming. Memories recur, however, in the form of nightmares and flashbacks. Anger is controlled in an especially rigid manner. There is a pervasive sense of sadness and shame (Gelinas 1983; Goodwin 1985, 1988, 1989; Herman 1981).

Despite suicidal thoughts that date back to grade-school years, and despite fears that their auditory and visual flashbacks are precursors of insanity, individuals often cope with this level of symptomatology by themselves. Symptoms often reach psychiatric attention only when there is an intercurrent emotional stress, medical illness, or both.

The prominent symptoms of anxiety and depression in these abuse survivors can warrant diagnoses of dysthymia or panic disorder. Briere (1989) has noted that persons who have experienced childhood sexual abuse are 10 times more likely than are persons who have not experienced such abuse to be given a diagnosis of anxiety disorder. Because these individuals fear that their symptoms are psychotic, they may be confusingly diagnosed as having brief psychotic reactions as well. The following case examples illustrate these diagnostic problems.

## ➤ Case Example 1

Ms. D was a 45-year-old unmarried South American scientist who had struggled for many years to gain refugee status in this country. She was referred for psychiatric evaluation when she reported to co-workers that neighbors were monitoring her movements and disparaging her sexuality, perhaps for political reasons. She described living in a constant state of terror and confusion, which she compared to her feeling at age 8 when she was followed by a neighbor who reached under her dress and digitally penetrated her. When she had told her mother about the incident, her mother had not believed her.

Once the evaluator had gained her trust by believing that she must have good reasons to have panicked, Ms. D consented to a physical examination that revealed heart failure due to rheumatoid heart disease. Time-limited psychotherapy focused on the childhood trauma as one source of her distrust of neighbors and her fear that there was a problem with her sexuality. Her difficulties in trusting her own perceptions and asking for help had been heightened in childhood by her parents' clandestine participation in a revolutionary group, as well as by the patient's memories of her mother's disbelief when she ran to her for help after the sexual assault. As psychotherapy proceeded, Ms. D was able to obtain the assistance she needed to resolve both her bureaucratic and her medical problems.

> **Case Example 2**

A 35-year-old married Anglo-American male professional presented for psychiatric evaluation when his panic attacks failed to disappear after definitive treatment of newly diagnosed familial thyrotoxicosis, a hereditary endocrine condition. His diagnosis had precipitated a move back to his hometown and consequent increased contact with his mother, who had physically abused him throughout childhood and into adulthood. His mother's habit of punching her children in the face and head with fists and other objects had been excused in the family on the basis of her suffering from thyrotoxicosis as well. Several of the patient's brothers had engaged in fist and knife fights with each other, and one, also a highly trained professional, had recently been convicted for physically assaulting his wife.

The patient agreed to the use of medication to treat his anxiety. He did not, however, agree to psychotherapy, because he felt that personal exploration of his parents' treatment of him would mean the loss of any hope that they might make reparation to him and provide him with a nurturant relationship.

Alice Miller (1981) has drawn attention to the tendency of abused children to gravitate toward demanding creative or helping occupations. Unfortunately, these are often also highly stressful fields. The presence of ameliorating functional strengths may be viewed by abuse survivors as making ongoing therapy optional rather than a survival issue. However, it is often helpful, in a brief diagnostic encounter, for the mental health professional to define some of the specific links between childhood maltreatment and prominent crisis symptoms or issues. This can assist the abuse survivor to recognize specific triggering vulnerabilities and to understand the shame about basic needs that may interfere with finding and using necessary assistance. Once abuse survivors can recognize and understand their posttraumatic symptoms, these symptoms no longer act as yet another focus for shame, self-blame, and resistance to treatment.

## ▌ Borderline Conditions

It is not surprising that in many situations the presence of a physically or sexually assaultive caretaker in childhood coincides with other adversities in the child's environment. The assaultive caretaker or the child or children abused by the caretaker may suffer emotional or substance use disorders; in addition, the caretaker may assault other family members while the child looks on. The child's needs in infancy or later medical, educational, or emotional needs may be experienced as overwhelming by a family in chaos and may trigger further neglect and abuse. An assaultive parent usually experiences difficulties with many relationships, which may disrupt any opportunities the child finds for acquiring long-term adequate extraparental caretakers and social supports.

A common sequela of this type of abuse is a complicated history of medical, psychiatric, and legal involvements. Here, sensory repetitions and behavioral reenactments of the variety of child abuse experienced are so multiple as to defy a single diagnosis or misdiagnosis. At times, the sensory reexperiencing of the pelvic pain of sexual abuse or the head pain of battering may produce a medical diagnosis or a diagnosis of somatization disorder. When the reexperiencing of the gagging and vomiting associated with forced fellatio comes to the forefront, a diagnosis of bulimia may be made. Attempts to use substances for numbing may lead to an alcohol or substance use disorder.

Reenactments of child abuse through self-mutilation and through revictimizing or reabusing others may lead to a diagnosis of borderline personality disorder. Perry et al. (1990) found that many patients with borderline personality disorder had experienced childhood trauma. Dissociative defenses also may interfere with self-protection. Survivors may come to treatment with diagnoses of secondary interpersonal trauma, such as rape or battered-spouse experiences, or with a history of having been assaulted by a therapist, only to disclose later their childhood maltreatment.

The combination of dissociative symptoms with high levels of depression, anxiety, and mistrust may lead to a diagnosis of psychosis. Subtle neurosensory and other physical sequelae of abuse complicate the picture. Van der Kolk et al. (1991) pointed out that although childhood trauma contributes to the initiation of self-destructive behavior, it is the lack of secure attachments—prolonged separations from primary caregivers, or feelings of being unloved—that helps maintain the self-destructive behavior. In addition, assaultive parents may suffer conditions such as manic-depressive illness, major depression, genetic risk for alcoholism, or antisocial personality disorder, for which their abused children are also at risk.

➤ **Case Example 3**

A 50-year-old divorced disabled woman of Central European origin, during psychotherapy, disclosed prior incest. At age 35, after she had had an auto accident, temporal lobe seizures had been diagnosed. At age 45, after a divorce, major depression had been diagnosed. Neither condition responded well to medication. Fifteen years after the onset of symptoms, the following childhood history was elicited:

Her father, who had an alcoholic condition and manic-depression, abused her, her sister, and her mother physically and sexually until she was removed to foster care at age 6. His principal method for punishing her had been to strangle her until she passed out. She had witnessed him raping her mother and fellating her infant sister. Her father usually slept with her, engaging in both vaginal and anal intercourse. At the time she was removed to care, his principal delusion was that Martians were poisoning the food supply. The patient's memories were confirmed by protective service records, by medical records for her, her sibling, and her father, and by records of divorce litigation. Her mother had been judged too depressed to care for the children, and the patient was separated from her sister and raised in three foster homes. In one foster home she was severely scapegoated, and in another she was sexually fondled by the foster father. She was also sexually abused by a teacher and emotionally abused in her marriage.

In reviewing the natural history of her symptoms, it became apparent that suicidality, depression, sexual dysfunction, anxiety, an eating disorder, and somatic symptoms had been present since childhood. Her seizures, also present since childhood and definitively worked up once the trauma history was available, seemed to include both psychomotor and dissociative episodes. After 48 sessions in a therapy group designed for survivors of

multimodalchild abuse, her symptoms declined and her functioning improved.

Successful treatment plans provide adequate team coverage of all
symptoms by using the multiple modalities necessary. These modalities include

➤ Hospital care
➤ Medication
➤ Emergency care
➤ Specific treatment for sexual, eating, and addictive disorders
➤ Family intervention
➤ Medical care
➤ Rehabilitation
➤ Exercise
➤ Group and individual psychotherapy

It is important not to label these patients "dependent" or "needy,"
because this may obscure real deficits in their capacity to experience
their own real needs and to begin to meet them. It is also important
not to label them "manipulative," because this implies an excess of
interpersonal sophistication, which is the reverse of the actual case.
A deficit of interpersonal experience has resulted not only from imposed isolation but also from their own protective retreat to dissociated internal worlds.

The therapist's task is to facilitate recall of childhood experiences
without preconceptions about the truth or falsehood of what emerges.
Accounts of overwhelming or violent incidents often emerge only after
years of treatment and may be renounced or minimized if they are too
quickly challenged. Although it is true that the patient may be con-
cealing symptoms of compulsive violence, sexual addictions, or abuse
of children, these symptoms are usually understood in the end as consequent to the childhood maltreatment history rather than as an explanation for disclosing that history.

A core theoretical difference exists between therapists using a
model based on the works of Klein, Kernberg, and Mahler and those
using trauma theory. The former tend to understand the patient's
symptoms and problems with relationships as aberrations of love and
attachment manifesting in a regressive form; those working from
trauma theory understand the same manifestations as relating to

repetitive reenactments and compulsive defenses against life-threatening assaults. Within this trauma framework, the fundamental aim of the abuse survivor is to protect the self and others from the felt ongoing danger of such assaults. A trauma focus emphasizes the patient's suppression of complaints and concealment of suffering, in contrast to the psychodynamic approach to complaints, which tries to illuminate the sources of those that do become audible.

Vamik Volkan (1987) provides a detailed case history of such a patient that illustrates the advantages and disadvantages of dynamic therapy uninformed by trauma theory. In this case, analytic treatment was helpful, in part, because of its frequency and intensity. Sexual and aggressive impulses came under progressively improved control. The young woman patient forged a relationship with the analyst that far surpassed the abused-child–persecutor–rescuer patterns of her past. What was absent was detailed exploration of her maltreatment history (it remained unclear whether abuse had persisted into adulthood and whether other family members were being abused). The patient's hints about intrafamilial sexual abuse were not pursued, and sexual exploitation by a previous therapist continued during the analysis. Also missing was a specific focus on the patient's posttraumatic and dissociative symptoms, which in this case rose to the level of alter ego fragments and remained unintegrated at the end of treatment.

Volkan's patient might be better described as having a Disorder of Extreme Stress Not Otherwise Specified (Spitzer et al. 1989), or as having Complex Post Traumatic Stress Disorder (Herman 1992), rather than as having the dual diagnosis of borderline personality disorder and posttraumatic stress disorder that DSM-IV recommends (American Psychiatric Association 1994).

The category of extreme or complex stress would allow differentiation of the multiple and severe symptoms found in some traumatized persons from the symptoms that characterize personality disorders. Such a differentiation would facilitate data collection about phenomenology, natural history, and optimal psychotherapeutic approaches.

## Dissociative Disorders

Occasionally abuse is inflicted on children not because of a nondeliberate clustering of adversities, but because children fall into the hands of someone who takes pleasure in inflicting physical and emotional pain. Children who have been previously abused are at particular risk for being unable to recognize, to complain about, or to extricate themselves from sadistic abuse. However, it is also true that certain sadistic abusers, well practiced in violence, are capable of abusing even the most emotionally healthy child or adult.

Sadistic abusers of children are often found among the perpetrators of extreme family violence, among political torturers, in prostitution and pornography rings, among criminal gangs, and among pseudoreligious cults. Behavioral signs and histories of persons who have been sadistically abused include

- Reports of great intensity and variety of types of violence during maltreatment
- Infliction of "unnecessary" injury or humiliation during abuse
- Elaborate and detailed planning of abuse
- Death threats during abuse

Survivors of such abuse may have been forced to witness the killing of animals or may have been duped into believing that they were about to be killed. Other reported characteristics are the use of bondage or incarceration and the presence of multiple perverse acts (DSM-III-R [American Psychiatric Association 1987]).

In sadistic abuse, multiple perpetrators acting in concert have often been implicated. In multimodal abuse the child experiences both physical and sexual abuse, but at various times and from various caretakers. In sadistic abuse, physical and sexual abuse tend to occur simultaneously because of the abusive person's dependence on witnessing pain in order to experience sexual arousal or discharge.

Dissociation is the most typical response of a child who experiences sadistic abuse. Such children may depersonalize and appear robotic or "not there." The child may leave the body, escape into fantasy, or devise imaginary playmates or alter egos to endure the abuse, to maintain some capacity for healthy living, or both.

Dissociation appears during sadistic abuse for a number of reasons. First, as previously noted, dissociation varies directly with the severity of abuse, and this is the most severe type of abuse. Second, sadistic abusers, because they are experienced in child abuse and because they risk more in terms of criminal prosecution, may deliberately manipulate the trance states that are common in children abused in this way. Whether deliberate or accidental, threats made to children in trauma-induced trances or statements about their help-lessness or blame may be absorbed uncritically by the dissociated child and may enhance the abusive person's chances of escaping un-detected.

Self-mutilation is a symptom often reported in victims of sadistic child abuse (Goodwin 1993). It often mimics the predilections of sa-dists: delicate cutting, poisoning, cigarette burns, and painful inser-tion of objects into orifices.

### ➤ Case Example 4

Elsa was a 32-year-old divorced, disabled Anglo-American whose diagnosis had been schizophrenia throughout most of her 20-plus psychiatric hospitalizations. Other past diagnoses included ano-rexia nervosa, major depression, borderline personality disorder, and polysubstance abuse. Since the onset of illness in her late teens, she had sustained almost as many medical as psychiatric admissions, presenting typically with dehydration and urinary re-tention.

After the death of a favorite aunt, what had seemed to be the marginal adjustment of a person with schizophrenia collapsed to reveal a patchwork of dissociative mechanisms. She had kept the dead aunt as an imaginary companion and was able to sort out over time about 30 other imaginary entities. On initiating trauma-based treatment, she seemed to be oscillating among three basic ego states: 1) "the other Else," a compliant, dependent adult who contained many of the posttraumatic somatic symptoms, 2) "El-lie," an angry 7-year-old who remembered multimodal abuse from various family members and sadistic abuse from her grandfather, and 3) "Elinor," an adult without emotions who appeared when it was necessary to deal with emergencies. Much of the additional self-fragmentation included 1) ego states that encapsulated a par-ticular posttraumatic symptom, such as vomiting, 2) ego states that maintained islands of functioning, such as housekeeping, re-ligious activities, driving, maintenance of both heterosexual and homosexual relationships, and so on, and 3) ego states that held memories and feelings related to specific incidents of childhood maltreatment (for example, a 3-year-old self-fragment that always cried). When this crying state and the one that vomited were in control together, the dehydration episodes would occur.

The last set of self-states to emerge were those that represented identifications with her abusers. These were involved in destroying her clothes, favorite objects, and writings, in keeping up a stream of emotionally abusive comments, in engaging in various illegal acts, in interfering with supportive relationships and treatment, and in mutilating her body through a variety of methods: burning, banging, cutting, and genital manipulation using ice picks and screwdrivers. These internal persecutors also organized suicide attempts.

The sexual abuse from Elsa's maternal grandfather had begun in infancy and lasted until his death when she was still prepubertal. Two of her sisters also disclosed sexual abuse from their grandfather, and their mother had a dense amnesia from her childhood. Sadistic elements included locking up, inserting objects, gang rapes in which Elsa's grandfather involved his brothers as coperpetrators, and "hunts" for the child through wooded areas.

The patient's use of medical and psychiatric emergency visits markedly decreased following diagnosis. Even with specific diagnosis and treatment, however, she remained polysymptomatic and required a complex treatment plan that included individual therapy, medication, medical care, home health care, about 20 days of hospitalization per year, and family intervention. Use of hypnotic techniques was also helpful in preventing dissociative lacunae, predicting self-harm, and managing her eating disorder.

Victims of sadistic abuse often appear to get worse after accurate diagnosis removes the veil of dissociation to reveal previously concealed symptoms. However, strengths are revealed as well. For example, no one who had treated this woman for schizophrenia knew of her complex sexual involvements and extensive travel.

The goal of protecting such patients from further sadistic involvements may be unrealistic. This patient had become involved in adulthood both with a pseudoreligious sadistic cult and with a criminal gang. Confronted with a no-self-harm contract, she said, quite seriously, that when she was able to sign it, she would be well, so it was foolish to require it as a precondition of treatment.

## Assessment

If continued research confirms the role of child maltreatment in shaping psychopathology, clarifying this aspect of a patient's history will become routine in each evaluation, even though, in many cases, treatment will not focus on this area. The importance of diagnosing posttraumatic symptoms may often lie in clearing away confusing elements so that an underlying comorbid psychiatric, metabolic, or neurological condition can be discerned or in understanding and overcoming resistance to treatment. Mood disorders, anxiety attacks, substance use disorders, and antisocial behavior are common coexisting mental health problems associated with the more severe post-child-abuse syndromes. These entities have often been shown to have familial clustering, as has dissociation (Braun 1986, 1990). It is likely that both genetic vulnerability and exposure to violence or other factors are necessary to the evolution of severe syndromes involving multiple symptoms.

Preliminary indicators suggest that any patient with psychiatric problems—particularly those with sexual or aggressive dyscontrol, multiple symptoms, dissociative symptoms, or intolerably high levels of emotional or psychosomatic pain—should be interviewed systematically about childhood maltreatment and violence history.

In the past, questioning about maltreatment has not been routine in psychiatric practice or in other aspects of health care (American Medical Association 1992). In a chart review of consecutive admissions to a public psychiatric hospital, Goodwin and co-workers (1990) found that parental psychopathology was noted as present or absent in less than 60% of charts. Childhood maltreatment—neglect, witnessed violence, and physical and sexual abuse—were mentioned only rarely. In reviewing the chart of a young African-American man hospitalized 14 times for borderline personality disorder, records were found of admissions before age 8 for two injuries resulting from "catching" his hands and arms in a washer-wringer and one hospitalization for severe genital bruising. Yet, though readily available in the chart, these had never been mentioned in his psychiatric evaluations.

## Facilitating Adult Memory for Childhood Abuse and Neglect

Childhood maltreatment is often an open secret, confirmed (sometimes proudly) by family members or witnessed in family sessions and documented in medical and legal records. Even in incest cases, where secrecy is a central concern, Herman and Schatzow (1987) found that over two-thirds of adults who described such abuse were able rather easily to find witnesses or material evidence to confirm their hazy and blocked memories. Helping the symptomatic person recognize and integrate data that shed light on memories of maltreatment is an important aspect of assessment.

Does remembering hurt? In a small study of female psychiatric patients randomized to structured interview and noninterview groups, no evidence was found that patients queried about childhood sexual abuse stayed in the hospital longer, were readmitted more quickly, or were less likely to cooperate in outpatient care. Patients did describe the interview as stressful, but they also expressed relief and gratitude in their comments (Goodwin et al. 1988). Because so many adults maltreated in childhood are intensely and multiply symptomatic, it may be that these problems—although present for years—have been mistakenly thought to have been caused by the probing for childhood history that takes place during intervention. Chu (1992b) emphasized that efforts to build an adequate psychotherapeutic relationship should precede the reworking of painful memories and exploring past traumatic experiences.

When physicians learn about ongoing child abuse or a serious threat to an adult's life, such as a communicable disease or a threat of violence, there is a responsibility to protect—a responsibility that often conflicts with the duty to maintain confidentiality. If a written violence history is used, an informed-consent statement can be included, explaining the situations in which the physician would have to disclose information to law enforcement. In some practices this type of written agreement is routine in all cases. Most patients can understand a simple statement that when they are in physical danger or are placing someone else in physical danger, it is an emergency situation, for which additional help will need to be called in.

## Sample History

The 10 questions in Table 7–1 constitute an informal approach to determining the importance of child maltreatment in a particular case. Such screening seeks to define major distortions in the childhood environment and the presence of hallmark posttraumatic and dissociative symptoms. Once a suspicion is raised, the next step is more extensive testing. It should include 1) a systematic violence history, 2) a detailed sexual history, 3) a family genogram, 4) testing for posttraumatic, affective, borderline, somatic, and dissociative symptoms, and 5) a life history of symptoms, including those related to eating, sexuality, substance abuse, and reenacted violence. The Dissociative Disorders Interview Schedule (Ross 1989) is an example of a structured instrument that is useful at this stage.

# Overview of Treatment

As indicated by the case examples, these are often complex cases requiring a step-by-step approach. It is often helpful to list the (usually) multiple types of childhood maltreatment, the multiple symptoms and diagnoses, and the multimodal treatment approaches that will be employed.

How is the process different from that in other complex cases? One way to organize the differences is to review the special interventions used for children when ongoing child maltreatment is disclosed. The therapist secures for the child a physical examination and a complete investigation of the alleged maltreatment. The therapist supports the child through requisite legal procedures, tries to understand the family environment, and identifies and treats posttraumatic and comorbid symptoms and disorders. Similar emphases are important when such memories surface in adulthood.

| Table 7–1. | Ten questions to facilitate child maltreatment disclosure |
|---|---|

1. In a conflict, have you ever been pushed or shoved? Hit with a fist, kicked, or bitten? Threatened with a weapon?
2. In a conflict, have you ever pushed or shoved? Hit with a fist, kicked, or bitten? Threatened with a weapon?
3. Do you have any scars on your body from someone trying to hurt you on purpose? From you trying to hurt yourself?
4. Have you ever been tied down or locked up?
5. When you were a child, did anyone do anything to you that you thought was sexual that made you feel uncomfortable?
6. Have you ever been hit with an object? What object?
7. As a child, did you ever worry about the mental state of a caretaker? Run away from home? Think about suicide?
8. Do you have nightmares or bad dreams about something bad that happened to you?
9. Do you ever use drugs or alcohol to get numb?
10. Have you ever tranced out, lost time, or left your body?

Careful attention to somatic symptoms, basic bodily needs, and physical safety and protection will assist the adult patient in recognizing dissociative flights from the body and in becoming aware of the extent to which sensations and feelings have become divorced from cognitions. Hospitalization is often necessary to establish safety and restore basic functions. When amnesia is dense, physical examination can provide the first concrete indications of prior trauma. One young woman, by history virginal, was found on physical examination to have a marital introitus and, scarred into the mons, a pentagram. An older woman with the same negative sexual history showed evidence of prior deliveries, as well as excision of her clitoris and labia minora.

Lebowitz et al. (1993) offer a model of treatment-facilitated recovery from sexual trauma occurring during childhood. The recovery process they describe unfolds over progressive stages, which include safety, remembrance, integration, mourning, and reconnecting with others.

The initial or investigatory phase of treatment may include for adults the compiling of documents beginning with the birth certificate and including pediatric records, school records, and interviews with collateral informants. Some adults abused as children compile a life-book in journal or scrapbook format. Starting with one page devoted to each year of life, it is possible to recognize early in the process which years are obliterated by amnesia. Self-help resources such as *The Courage to Heal* (Bass and Davis 1988) or *Toxic Parents* (Forward 1990) are used by some adults in this exploration phase. It is sometimes helpful when treating patients with severe dissociation to use file cards to note flashbacks, dreams, symptoms, or memories (Zimrin 1986). If the patient is allowed to leave these confusing and frightening fragments locked in the therapist's desk between sessions, he or she often will allow knowledge to build gradually during sessions as file cards are amended and rearranged like pieces of a puzzle.

Often techniques of play therapy are helpful in reconstructing the patient's inner world. Indeed, Melanie Klein (1950) invented play therapy in the process of trying to help a young girl disclose sexual abuse by a schoolmate. Sand-tray play (Kalff 1980), a Jungian technique widely used with adults abused as children, is very similar to Melanie Klein's earliest approaches and offers the patient the opportunity to construct a miniature world with a variety of small objects. Art therapy, poetry therapy, and similar approaches are also used (Goodwin 1989).

Group therapy (Goodwin 1988) has been very helpful in reconstruction. Particularly with individuals who have been abused by multiple adults in group settings, group validation may be necessary to
revise images of the self and others that were distorted by repetitive
traumatic experiences reinforced by the presence of multiple adult
perpetrators.

Hypnosis and Amytal (amobarbital sodium) interviews are occasionally helpful, but they must be used with caution. It is essential to
understand the peculiarities of the trance state—the sense of paralysis, the easy access to autonomic functions and pain control, the lack
of critical appraisal of input, the heightened visual imagery, the suggestibility—and to help the adult abused as a child to recognize this
state and gain control over entry and exit. Before using such techniques for reconstruction, it is important to assess whether the posttraumatic state has in fact settled too much on the side of numbing,
making amnesia the primary block, or whether flashbacks and positive
symptoms are already flooding the system. When it is flooding that
underlies the patient's frustration about not knowing, then decreas-
ing the level of consciousness through hypnosis and introducing new
traumatic material may lead to worsened symptoms.

Familiarity with possible legal ramifications is as important in
dealing with adults as with children. If the person who committed the
abuse continues to have contact with children, or if the abused person's symptoms include being a child abuser or exposing children to
an abuser, a report to child protective services (CPS) may be necessary. Civil commitment procedures for abused persons who are compulsively suicidal or homicidal may also be needed. Experiences such
as adult rape or spousal battering may have to be addressed through
criminal or civil court actions, including restraining orders and divorce. For those reabused by therapists, physicians, or any other
health care providers, complaints to licensing agencies or to law enforcement may be required in certain states.

The abused person's symptoms in the realm of substance use and
antisocial acts may lead to legal problems. An example would be the
case (an actual one) of an abused person whose severe anxiety led to
self-medication with alcohol and a delusion that she had an undiag-
nosed heart problem. These problems in turn led to medical visits so
frequent and perturbing that her physician obtained a restraining order, which she promptly violated. By the time her anxiety was traced
back to her multimodal child abuse and she was persuaded to undergo

appropriate treatment for this and her underlying mood and alcohol disorders, there were many legal knots to untie. An extreme scenario of this type is the abused person who murders the abuser (Kleiman 1988).

Even when childhood maltreatments occurred far in the past, there may continue to be legal remedies. In some states, laws that take into consideration a delayed recognition of trauma have reset the statute of limitations to begin at the moment of recall rather than at the moment of injury. (See "Legal Commentary" in this chapter.) There is no statute of limitations on murder; therefore, persons who have experienced sadistic abuse that involved being a witness to murder need to be encouraged to report it to law enforcement. Units dealing with vice or gang crimes are accustomed to assembling old information, often anonymously received, to elucidate long-standing patterns of crime.

Understanding the patient's family dynamics can be crucial to management. Maltreatment often continues into adulthood, and it can preclude both adequate treatment and symptomatic improvement. Chu (1992a) described revictimization in adults with histories of child maltreatment. Therapists may assist patients to recognize and disrupt this process. Curtailing interaction with abusive family members may be a necessary first step in treatment. However, a break with family can be an overwhelming recommendation for a disabled adult with chronic psychiatric symptoms for whom family is the only apparent asset. Several years ago I diagnosed multiple personality disorder in a 28-year-old man who reported continuing sexual involvement with a family member. Neither adult coerced protective services nor civil commitment provided a way out for this person. He remains ill and in the relationship.

The middle phase of treatment involves systematically identifying trauma-related symptoms and tracing them back to the overwhelming childhood events—remembered now with feeling and sensation—and with the associated childhood fantasies. Because this process allows the abused person some relief from fears and phobias, low self-esteem, repetition compulsions, chronic anger, dissociative numbing, and unintelligible body symptoms, the patient's repetitive crises become less frequent and more manageable (Putnam 1989). Ultimately the patient becomes able to distinguish feelings of pleasure and displeasure from the massive dysphoria connected with the reconstructed childhood maltreatment. At this point he or she has the wherewithal to learn about his or her own wishes, ideals, ambitions, and appetites. Once symptoms are controlled and the reconstruction of the past is complete, the therapeutic work can focus on end-phase therapeutic issues of how to live a life now reclaimed as her own.

## Research: Strategies and Obstacles

Longitudinal follow-up study is one ideal strategy for elucidating the effects of child maltreatment on adult psychopathology (Finkelhor 1984). One defines a sample of abused or neglected children, matches these children to nonmaltreated control groups, follows both groups into adulthood, and compares the frequencies and types of psychopathology. Early results are beginning to be available now from a National Institute of Mental Health (NIMH) study designed in this way (Putnam 1989). Such studies are expensive and cumbersome, especially with child subjects who must be followed for many years. Some of the most useful studies—Lenore Terr's (1979) follow-up of abducted schoolchildren, Michael Rutter's (1985) study of British foster children, and the study on sexually abused children done by Gomez-Schwartz et al. (1990)—have been able to follow the child subjects only into adolescence. There is clinical evidence that this study period is not long enough. Studies done with adults who experienced incest as children often show higher symptom frequencies than do studies done with children (Goodwin 1989). Follow-up studies can help here; populations unambiguously defined as maltreated in childhood are recontacted years later and reassessed (Williams 1992).

One strategy that might bypass the expense involved in initiating longitudinal studies would be to piggyback a maltreatment question onto existing studies. However, problems of ascertainment make this strategy difficult. The secrecy that surrounds child abuse is so profound that professionals have not screened for it routinely, adults who commit abuse have not asked for help, and abused children have not complained.

This problem of ascertainment plagues all research designs. The evidence has shown that, on balance, the problem is one of children or adults minimizing their abuse, not exaggerating it. Researchers have learned to limit the minimizing 1) by asking about specific actions (Straus et al. 1980) and about specific body parts (Lewis et al. 1985) rather than talking abstractly about "abuse" and 2) by using interviewers who are likely to be seen as trustworthy by the informants and who are able to spend a great deal of time building a relationship during the interview (Wyatt and Powell 1988). Dill et al. (1991), in studying the methods of obtaining abuse histories, found that a standard psychiatric intake interview at admission for inpatient treatment was less reliable than a subsequent confidential self-report survey about various forms of early childhood trauma. The data confirm the notion that some patients may choose not to disclose their painful histories until they become more comfortable with their therapists.

Another way to bypass the problem of ascertainment in intrafamilial child abuse is to study extrafamilial maltreatment, where secrecy may be less profound. Lenore Terr (1979) studied children abused by strangers who had committed crimes in addition to the abuse. Bergmann and Jucovy (1982) studied children of the Holocaust, whose abuse occurred in the context of political persecution. Another less difficult way to study the effects of human-induced trauma is to look at children traumatized in medical settings (Terr 1991).

Sampling is another difficulty that plagues all research designs. Children who have experienced intrafamilial abuse differ in multiple ways from children not so abused. These differences probably extend over multiple generations (Oliver 1988). It is difficult to find a control population that differs only on the abuse variable. When foster children are studied, for example, both the effects of their child maltreatment (which may be quite variable in both type and severity) and the effects of removing the children from their parents are seen.

Another problem in selecting a control population is finding a sample that has not been abused. Many studies indicate that more than 90% of American children are physically disciplined (Straus and Gelles 1986; Straus et al. 1980). Specific questioning is needed to differentiate "normal spanking" from physical discipline that involves hitting with objects, undressing, hitting on the head or face, or leaving bruises and other physical injuries.

The best evidence is that psychiatric populations have experienced even more abuse than the general population. Because of this, one must question studies that compare symptoms of sexually abused children to symptoms of children in a general psychiatric population; we cannot assume that the "control" psychiatric population is less abused if we take into account all types of maltreatment and severity factors.

Cross-sectional studies compare histories of child maltreatment and specific psychiatric symptoms in two groups of adults. These studies test the hypothesis that these two phenomena will cluster together. One looks not only for higher frequencies of abuse history in clinical as opposed to nonclinical samples, but also for correlations between severity of target symptoms and severity of prior maltreatment, which should be found in nonclinical populations as well.

Cross-sectional studies establish nonrandom patterns of clustering, but they do not define causation. For example, psychiatric patients with more severe childhood histories of abuse or neglect may show more severe symptoms for many reasons other than that their severe symptoms were caused by the maltreatment. More aberrant constitutional factors in the child may have provoked both more intense maltreatment by parental caretakers and more severe symptoms. Genetically transmitted illnesses may have produced greater abnormalities both in the caretaking behaviors of parents and in the symptom patterns of the index patients.

Ultimately, we need to study the effects of specific therapies on children who have experienced maltreatment. Currently available clinical data suggest that the treatment of choice would be psychotherapies that focus on the nature of the childhood maltreatment and its specific connections to present symptoms. Intervention studies in this area need to include 1) credible placebo psychotherapies and 2) methodological strategies for blinding both patients and therapists to the hypothesis and to the presence of presumed active treatment.

One clinical factor that favors the outcome study approach is the sheer severity of symptoms. Moderate amelioration should be detectable even in small samples. For example, in an ongoing study of incest survivors with at least one prior psychiatric hospitalization, we intervened with a 12-session abuse survivors group. The first 10 patients had logged 37 emergency visits in the 2 years preceding entry into the group. On a 2-year posttreatment follow-up, they had logged only 12 such visits. Even in this tiny sample, the effectiveness of specific treatment was strongly suggested (Goodwin et al. 1992).

This example also illustrates that because the natural history of childhood maltreatment involves lifelong proneness to symptoms, studies of treatment response can measure symptom prevention as well as symptom relief. Further research on natural history is especially important in designing recommendations for the initial acute treatment and management of maltreated children by human service agencies and by mental and physical health services, as well as in designing therapeutic recommendations for survivors.

## Summary

In this chapter I review, with case illustrations, three presentations of adult psychopathology associated with different types of child maltreatment, as well as techniques for recognizing and treating these conditions. Maltreatment syndromes often coexist with other psychiatric disorders. More research is recommended to establish the etiological role of childhood maltreatment and the efficacy of specific psychotherapeutic approaches.

## Legal Commentary

### ▌ Issues Related to Abused Persons, Other Family Members, and Offenders

One legal issue facing adult survivors of child maltreatment is whether to pursue judicial relief via a civil or criminal action against the person or persons who abused them. Traditionally, U.S. courts have been reluctant to entertain lawsuits brought by minor children against their parents. This doctrine of "parental immunity," however, has never been absolute. Courts have permitted actions against parents who maliciously, intentionally, or recklessly inflict injuries on their children. Children have been permitted to file tort actions against noncustodial parents, stepparents, and other relatives standing in the place of parents. Significantly, some courts have specifically permitted children to recover damages against parents when the parents were protected by insurance. (Many of these cases involve the child's being injured as a result of the parent's negligent operation of a motor vehicle.)

Today, most states have in some way abrogated or modified the doctrine of absolute parental tort immunity. In addition, several states have created special civil causes of action for injuries due to child abuse. Yet lawsuits by children (brought during their minority or after they become adults) against parents based on child abuse are still relatively rare, and there are very few case precedents. Appellate courts are only beginning to review lower court judgments made on behalf of children as a result of their parents' abuse. In addition to the basic assault and battery civil tort action grounds, abuse survivors are making claims such as the intentional or negligent infliction of emotional distress, as well as an implied cause of action based on the violation by the perpetrator of a criminal abuse statute.

In recent years, litigation filed by and on behalf of physically abused and molested children has become more commonplace. These lawsuits have sought monetary awards to compensate for injuries (both physical and emotional) caused by physical and sexual abuse. In many of these cases, there has been evidence of considerable emotional pain and suffering to the child and the protective (nonabusing) parent. Such evidence has included an expert diagnosis of the child's problems, a description of the treatment provided and still required, and the prognosis for the child's future. One form of evidence that has been helpful in establishing a child's injuries resulting from abuse involves testimony regarding the extent of violence that was involved as part of the abuse.

There has been a growing interest among adult survivors of childhood sexual abuse in seeing their previously unpunished molesters prosecuted, as well as in bringing civil damage lawsuits against their abusers. Because these recovering abuse survivors are often in their 20s, 30s, or even older, they face a special burden in filing legal actions: the laws of the state known as statutes of limitations. These statutes place time limits on the period in which both criminal and civil court cases can be commenced. Many of these abuse survivors have held on to the secret of their abuse for years (or they have suppressed the knowledge of it), and recognition of the impact of the abuse has occurred only through psychotherapy.

States generally "toll" (suspend) the statute of limitations during the period that the abused person is a minor (or in some states up to the age of 21); therefore, the permissible period for bringing a legal action—generally 3 to 5 years—begins at age 18, 19, 20, or 21. Many state laws have lengthened the period of time after the sexual abuse occurred in which an alleged survivor can begin a court action. However, the greater the number of years between the alleged abuse and the time of the court action, the more difficult it will be to convince a district attorney to prosecute or to convince a jury of the accused's guilt.

Sometimes even this extension of the statute of limitations will be of little use, because, for example, the survivor may now be 27 and the sexual abuse last occurred when she was 12. In such situations, courts have permitted four exceptions to the absolute barring of the lawsuit because of the statute of limitations.

The first is situations in which the person committing the abuse conceals the child's injuries or obstructs the survivor from filing a legal action. The second is cases in which a lawsuit was not filed as a result of duress from the person committing the abuse, such as death threats made against the person being abused if she seeks legal relief. The third is cases in which the survivor of abuse has remained under a severe mental disability that prevented him from functioning at all in society and thus pursuing his legal remedies. The fourth exception, and the most common (and controversial) one, involves claims that the abused person was unable to discover her injury because of its inherently unknowable nature or because of subconscious repression. Attorneys for such survivors have begun to use the psychological concept of *delayed discovery* in childhood sexual abuse lawsuits. States are increasingly amending their laws so that the statute of limitations begins to run only from the time of the "discovery" of the abuse (or the date that the survivor should have discovered that the abuse occurred). Increasingly, judges are being asked to rule that the statute of limitations period should begin to run only from the date on which the survivor himself recognized facts that he long ago allegedly suppressed in his memory.

Despite this psychiatric theory, and the fact that delayed lawsuits by alleged survivors of childhood sexual abuse are on the rise, relatively few adult incest survivors have been successful in litigating their civil childhood molestation claims against parents or other family members. The most common barrier, in the absence of laws addressing this problem, has been the affirmative defense of the lapse of the statute of limitations. A more basic problem has been that even if the court allows the lawsuit to proceed, few old cases of sexual abuse will include corroborative evidence, such as medical records, testimony of witnesses or other persons documented to have been abused, or written admissions by those who committed the abuse.

## ▌ Guidance for Mental Health Professionals and Practitioners

One issue that will continue to be at the forefront of the delayed-discovery legal claims is the validity of such recollections. There is much debate in the scientific community about whether allegedly long-suppressed memories are accurate or whether they could have been planted in a patient's mind by therapists or other family members. Some memories may have surfaced through the use of hypnosis, and although this evidence would probably be barred in a criminal case, it is more likely to be allowed in a civil lawsuit.

Mental health professionals are likely to be called as expert witnesses to testify about the reliability of the disclosure of allegedly long-suppressed sexual abuse. They may be asked for opinions about whether it is possible to convincingly fabricate detailed memories of alleged childhood molestation experiences. They may be asked to explain why such memories are repressed or otherwise unavailable. They may be asked to provide a summary of the findings of related scientific research on the reliability of long-term memory and the ability of interviewers or therapists to exercise the power of suggestibility over a vulnerable individual. These are subjects about which there is likely to be considerable professional disagreement for many years to come. (See Appendix H for legal resources.)

# References

American Medical Association: Violence against women, relevance for medical practitioners. Council on Scientific Affairs, JAMA 267:3184–3195, 1992

American Psychiatric Association: Diagnostic and Statistical Manual of Mental Disorders, 3rd Edition. Washington, DC, American Psychiatric Association, 1980

American Psychiatric Association: Diagnostic and Statistical Manual of Mental Disorders, 3rd Edition, Revised. Washington, DC, American Psychiatric Association, 1987

American Psychiatric Association: Diagnostic and Statistical Manual of Mental Disorders, 4th Edition. Washington, DC, American Psychiatric Association, 1994

Balmary M: Psychoanalyzing Psychoanalysis. Baltimore, MD, Johns Hopkins University Press, 1979

Bass E, Davis L: The Courage to Heal. New York, Harper & Row, 1988

Beck J, van der Kolk B: Reports of childhood incest and current behavior of chronically hospitalized psychotic women. Am J Psychiatry 144:1474–1476, 1987

Berger A, Knutson J, Mehm J, et al: The self-report of punitive childhood experiences among young adults and adolescents. Child Abuse Negl 12:251–262, 1988

Bergmann M, Jucovy M: Generations of the Holocaust. New York, Basic Books, 1982

Braun B: Dissociative disorders as a sequel to incest, in Incest-Related Syndromes of Adult Psychopathology. Edited by Kluft R. Washington, DC, American Psychiatric Press, 1990, pp. 227–446

Braun B: Treatment of Multiple Personality Disorder. Washington, DC, American Psychiatric Press, 1986

Briere J, Runtz M: Symptomatology associated with childhood sexual abuse in a nonclinical adult sample. Child Abuse Negl 12:51–59, 1988

Briere J: Therapy for Adults Molested as Children: Beyond Survival. New York, Springer, 1989

Brown G, Anderson B: Psychiatric morbidity in adult inpatients with childhood histories of sexual and physical abuse. Am J Psychiatry 148:55–61, 1991

Bryer J, Nelson B, Miller J, et al: Childhood sexual and physical abuse as factors in adult psychiatric illness. Am J Psychiatry 144:1426–1430, 1987

Carmen E, Reiker P, Mills T: Victims of violence and psychiatric illness. Am J Psychiatry 141:378–383, 1984

Chu J: The revictimization of adult women with histories of child abuse. Journal of Psychotherapy Practice and Research 1:259–269, 1992a

Chu J: The therapeutic roller coaster: dilemmas in the treatment of child abuse survivors. Journal of Psychotherapy Practice and Research 1:351–371, 1992b

Chu J, Dill D: Dissociative symptoms in relation to childhood physical and sexual abuse. Am J Psychiatry 147:887–892, 1990

Craine L, Henson C, Colliver J, et al: Prevalence of a history of sexual abuse among female psychiatric patients in a state hospital. Hosp Community Psychiatry 39:300–304, 1988

Dill D, Chu J, Grob M, et al: The reliability of abuse history reports: a comparison of two inquiry formats. Compr Psychiatry 32:166–169, 1991

Elliott D, Briere J: Sexual abuse trauma among professional women: validating the Trauma Symptom Checklist-40 (TSC-40). Child Abuse Negl 16:391–398, 1992

Finkelhor D: Child Sexual Abuse: New Theory and Research. New York, Free Press, 1984

Forward S: Toxic Parents. New York, Bantam, 1990

Gelinas D: The persisting negative effects of incest. Psychiatry 46:312–332, 1983

Gomez-Schwartz B, Horowitz J, Cardarelli A: Child Sexual Abuse: The Initial Effects. Newbury Park, CA, Sage, 1990

Goodwin J: Post-traumatic symptoms in incest victims, in Post-traumatic Stress Disorder in Children. Edited by Eth S, Pynoos RS. Washington, DC, American Psychiatric Press, 1985, pp 155–168

Goodwin J: Post-traumatic symptoms in abused children. Journal of Traumatic Stress 1:475–488, 1988

Goodwin J: Sexual Abuse: Incest Victims and Their Families. Chicago, IL, CV Mosby-Yearbook, 1989

Goodwin J: Rediscovering Childhood Trauma: Historical Casebook and Clinical Applications. Washington, DC, American Psychiatric Press, 1993

Goodwin J, Attias R, McCarty T, et al: Reporting by adult psychiatric inpatients of childhood sexual abuse. Am J Psychiatry 145:1183, 1988

Goodwin J, Cheeves K, Connell V: Borderline and other severe symptoms in adult survivors of extreme incestuous abuse. Psychiatric Annals 20:22–32, 1990

Goodwin J, Wilson N, Connell V: Natural history of severe symptoms in borderline women treated in an incest group. Dissociation 5:221–226, 1992

Havens L: Participant Observation. New York, Jason Aronson, 1976

Herman J: Father-Daughter Incest. Cambridge, MA, Harvard University Press, 1981

Herman J, Perry J, van der Kolk B: Childhood trauma in borderline personality disorder. Am J Psychiatry 140:490–495, 1989

Herman J, Russell D, Trocke K: Long-term effects of incestuous abuse in childhood. Am J Psychiatry 143:1293–1296, 1986

Herman J, Schatzow E: Recovery and verification of memories of childhood sexual trauma. Psychoanalytic Psychology 4:1–4, 1987

Herman J: Complex PTSD: a syndrome in survivors of prolonged and repeated trauma. Journal of Traumatic Stress 5:377–391, 1992

Jacobson A: Physical and sexual assault histories among psychiatric outpatients. Am J Psychiatry 146:755–758, 1989

Jacobson A, Richardson B: Assault experiences of 100 psychiatric inpatients: evidence of the need for routine inquiry. Am J Psychiatry 144:908–913, 1987

Kalff DM: Sandplay. Boston, MA, Sigo, 1980

Khan M: Introduction, in Through Pediatrics to Psychoanalysis: Collected Papers. Edited by Winnicott DW. New York, Basic Books, 1975, pp i–xxx

Kleiman D: A Deadly Silence. New York, Atlantic, 1988

Klein M: The Psychoanalysis of Children. London, Hogarth Press, 1950

Lebowitz L, Harvey M, Herman J: A stage-by-dimension model of recovery from sexual trauma. Journal of Interpersonal Violence 8:378–391, 1993

Lewis DO, Moy E, Jackson LD, et al: Biopsychosocial characteristics of children who later murder: a prospective study. Am J Psychiatry 142:1161–1167, 1985

Miller A: Prisoners of Childhood: The Drama of the Gifted Child and the Search for the True Self. New York, Basic Books, 1981

Miller A: Thou Shalt Not Be Aware: Society's Betrayal of the Child. New York, Meridian, 1984

Modell A: Other Times, Other Realities: Toward a Theory of Psychoanalytic Treatment. Cambridge, MA, Harvard University Press, 1990

Oliver J: Successive generations of child maltreatment. Br J Psychiatry 153:543–553, 1988

Perry J, Herman J, van der Kolk B, et al: Psychotherapy and psychological trauma in borderline personality disorder. Psychiatric Annals 20:33–43, 1990

Putnam FW: Diagnosis and Treatment of Multiple Personality Disorder. New York, Guilford, 1989

Ross CA: Multiple Personality Disorder. New York, Wiley, 1989

Russell D: The Secret Trauma: Incest in the Lives of Girls and Women. New York, Basic Books, 1986

Rutter M: Developmental psychopathology: issues and perspectives, in Depression in Young People. Edited by Rutter M, Izard CE, Read PB. New York, Guilford, 1985, pp 3–37

Saunders B, Villeponteaux L, Lipovsky J, et al: Child sexual assault as a risk factor for mental disorders among women: a community survey. Journal of Interpersonal Violence 7:189–204, 1992

Saxe G, van der Kolk B, Berkowitz R, et al: Dissociative disorders in psychiatric inpatients. Am J Psychiatry 150:1037–1042, 1993

Scurfield RM: Post-trauma stress assessment and treatment overview and formulations, in Trauma and Its Wake: The Study and Treatment of Post Traumatic Stress Disorder. Edited by Figley CR. New York, Brunner/Mazel, 1985, pp 219–256

Shengold L: Soul Murder: The Effects of Childhood Abuse and Deprivation. New Haven, CT, Yale University Press, 1989

Spitzer R, Pelcovitz D, Kaplan S: Disorders of extreme stress. Paper presented at the 142nd annual meeting of the American Psychiatric Association, San Francisco, CA, May 1989

Stover E, Nightingale E: The Breaking of Bodies and Minds. New York, Freeman, 1985

Straus M, Gelles R: Societal change and change in family violence from 1975 to 1985 as revealed by two national surveys. Journal of Marriage and the Family 48:465–479, 1986

Straus M, Gelles R, Steinmetz S: Behind Closed Doors. New York, Anchor, 1980

Summit R: The child sexual abuse accommodation syndrome. Child Abuse Negl 7:177–193, 1983

Terr L: Children of Chowchilla. Psychoanal Study Child 34:547–623, 1979

Terr L: Childhood traumas: an outline and overview. Am J Psychiatry 148:10–20, 1991

van der Kolk B: Psychological Trauma. Washington, DC, American Psychiatric Press, 1987

van der Kolk B, Perry J, Herman J: Childhood origins of self destructive behavior. Am J Psychiatry 148:1665–1671, 1991

Volkan V: Six Steps in the Treatment of Borderline Personality Organization. Northvale, NJ, Jason Aronson, 1987

Williams LM: Adult memories of chldhood sexual abuse: preliminary findings from a longitudinal study. The Advisor 5:19–21, 1992

Wyatt GE: The sexual abuse of Afro-American and White American women in childhood. Child Abuse Negl 9:507–519, 1986

Wyatt G, Powell G: Lasting Effects of Child Sexual Abuse. Newbury Park, Sage, 1988

Yesavage J, Werner P, Becker J, et al: Inpatient evaluation of aggression in psychiatric patients. J Nerv Ment Dis 169:299–302, 1981

Zimrin H: A profile of survival. Child Abuse Negl 10:339–349, 1986

# CHAPTER 8

## Memories of Childhood Trauma: Therapeutic Considerations for Assessment and Treatment

*Stephen J. Ceci, Ph.D.*
*Maggie Bruck, Ph.D.*

In recent years there has been an outpouring of mass-allegation day care cases, the first and best known of which was the McMartin Preschool case in Manhattan Beach, California. Since McMartin, there have been mass-allegation day care cases in virtually every United States city of any size. A number of these cases have been the subject of television and print media accounts (e.g., the Kelly Michael case in New Jersey; The Country Walk case in Miami, FL; the Little Rascals case in Edenton, NC; the Akiki case in San Diego, CA; the Fijnje case in Florida). Cases such as these, though differing from each other in some respects, present a similar galaxy of factors relating to children's testimony. In all these cases, as well as hundreds like them, the key witnesses for the prosecution were pre-

This research was supported in part by grants to the first author from the National Institutes of Child Health and Human Development (RO1 HD 25775) and by a grant to the second author from the Natural Sciences and Engineering Research Council. The authors have drawn on several of their past articles in writing the present chapter, particularly a Social Policy Report for the Society for Research in Child Development (Ceci and Bruck 1993b) and an article in the Psychological Bulletin (Ceci and Bruck 1993a).

schoolers at the time the alleged abuse took place; furthermore, their disclosures were not made immediately following the alleged event, but after a long delay. The children's disclosures often were preceded by intensive interviewing, both by professionals (e.g., child protective services [CPS] workers, law enforcement personnel, and therapists) and by nonprofessionals (e.g., parents and grandparents). In all these cases, the children were the only witnesses to the alleged events. Diagnostic physical evidence was lacking, and all the defendants maintained their innocence, even after some codefendants were convicted. The major issue before the jury in all these cases was whether to believe the children.

These cases have changed the course of research and thinking about children's memory as well as research about how to elicit reports of early abuse from adults, how to devise new experimental paradigms, and how to challenge and extend previous research on the reliability of both young children's and adults' statements. In turn, this new research has raised questions and concerns for those who elicit reports from children and adults, including therapists, social workers, and law enforcement professionals.

In this chapter we provide a synopsis of the most recent social science research on the aspect of children's testimony that was at the center of the mass-allegation day care cases: preschoolers' presumed suggestibility. We then present some tentative thoughts about the therapeutic and forensic implications of this research with adults.

## Research on Children's Suggestibility: Past and Present Trends

The scientific study of children's suggestibility dates back nearly a century. A comprehensive review of this research can be found in Ceci and Bruck (1993a), and we do not repeat that analysis here; rather, we highlight some of the more consensual conclusions from this review.

Beginning with the early experiments of Binet and his European colleagues (Binet 1900; Lipmann 1911; Stern 1910; Varendonck 1911), and concluding with empirical studies in the 1920s and 1930s (Messerschmidt 1933; Otis 1924; Sherman 1925), early researchers viewed children as extremely susceptible to leading questions and unable to resist an interviewer's suggestions. Against this background,

M. R. Brown (1926), a legal scholar, wrote, "Create, if you will, an idea of what the child is to hear or see, and the child is very likely to see or hear what you desire" (p. 133).

Although the conclusions of these early researchers were confirmed by studies conducted right up until the 1980s, modern researchers have been ambivalent about generalizing from them to the forensic arena because not a single study in the first 80 years of this century included preschoolers, the fastest-growing age group of witnesses in contemporary United States courts. Since 1980, approximately 30 studies of children's suggestibility have included a preschool sample.

Another basis of ambivalence about the early studies was that most of them involved children's memory for events that were forensically irrelevant. In most of this earlier literature, researchers examined the influences of a single misleading suggestion or a leading question on children's reports of neutral, nonscripted, and often uninteresting events that occurred in a laboratory setting. For example, children would be shown a movie or read a story. Then later they would be asked questions about what happened. Some of these questions would be misleading (e.g., "What color was the boy's hat?" when in fact the boy was not wearing a hat).

A common finding in most of these studies was that there was a correlation between the age of the subject and accurate responses to suggestive or misleading questions; younger children were more prone than older children or than adults to accept the suggestions in misleading questions. Thus, in the example above, younger children would be more likely to reply that the hat was "yellow" or "red," whereas older children or adults would be more likely to reply that the boy was not wearing a hat. Although these results may be important for theoretical reasons, they have limited practical and legal relevance to cases in which the child is a participant rather than a bystander. They also have limited relevance to cases in which the child is involved in repeated interviews that are highly suggestive and in which the child is asked to recall salient, emotionally charged, and highly stressful events—such as sexual molestation—rather than peripheral events.

Recently a number of researchers have developed new paradigms containing some important elements of the contexts that bring child witnesses to court. This section includes discussion of two major lines of recent research, each of which illustrates a different paradigm: increasing the salience of the experienced events about which children will be interviewed, and increasing the salience of interviewing techniques. A third important line of recent research, the use of anatomically detailed dolls, is the topic of a study described within the topic of increasing the salience of interviewing techniques.

## ▌ Increasing the Salience of Events

As discussed above, earlier studies were not forensically relevant, because they did not examine how children respond to questions about events that involved their own bodies or about other salient events that occurred in personally experienced and stressful situations. In response, a number of researchers have designed studies in which children are asked misleading questions about being touched during different types of medical procedures.

For example, Saywitz et al. (1991) examined 5- and 7-year-old girls' memories of medical examinations. Half of each age group had a scoliosis exam, and the other children had a genital exam. Some children were interviewed 1 week later, some 4 weeks later; all were asked suggestive and nonsuggestive questions that were related to abuse (e.g., "How many times did the doctor kiss you?") or not related to abuse (e.g., "Didn't the doctor look at your feet first?"). Although the older children were initially more accurate than the younger children on most questions, some of these age differences disappeared after the 4-week delay. Most important, although there were age differences in response to the suggestive abuse questions, very few children of either age gave incorrect responses; the 7-year-old children never made a false report of abuse, and the 5-year-olds did so only 4 times, although they were given 215 opportunities.

Saywitz et al. (1991) concluded that children's inaccurate reports involved mainly errors of omission rather than of commission. The majority of children in the genital examination condition did not disclose genital contact unless asked specific questions about this (e.g., "Did the doctor touch you here?"). In the scoliosis condition, when children were asked such specific questions, 2.86% of them falsely affirmed vaginal touch and 5.56% falsely affirmed anal touch. In reviewing this study, Goodman and Clarke-Stewart (1991) conclude that

> Obtaining accurate testimony about sexual abuse from young children is a complex task. Part of the complexity rests in the fact that

there are dangers as well as benefits in the use of leading questions with children. The benefits appear in the finding . . . that leading questions were often necessary in order to elicit information from children about actual events they had experienced (genital touching). . . . The children. . . . were generally accurate in reporting specific and personal things that had happened to them. If these results can be generalized to investigations of abuse, they suggest that normal children are unlikely to make up details of sexual acts when nothing abusive happened. They suggest that children will not easily yield to an interviewer's suggestion that something sexual occurred when in fact it did not, especially if nonintimidating interviewers ask questions children can comprehend (pp. 102–103).

Thus, according to researchers such as Goodman and her colleagues, earlier studies of children's suggestibility probably overestimated the extent to which they are suggestible:

There is now no real question that the law and many developmentalists were wrong in their assumption that children are highly vulnerable to suggestion, at least in regard to salient details. Although some developmentalists may be challenged to find developmental differences in suggestibility in increasingly arcane circumstances, as a practical matter who really cares whether 3-year-old children are less suggestible about peripheral details in events that they witnessed than are 4-year-old children? Perhaps the question has some significance for developmental theory, but surely it has little or no meaning for policy and practice in child protection and law (Melton 1992, p. 154).

However, not all reports of children's recollections of medical procedures are consistent with these conclusions. For example, in contrast to the Saywitz et al. (1991) findings that false reports in response to suggestive questions were relatively infrequent, Baker-Ward et al. (1993) and Ornstein et al. (1992) found that when children were later questioned about their memories of a visit to the pediatrician, 3-year-olds were more prone than 6-year-olds to make false claims in response to suggestive questions about silly events involving body contact (e.g., "Did the nurse lick your knee?"). In one study (Gordon et al. 1991), the 3-year-old children's responses to these silly questions was at the level of chance when questioned 12 weeks after their examination. Of course, unlike the Saywitz et al. (1991) study,

Ornstein's studies do not include explicit questions about sexual touching. Later in this chapter, we will discuss some of our own research that does include these types of questions; as will be seen, our results indicate that young children can be quite inaccurate in reporting bodily touching.

## ▌ Increasing the Salience of Interviewing Techniques

Although it is very difficult to create experimental conditions that mimic those present in child witness interviews (stressful episodes, with repeated and suggestive questioning over prolonged periods of time), researchers are beginning to examine how children's reports are influenced by the repetition of suggestions in multiple interviews before and after an event. In addition, researchers have focused on the interviewer and the effects that a particular interviewer's bias may have on the reports elicited from young children. We confine our discussion here to five studies recently carried out with our colleagues at Cornell and McGill universities, because these studies were designed specifically to address these issues; see Ceci and Bruck (1993a) for discussion of additional studies. In focusing on our own studies, we necessarily present a particularized view, colored by our own hypotheses, assumptions, and values.

We designed these studies on the basis of materials collected over the past decade from court transcripts, therapy sessions, and law enforcement interviews involving children in cases similar to the McMartin case, in which there was a strong suspicion of abuse (Ceci and Bruck 1993a; transcripts in Ceci and Bruck 1995). The materials we have collected reveal that a child's first "disclosure" about abuse often occurs when an interviewer pursues a single hypothesis about the basis of the child's difficulties. The bias is conveyed through a number of suggestive interviewing techniques, which include repetition of misleading information, repetition of questions, and stereotype induction. Sometimes in these interviews, anatomically detailed dolls are used to elicit children's reports of abuse. In other cases, the interviewer may use fantasy inductions and "self-empowerment" techniques. Each of these techniques sometimes produces a "disclosure" from the child, which is then pursued in law enforcement, CPS, or therapeutic interviews. In the next sections we summarize studies that examine the effects of some of these components of biased interviewing styles. But first we examine the more general phenomenon of interviewer bias.

## Study 1: The Effect of Interviewer Bias on Children's Reports

Forensic interviews should entail hypothesis testing. Just as scientists try to arrive at the truth by ruling out their rival hypothesis and by attempting to falsify their favored hypothesis (Ceci and Bronfenbrenner 1991; Dawes 1992; Popper 1962), forensic interviewers should also attempt to rule out rival hypotheses, rather than attempting to exclusively confirm favored ones. However, because of situational pressures (e.g., because caseworkers must sometimes make immediate determinations of potential danger to a child), it is impractical for interviewers to attempt to test every conceivable hypothesis. But, as the following study shows, failure to test a rival hypothesis can result in reporting errors.

In this study (Ceci et al., in press), we examined how an interviewer's hypothesis can influence the accuracy of young children's reports. Preschoolers played a game similar to "Simon Says." One month later they were interviewed by a trained social worker. Before the interview, the interviewer was given a written report containing two types of information about the play episode: accurate information and erroneous information. For example, if the event involved one child touching her own stomach and then touching another child's nose, the interviewer would be told that the child touched her own stomach and then touched the other child's toe. The interviewer was not told that some of the information in the report was inaccurate. She was merely told that these actions might have occurred during the play episode. She was asked to conduct an interview to determine what each child could recall about the original play episode. The only instruction given to the interviewer was that she should begin by asking the child for a free narrative of what had transpired and that she should try to avoid all forms of suggestions and leading questions. Otherwise, she was allowed to use any strategies that she felt necessary to elicit the most factually accurate recall from the child.

The information provided on the one-page sheet influenced the interviewer's hypothesis (or beliefs) about what had transpired and powerfully influenced the dynamics of the interview: the interviewer eventually shaped some of the children's reports to make them consistent with her hypothesis, even when it was inaccurate. When the interviewer was accurately informed, the children correctly recalled 93% of all events. However, when she was misinformed, 34% of those 3–4 years old and 18% of those 5–6 years old corroborated one or more events that did not occur but that the interviewer falsely believed had occurred. Interestingly, it was our impression that the children seemed to become more credible as their interviews unfolded. Many children initially stated details inconsistently or reluctantly, but as the interviewer persisted in asking leading questions about nonevents that were consistent with her hypothesis, a significant number of these children abandoned all contradictions and hesitancy and endorsed the interviewer's erroneous hypothesis.

Because the interviewers were trained professionals, we believe that the types of interactions observed in this study may be similar to those occurring in interviews between young children and parents, teachers, and professionals who are not given explicit training in how to generate and test alternative hypotheses. Our review of the materials from some publicized cases, such as McMartin, reveals that professional interviewers often steadfastly stick with one line of inquiry even when children continue to deny that the questioned events ever occurred (for examples see Ceci and Bruck 1995).

## Study 2: The Effects of Stereotype Induction and Repeated Suggestions on Young Children's Reports

What follows is an abbreviated version of a study designed to assess the influence of combining repeated suggestions and a negative stereotype over long periods of time. For ease of exposition, we describe here only two of the experimental conditions in that study.

A stranger named Sam Stone paid a 2-minute visit to preschoolers (ages 3–6) in their day care center (Leichtman and Ceci 1995). Following his visit, the children were asked for details about the visit on 4 different occasions over a 10-week period. On each of these occasions, the interviewer refrained from using suggestive questions; she simply encouraged children to describe Sam Stone's visit in as much detail as possible. One month later, the children were interviewed a fifth time by a new interviewer, who first elicited a free narrative about the visit. Then, using probing questions, she asked about two nonevents, which involved Sam Stone doing something to a teddy bear and a book. In reality, he never touched either item.

When asked in the fifth interview, "Did Sam Stone do anything to a book or a teddy bear?" most children accurately replied "No." Only 10% of the youngest (3- to 4-year-old) children's answers contained claims that Sam Stone did anything to a book or a teddy bear. When asked if they actually saw him do anything to the book or the teddy bear, as opposed to "thinking they saw him do something," or "hearing that he did something," only 5% of their answers contained claims that anything occurred. Finally, when these 5% were gently challenged ("You didn't really see him do anything to the book or the teddy bear, did you?"), only 3% still insisted on the reality of the fictional event. None of the older (5- to 6-year-old) children reported that they had seen Sam Stone do either of the fictional actions.

Another group of preschoolers was presented with a stereotype of Sam Stone before he ever visited their school. This was done to mimic the sort of stereotypes that some child witnesses have acquired about actual defendants. (In actual cases, for example, some children have been told repeatedly that the defendant did "bad things.") Each week, beginning a month prior to the visit, the children in our study were told a new Sam Stone story in which he was depicted as very clumsy. For example: "You'll never guess who visited me last night. [pause] That's right. Sam Stone! And guess what he did this time? He asked to borrow my Barbie and when he was carrying her down the stairs, he tripped and fell and broke her arm. That Sam Stone is always getting into accidents and breaking things!"

Following Sam Stone's visit, these children were interviewed four times over a 10-week period. These interviews contained erroneous suggestions—for example, "When Sam Stone ripped that book, was he being silly or was he angry?" At the last interview, these children were asked for a free narrative about Sam's visit and then were asked probing questions about the two nonevents.

In this final interview, 72% of the youngest preschoolers claimed that Sam Stone did one or both misdeeds, a figure that dropped to 44% when they were asked if they actually saw him do these things. It is important to note that 21% continued to insist that they saw him do these things, even when gently challenged. The older preschoolers, though more accurate, included 11% of children who insisted they saw him do the misdeeds.

Some researchers have stated the opinion that the presence of perceptual details in reports is one of the indicators of an actual memory, as opposed to a confabulated one (Raskin and Yuille 1989;

Schooler et al. 1986). In this study, however, the presence of perceptual details was no assurance that the report was accurate. In fact,
children in the stereotype-plus-suggestion condition produced a surprising number of fabricated perceptual details to embellish their
false accounts of nonevents—for example, claiming that Sam Stone
took the teddy bear into a bathroom and soaked it in hot water before
smearing it with a crayon. The difference in the quality of reports obtained in this study from others in the suggestibility literature may
reflect the conditions under which the reports were obtained. As mentioned earlier, in most past studies, children's erroneous reports were
made in response to a single misleading question, posed after a brief
delay following the event in question. In contrast, in the present study,
children's false reports were a product of repeated erroneous suggestions over a relatively long period of time, coupled with a stereotype
that was consistent with these suggestions.

It is one thing to demonstrate that children can be induced to
make errors and include perceptual details in their reports, but it is
another to show that their faulty reports are convincing to others. To
examine the believability of the children's reports, we showed video-
tapes of their final interview to 119 researchers and clinicians who
work on children's testimonial issues. These researchers and clinicians were told that all the children observed Sam Stone's visit to their
day care centers. They were asked to decide which of the events reported by the children actually took place and then to rate the overall
credibility of each child.

The majority of the professionals were inaccurate. Analyses indicated that these experts—who conduct research on the credibility of
children's reports, provide therapy to children suspected of having
been abused, or carry out law enforcement interviews with children—
generally failed to detect which of the children's claims were accurate,
despite being confident in their judgments. Because so many of the
children claimed that Sam Stone ripped the book, soiled the bear, or
both, it is understandable that many of the experts reasoned that
these events must have transpired. But their overall credibility ratings
of individual children were also highly inaccurate, with the very children who were least accurate being rated as most accurate. We believe
that the highly credible yet inaccurate reports obtained from the children resulted from a combination of repeated interviews with persistent and intense suggestions that built on a set of prior expectations
(i.e., a stereotype). In a similar way, it may become difficult to sepa-

rate credibility from accuracy when children, after repeated interviews, give a formal videotaped interview or testify in court.

## Study 3: Influencing Children's Reports of a Pediatric Visit

In evaluating the reliability of a child witness who reports personally experienced events involving his or her own body, especially when the experience involves some degree of distress, some might argue that the Sam Stone data are not germane. In cases in which the event involves a child's own body, is somewhat stressful, and is predictable, children may be less prone to suggestion than were subjects in the Sam Stone study.

To determine whether children could be misled under such circumstances, we examined the influence of postevent suggestions on children's reports about a pediatric visit in which they were examined (Bruck et al. 1995). The study had two phases. In the first phase, in which 5-year-old children visited their pediatrician for an annual checkup, a male pediatrician examined the child. Then the child met a female research assistant, who talked about a poster that was hanging on the wall in the examining room. Next the pediatrician gave the child an oral polio vaccine and a DPT (diphtheria-pertussis-tetanus) inoculation. Then the research assistant gave the child one of three types of feedback about how the child had acted when receiving the inoculation. One group was given pain-affirming feedback: they were told that it seemed as though the shot really hurt them, but that shots hurt even big kids (hurt condition). A second group was given pain-denying information; these children were told that they had acted as if the shot did not hurt much and that they were really brave (no-hurt condition). Finally, a third group was merely told that the shot was over (neutral condition). After the feedback, the research assistant gave each child a treat and then read the child a story. One week later, a different assistant visited the children and asked them to indicate through the use of various rating scales how much he or she had cried during the shot and how much the shot had hurt.

The children's reports did not differ as a function of feedback condition. Thus, we found that children could not be influenced to make inaccurate reports concerning significant and stressful procedures involving their own bodies. These results are similar in spirit to those of Saywitz et al. (1991), who also provided children with suggestions about stressful, personally experienced events in a single interview and discovered that children can be quite resistant to erroneous suggestions about their own bodies. In the second phase of our study, we reinterviewed the children four more times, approximately a year after the shot. During these interviews, children were provided with repeated suggestions about how they had acted when they received their inoculations. Thus, as in the first phase of the study, some children were told that they were brave when they got their shot, whereas other children were not given any feedback. (For ethical reasons, we provided only "no-hurt" and "neutral" feedback in this phase of the study: we felt that providing "hurt" feedback might induce false or unpleasant memories about visiting the doctor.) When the children were visited for a fourth time and asked to rate how much the shot had hurt and how much they had cried, there were large suggestibility effects. Those who had been repeatedly told that they had acted brave when they had received their inoculation a year earlier reported significantly less crying and less hurt than children who were given no feedback. Thus, these data indicate that under certain circumstances, children's reports of stressful events involving their own bodies can be distorted, under certain circumstances.

In the second phase of this study, we also tried to mislead children about the people who performed various actions during the original inoculation visit. Some children were falsely reminded, on three occasions, that 1 year previously the pediatrician had given them treats, had shown them the poster, and had read them a story. Some children were falsely reminded on three occasions that the research assistant had given them the inoculation and the oral vaccine. Control-group children were merely reminded that "someone" did these things. On the basis of conclusions of other researchers (e.g., Fivush 1993; Melton 1992), it was hypothesized that children should not be suggestible about such important events and that they should be particularly immune to suggestions that incorporate shifts of gender. The male pediatrician had never given them treats or read them a story, and the female research assistant had never performed any medical procedures.

Contrary to these predictions, the children were misled. In the fourth interview, when asked about their doctor's visit in the previous year, 67% of the children (versus 27% of the control-group children) who were given misleading information about the pediatrician reported that the pediatrician showed them the poster, gave them treats, or read them a story. For children who were falsely told that the research assistant had given them the shot and the vaccine, 50% (versus 16% of the control-group children) succumbed to at least one of these two suggestions. Interestingly, 38% of the children who were falsely told that the research assistant gave them both the oral vaccine and the inoculation also said that the research assistant had performed other scripted events that not only had never occurred but also had never been suggested—for example, they reported that the research assistant had checked their ears and nose. None of the control-group children made such inaccurate reports. Thus, our suggestions influenced not only children's reports of personally experienced, salient events, but also their reports of nonsuggested scripted events that were related to the suggested events.

These data indicate that under certain circumstances, children's reports concerning stressful events involving their own bodies can be influenced. The two factors that were most critical to this pattern of results were the intensity of the suggestions (repeating the suggestions over multiple interviews) and the timing of the suggestions (the long delay between the original event and interview about the event). These same two factors are characteristic of the conditions under which children made allegations of sexual abuse in many of the cases described at the beginning of this report.

The results of this study are consistent with the Sam Stone study, even though the nature of the events about which children were misled was different. In the Sam Stone study, repeated suggestions and stereotypes led to convincing fabrications of nonoccurring events. In the pediatrician study, misleading information given in repeated interviews after a long delay following a target event influenced children's reports of personally experienced, salient events.

## Study 4: The Suggestibility of Anatomically Detailed Dolls

Anatomically detailed dolls are frequently used by professionals—including child therapists, police, child protection workers, and attorneys—in interviewing children about suspected sexual abuse. According to recent surveys, 90% of field professionals use anatomically detailed dolls at least occasionally in their investigative interviews with children suspected of having been sexually abused (Boat and Everson 1988; Conte et al. 1991). Although no national figures

are available, it appears that expert testimony is often based on observations of children's interactions with such dolls (Mason 1991). We
include a discussion here of anatomically detailed dolls because a
number of commentators have raised questions about whether the
dolls are suggestive (e.g., McGough 1994; Raskin and Yuille 1989).

One rationale for the use of anatomically detailed dolls is that
they allow children to manipulate objects reminiscent of a sexual
event, thereby cuing recall and overcoming language and memory
problems. Another rationale is that their use is thought to overcome
embarrassment and shyness. The dolls have also been used as projective tests. Some claim that a child's actively avoiding these dolls, showing distress if they are undressed, or showing unusual preoccupation
with their genitalia is consistent with the hypothesis that the child has
been abused (Mason 1991).

The use of anatomically detailed dolls has raised skepticism, however, among researchers and professionals alike. Two related arguments are frequently invoked against their use. The first is that the
dolls are suggestive—that they encourage the child to engage in sexual play even if the child has not been sexually abused (Gardner 1989;
Terr 1988). A child may insert a finger into a doll's genitalia, for instance, simply because of its novelty or availability, much the way a
child may insert a finger into the hole in a doughnut. Another criticism is that it is impossible to make firm judgments about children's
abuse status on the basis of their doll play because there are no normative data on nonabused children's doll play.

In several studies, researchers have compared the doll play of sexually abused and nonabused children. In addition, there have been a score
of studies examining the doll play of nonabused children. Reviews of this
literature (Berry and Skinner 1993; Ceci and Bruck 1993a; Wolfner et al.
1993) indicate that many of the studies are methodologically inadequate
and do not allow for firm interpretations about the potential usefulness
or risks of using dolls. Furthermore, some data indicate that some of the
play patterns thought to be characteristic of abused children, such as
playing with the dolls in a suggestive or explicit sexual manner or showing reticence or avoidance when presented with the dolls, also occur in
samples of nonabused children (see Ceci and Bruck 1995 for a review).
Finally, other data indicate that the dolls, though not suggestive, do not
improve reporting, particularly among younger children (e.g., Goodman
and Aman 1990).

A recent study of 3-year-old children's interactions with anatomically detailed dolls highlights each of these results (Bruck et al. 1995b). The children in this study visited their pediatrician for their annual checkup. The pediatrician conducted genital examinations with half the children; the remaining children did not receive genital examinations. Immediately after the examination, the child was interviewed by a research assistant. Pointing to the buttocks and then to the genital areas of an anatomically detailed doll, the assistant asked each child, "Did the doctor touch you here?" Later in the interview, the child was asked to use the doll to show how the doctor had touched his or her buttocks and genitals.

Children were quite inaccurate across all conditions. Only 45% of the children who received genital examinations correctly answered "Yes" to the question "Did the doctor touch you here [on buttocks or genitals]?" Only 50% of the children who did not receive genital examinations correctly replied "No" to these questions. Further, the children's accuracy did not improve when they were given the dolls and asked to show how the doctor had touched them. Only 25% of the children who had received genital examinations correctly showed how the pediatrician had touched their genitals and buttocks. (A significant number of girls in this condition were inaccurate, because they inserted their fingers into the anal or genital cavities of the dolls—which the pediatrician never did.) Only 45% of the children who did not receive genital examinations were accurate in not showing any touching; that is, 55% of the children who did not receive genital examinations falsely showed either genital or anal touching when given the dolls. This pattern was most prevalent among the girls in this group; 75% of the girls who did not receive a genital examination falsely showed that the pediatrician touched their genitals or their buttocks.

Because the data on the potential usefulness of dolls are equivocal at best, we feel that an important confound in the literature deserves mention: the context for the presentation of the dolls in these research settings is very different from that of actual forensic and clinical settings. Transcripts of therapy sessions with children suspected of having been sexually abused reveal interviewers employing various practices: naming the dolls after defendants; berating the dolls for alleged abuses against the child (e.g., shaking a finger at the male doll who has been named after the defendant, and yelling, "You are naughty for hurting Jennifer!"); assuming the role of fantasy characters in doll play; and creating a persistent atmosphere of accusation. In the research settings in which the use of anatomical dolls has been studied, nonabused children were never subjected to such highly suggestive experiences before being interviewed with the dolls, and they were not given prior motivation to play with the dolls suggestively or aggressively. On the other hand, children who were alleged to have been abused had sometimes been exposed to the dolls repeatedly before coming to the research setting; perhaps these interviews had involved repeated suggestions from parents and interviewers about various sexual themes. That their play with the dolls differed from that of nonabused children who lacked this prior experience could be attributed to the abused children's prior therapeutic or investigatory experiences, rather than to any inherent way in which abused children might be expected to play with the dolls.

Unfortunately, no study has examined the suggestive attributes of anatomical dolls and has controlled for the preexperimental experience as a potentially serious confound. We simply do not know how nonabused children would behave with the dolls were they to have suggestive experiences before the experimental interview. Conversely, we also do not know how abused children play with the dolls in their first investigatory interview, because the children in these studies have often been interviewed more than once, and some have been exposed to the dolls at least once, before the experimental interview.

On the basis of our literature review (Ceci and Bruck 1993a, b), we concluded that the inconsistent findings point to the need for additional research and to the need for the development of explicit procedures to govern the use of anatomically detailed dolls by interviewers. Until such research is available, the dolls ought to be used with great caution. Recently, Berry and Skinner (1993) were even less supportive of doll use, as were Wolfner et al. (1993):

> We are left with the conclusion that there is simply no scientific evidence available that would justify clinical or forensic diagnosis of abuse on the basis of the dolls. The common counter is that such play is "just one component" in reaching such a diagnosis based on a "full clinical" picture. . . . [Doll] play cannot be validly used as a component, however, unless it provides incremental validity, and there is virtually no evidence that it does." (p. 9)

### Study 5: Source Monitoring Errors

Some of the suggestive interviewing techniques that we have described are quite salient; their presence can be easily isolated in transcribed interviews. Less salient and less easily detectable suggestions, however, can also exert a significant influence on children's report accuracy. In this section we focus on source monitoring errors.

Source monitoring is a task that we perform continuously and often unconsciously. It involves identifying the origins of our memories in order to elucidate them or to validate them. For example, it involves remembering when or where an event occurred, identifying the speaker of a remembered utterance, keeping track of who did what, and monitoring the origins of our experiences. Source monitoring generally refers to the monitoring of events that actually occurred. A more specific term, reality monitoring, is used to refer to the determination of whether an event was imagined or real. These are sometimes indistinguishable in cases in which the task involves trying to remember whether something actually happened to us or whether someone said that something happened to us.

Source monitoring was initially studied in the context of adult memories, because adults occasionally misidentify the sources of their recollections. They may, for example, remember someone telling them about an event when in actuality they had read about the event in a newspaper. But recently, a number of developmental psychologists have begun to examine source monitoring in children (Ackil and Zaragoza 1995; Poole and Lindsay 1995). In these studies, children experience an event, then later are told a number of details about the event, some of which did not occur. Later, when asked to recall the details of the original event, subjects often cannot monitor the source of the information; that is, they report that some of the nonoccurring details that were provided after the event actually happened during the event. This effect happens at all ages, but it seems that younger children make disproportionately more of these errors. Some recent work also suggests that these errors are true reflections of confusions; when subjects are warned before their final recall not to believe anything that was said to them after the event because it was not true, they continue to make source errors. And this pattern is most prominent for preschoolers (Lindsay et al., in press).

We wondered what would happen if preschoolers merely were asked to think about some event repeatedly, creating mental images each time they did so. In this fifth and final study, we briefly describe a program of research that involves three separate studies, though we confine our discussion here to only one of them (for details see Ceci et al. 1994a, 1994b). The events that we asked children to think about were both actual events that they experienced (e.g., an accident that required stitches) and fictitious events that they never experienced (e.g., getting their hand caught in a mousetrap and having to go to the hospital to get it removed).

Each week for 10 consecutive weeks, preschool children were individually interviewed by a trained adult. The adult showed the child a set of cards, each containing a different event. The child was invited to pick a card, and the interviewer would read it to the child and ask if the event ever happened to her or him. For example, when the child selected the card that read, "Got finger caught in a mousetrap and had to go to the hospital to get the trap off," the interviewer would ask, "Think real hard, and tell me if this ever happened to you. Can you remember going to the hospital with the mousetrap on your finger?" Each week the interviewer would ask the child to think real hard about each actual and fictitious event, with prompts to visualize the scene.

After 10 weeks of thinking about both real and fictitious events, these preschool children were given a forensic interview by a new adult. All these interviews were videotaped. The interviewer began by gaining rapport with the child, discussing events that were unrelated to the event in question, and giving the child the expectation that the interviewer wanted elaborated answers, not simple yes-or-no ones. Initially, the interviewer asked, "Tell me if this ever happened to you: Did you ever get your finger caught in a mousetrap and have to go to the hospital to get the trap off?" Following the child's reply, the interviewer asked for additional details (e.g., "Can you tell me more?" "What did you see or hear?" "Who was with you?" "How did it feel?"). When the child said that he or she had no additional details, the interviewer asked a number of follow-up questions that were based on the child's answers. For instance, if the child said that she did go to the hospital to get the mousetrap off, the interviewer asked how she got there, who went with her, and what happened at the hospital.

Although we had anticipated that asking children to think about events repeatedly would result in later confusions about whether they actually participated in the events, we had no expectation that this would result in the sort of highly detailed, internally coherent narratives that the children produced. In one study, 58% of the preschool children produced false narratives about one or more of the fictitious events, and 25% of the children produced false narratives about the majority of them. What was so surprising was the elaborateness of the children's narratives. They were very embellished; they would provide an internally coherent account of the context in which their finger got caught in the mousetrap as well as the affect associated with it.

We showed these videos to psychologists who specialize in interviewing children, and the results were sobering: professionals were fooled by the children's narratives. The professionals' opinions were not reliably different from the level of chance at detecting which events were real, because they did not expect that such plausible, internally coherent narratives could be fabricated by such young children. And we think they are right—if by fabrication we mean "a conscious attempt to mislead a listener about the truth as one understands it" (Ceci and Bruck 1993a). We are of the opinion, though we cannot prove it in any scientifically satisfying manner, that many of the children had come to believe what they were telling the interviewer. This is why they were so believable to professionals who watched them. They exhibited none of the telltale signs of duping, teasing, or tricking. They seemed sincere, their facial expressions and affect were appropriate, and their narratives were filled with the kind of low-frequency details that make accounts seem plausible. For example, one child in this study said, "My brother Colin was trying to get Blowtorch [an action figure] from me, and I wouldn't let him take it from me, so he pushed me into the woodpile where the mousetrap was. And then my finger got caught in it. And then we went to the hospital, and my mommy, daddy, and Colin drove me there, to the hospital in our van, because it was far away. And the doctor put a bandage on this finger [indicating]."

As can be seen, this child supplies a plausible account, not simply yes-or-no answers. Such an account might be very believable to someone asked to judge its authenticity.

One further bit of evidence supports our position that at least some of these children had come to believe that they actually experienced the fictitious events. Twenty-seven percent of the children in this study initially refused to accept debriefing, claiming that they remembered the fictitious events happening. When told by their parents that these events never occurred and they were merely imagined, these children often protested, "But it really did happen. I remember it!" Although such insistence in the presence of their parents is not proof that this subset of children believed what they were reporting about fictitious events, it does suggest that they were not duping us for any obvious motive, given that the demand characteristics were all tilted against their making such claims. We are presently pursuing this hypothesis with a new set of experiments.

To sum up, repeatedly thinking about a fictitious event can lead some preschool children to produce vivid, detailed reports that professionals are unable to discern from their reports of actual events. Although clearly the analogy to therapy is imperfect, such a study has relevance for the testimony of a child who has undergone a certain type of therapy for a long time, engaging in similar imagery inductions and "memory work."

## Summary of Current Literature

The five studies reviewed in this chapter highlight different paradigms that researchers are now employing to examine children's suggestibility. In our review of this literature (Ceci and Bruck 1993a), we found that results of the most recent studies, in contrast to older ones, are somewhat more contradictory about the reliability of children's reports. One can locate studies claiming that young children are as immune to suggestion as older children (e.g., Marin et al. 1979; Saywitz et al. 1991) and studies claiming that younger children are more suggestible than older children (Ceci et al. 1987; Cohen and Harnick 1980). Such mixed results have led to a confusing juxtaposition of headlines: "Study shows children are credible as witnesses" contrasted to "Research shows child witnesses unable to distinguish reality from fantasy."

A careful reading of the literature suggests, however, that there are reliable age differences in suggestibility: preschoolers' reports are more influenced by erroneous suggestions than are older children's. In our review of the suggestibility literature, we found 18 studies that compared preschoolers to older children or to adults; in 15 of 18 of these studies, suggestibility was greater among preschoolers than among older children or adults (see Table 2 in Ceci and Bruck 1993a).

To be sure, some researchers attach various caveats to this conclusion. For example, some have claimed that age differences in suggestibility are evident mainly for nonparticipant children (bystanders) (Rudy and Goodman 1991) and for peripheral, nonsalient events (Fivush 1993). And some researchers find that although young children may make some errors on suggestive questions with a sexual theme, on the whole they are highly resistant to such questions (e.g., Goodman et al. 1990; Saywitz et al. 1991). But our review of a fairly substantial literature suggests that young children are at greater risk for suggestion about a wide variety of topics, even those concerning sexual themes (Bruck et al. 1995b; Ceci and Bruck 1995).

Notwithstanding the above conclusion, it is clear that children—even preschoolers—are capable of recalling much that is forensically relevant. For example, as we have shown with some of our own studies, children in the control group recalled events flawlessly, indicating that the absence of suggestive techniques allows even very young preschoolers to provide highly accurate reports. There are a number of other studies that highlight the strengths of young children's memories (see Goodman et al. 1992 for a review). What characterizes many such studies is the neutral tone of the interviewer, the limited use of misleading questions (suggestions being limited to a single condition, if they are used at all), and the absence of the induction of any stereotype or any motive for the child to make a false report. When such conditions are present, it is a common (although not a universal) finding that children are much more immune to suggestive influences, particularly about sexual details.

It is also important to stress that even though suggestibility effects may be robust for younger children, they are not inevitable. Results sometimes vary dramatically between studies, and children's behaviors sometimes vary dramatically within studies. Thus, even in studies with significant suggestibility effects, there are always some children who are highly resistant to suggestion. We have seen this in our own studies as well as in transcripts of forensic and therapeutic interviews. In some cases, no matter how much an interviewer may try to erroneously suggest that a false event occurred, some children will consistently resist and not incorporate the interviewer's suggestion or point of view. On the other hand, although suggestibility effects tend to be most dramatic after prolonged and repeated interviewing, some children incorporate suggestions quickly, even after one short interview (e.g., Clarke-Stewart et al. 1989, as reported in Goodman and Clarke-Stewart 1991).

Although preschoolers are usually depicted as being the most suggestible, it is important to point out that older children and adults are also suggestible. For example, as described above, 7-year-olds' reports, after 1 year, of their visits to the pediatrician could be quite easily altered through suggestion. Clarke-Stewart et al. (1989), as reported in Goodman and Clarke-Stewart (1991), also found that 7-year-old children's reports and interpretations of a recently experienced event could be easily manipulated through suggestion. Also, Goodman et al. (1989) found that a substantial number of 7- to 10-year-old children incorrectly agreed with interviewers' suggestions about details of an event that had occurred 4 years earlier. Many of these misleading suggestions had sexual themes. Finally, suggestions can alter some fundamental aspects of adults' autobiographical memories (Loftus 1993). Thus, we cannot conclude that older children and adults are not suggestible, only that their level of suggestibility is less than that of preschoolers.

We reiterate, however, that the conditions created in these studies differ markedly from those that occur in actual therapy or in law enforcement investigations: these latter two contexts are seldom as sanitized of affect and free of motives as those in the research setting. The real-life situation may entail high levels of stress, assaults to the child's body, and loss of control. In some cases, children are interviewed and reinterviewed under emotionally charged circumstances, entailing the use of bribes and threats, and often in the presence of highly distressed parents; under such conditions, some children may finally utter reports that are simply consistent with the interviewer's expectations. In the McMartin case, interviewers were alleged to have coerced children's statements by praising them when they reported events that were consistent with the interviewer's beliefs and criticizing them for failing to do so (e.g., calling them "dumb"). Interviewers in both this case and other day care cases also told children that other children had already disclosed the details of the abuse, thus creating added pressure to assent to suggestions of abuse. Not surprisingly, interviewers in the McMartin case managed to elicit statements of abuse from 369 of nearly 400 children they interviewed (Sauer 1993), although only one child had made claims of abuse prior to the interviews. (This girl's accusations were so bizarre that the prosecution dropped them from the case [Sauer 1993].)

Elsewhere, we and others have used more emotionally laden events to examine issues related to the role of affect and bodily touching in producing misinformation effects, including suggestions about being kissed while naked, witnessing parents violating norms and hurting others to protect loved ones (see Ceci et al. 1993), and experiencing painful and/or embarrassing medical procedures (e.g., Goodman 1993; Ornstein et al. 1993). Although children's resistance to suggestions are sensitive to all these factors (and others), no study has attempted to incorporate all these factors into a single experiment.

It is highly unlikely, however, that we will ever mimic the assaultive nature of some acts or interviews that are experienced by children who have been abused or who have witnessed abuse. Thus we are far from being able to provide a definitive conclusion about the reliability of all child witnesses' reports. It is safe to conclude, however, that past pronouncements by some rather extreme advocates on both sides are simply unfounded. Children are neither as hypersuggestible and coachable as some prodefense advocates have alleged, nor as resistant to suggestions about their own bodies as some proprosecution advocates have claimed. They can be led, under certain conditions, to incorporate false suggestions into their accounts of even intimate bodily touching, but they can also be amazingly resistant to false suggestions and able to provide highly detailed and accurate reports of events that transpired weeks or months before. This mix of suggestibility and resistance to suggestion underscores the need for great caution in accepting the claims of those who would put either a prodefense or proprosecution spin on the data.

## Relationship Between Research and Clinical Practice

In this section we provide five examples of clinical practice concerning the interviewing of young children and evaluate these in light of the research that we have presented in this chapter. The purpose of this exercise to is show that there are some areas in which a clear disjunction exists between research and clinical practice, that there are some areas that call for a balance between science and humanitarian concerns, and finally that there are some areas in which some emerging research suggests how clinicians might cautiously use certain types of interview techniques.

Two examples illustrate this breach between the two perspectives. The first involves a survey of 212 mental health professionals about their assessment and validation procedures in sexual abuse cases (Conte et al. 1991). It was found that children had already been asked to tell their story an average of 2.3 times before talking to the professionals who were surveyed; only 27% of the respondents stated that they were the first person to talk with the child about the abuse. In discussing these findings, however, the authors do not seriously consider the impact of such interviewing practices:

> Little is currently known about the effects of such prior interviewing on the child's willingness to engage with yet another adult or on the quality of information obtained from the child. Although some professionals are likely to make much of the possible "contamination" that these prior interviewers have on the child's reports, there are virtually no data currently available suggesting that adults have the power through interviewing techniques to alter fundamentally a child's understanding of and ability to describe what events did or did not take place (Conte et al. 1991, p. 433).

We hope that work such as this chapter will inform clinicians that such data are available and that clinicians should carefully consider the degree to which interviewing practices may taint the report of their child clients.

A second example that illustrates the gulf between practice and research concerns the use of anatomically detailed dolls. Many professionals have no formal training or experience in the use of the dolls (Boat and Everson 1988) and may view some interactions of children with the dolls (e.g., placing a finger in the doll's anal cavity, tugging on its penis, or avoiding the dolls altogether) as indicative of sexual abuse even though there is no scientific support that such interactions are diagnostic of abuse. In a recent survey, for example, only 16% of mental health and law professionals stated that avoidance of the dolls was normal, and 80% rated digital penetration as abnormal (Kendall-Tackett 1991). Yet, as reviewed above, such behaviors are commonly observed in nonabused children.

Of more concern, perhaps, is the position of the American Psychological Association (APA) (1991) on the use of the dolls. The following statement was issued by APA's Council of Representatives:

> Neither the dolls nor their use are standardized or accompanied by normative data. . . . We urge continued research in quest of more and better data regarding the stimulus properties of such dolls and normative behavior of abused and nonabused children. . . . Nevertheless, doll-centered assessment of children, when used as part of a psychological evaluation and interpreted by experienced and competent examiners, may be the best available practical solution for a pressing and frequent clinical problem. (p. 1)

The APA's policy position seems contradictory in that it notes first that there are no standardized methods for doll interviews or normative data on nonabused or abused children's doll play but then asserts that experienced interviewers may nevertheless find doll-centered assessment the best available method for evaluating children suspected of sexual abuse. Even if one assumes that experienced examiners can avoid making false inferences from children's doll play and that such doll play can provide important clinical insights not obtainable from other sources, the APA should nevertheless codify this expert knowledge in such a way that researchers can accurately assess the incremental validity of doll-based assessments. Our reading of the literature is that at present such knowledge is more illusory than real. (See Wolfner et al.'s criticism [1993] of the lack of incremental validity of doll-based assessments.) Even if anatomical dolls are used as just one part of an assessment, other aspects of so-called developmentally sensitive assessments (e.g., play therapy, role-playing, techniques that induce visually guided imagery, self-empowerment training) may interact with the doll use to produce false positive assertions of abuse. Because the appropriate research has yet to be done, it is shortsighted to assume that the dolls do not present reliability risks. Although it could be the case that the use of dolls does provide important information, it could also be the case that this method leads to unacceptable levels of false positive reports. Only further research will tell.

Next we consider the implication for clinical practice of the studies on source monitoring errors. In many of the cases of alleged child sexual abuse that we have reviewed, children were in counseling for months or even years before testifying in a courtroom. Records of these therapy sessions, where they exist, document repeated imagery inductions, enjoinders to think hard, and repeated encouragement to reenact events with props. Some therapists asked the children to do "homework" or journal writing. These children were encouraged to go home and try to think "very hard" about some of the things that were difficult to talk about. Judging by the results of our studies in which children were simply asked to think about nonevents for a period of time, these therapeutic techniques raise some concerns.

Certainly our cataloguing of these techniques is a sensitive issue, because it raises in some people's minds the possibility that children who are repeatedly exposed to such techniques cannot be believed. Such a conclusion would, we believe, be premature until it can be demonstrated that children are this susceptible to source misattributions about sexual events. And even if they are just as vulnerable to such suggestions about sexual events, it does not mean that their claims are inevitably false, but only that they could be. For example, if a therapist simply asks a young child to think about certain events that may be beyond the experience and comprehension of children of that age, and if the child does come to produce a coherent, logical story, then perhaps the child is in fact faithfully reporting a memory.

But we also believe that the risk of using these techniques could be minimized under certain circumstances. If therapists regularly challenge children to make sure that they are telling the truth, and to check their own memories while engaging in visualization techniques, then again we might have some more faith in the validity of the child's report.

The worry is that these safeguards are not always attended to. Asking a child repeatedly to think about the time when he was abused, or to think about whether she was abused, is often used in concert with an array of other suggestive techniques (e.g., play therapy). These additional suggestive techniques may provide the details or the script for the child's emerging false memories. So we would not expect most 3-year-olds to have sufficient knowledge to describe oral-genital contacts if they are merely asked to repeatedly think about if someone touched them in a funny way. However, if this request is accompanied by a host of leading questions, then visually guided imagery may have a profound influence on the accuracy of the children's recall.

A second worry is that therapists and interviewers are often instructed not to challenge the authenticity of children's reports—that doing so will drive the child's emerging reports back underground. This is a sensitive issue, too, because frontline workers know from experience that the surest way to get a child to recant a disclosure is to express distrust or disdain. One must take seriously everything the child says. But there is a difference between taking a child seriously and believing everything the child says. No parents believe everything their child says, although most of us take our children's statements seriously. One can gently challenge the authenticity of a child's statement without calling into question the child's veracity. For example, one can say to a child who has made a disclosure after suggestive techniques: "OK, now let's talk about what really happened, OK? Now you must tell me only about the things that really happened, and not about the things that were only pretend."

Therapists who engage in such techniques are concerned that

some of their clients could develop elaborate pseudomemories that may not be detected as false by professionals. Clients are mistaken if they believe that a therapist, by virtue of clinical training, research acumen, or deep knowledge of the sequelae of childhood sexual abuse, can distinguish between accurate and inaccurate reports after the client has been put through relentless suggestions. If a child has been persistently rehearsed with suggestive techniques over long periods of time, there is no way one can be sure that the child's memory is genuine as opposed to co-constructed. This is particularly true if the child originally denied the reality of such memories. Simply put, there is no "Pinocchio Test"; the child's nose does not grow longer as the child's reports become less accurate.

Finally we discuss a dilemma whose resolution may ultimately involve balancing scientific and humanitarian concerns. Therapists face many dilemmas and choices in providing for children who may have been sexually abused. Often the favored treatment may conflict with forensic procedures. Let us take one example: how should a therapist proceed with a child client when there is reason to believe that this child may be asked to testify in a trial about matters that may be the subject of therapy (e.g., the sexual abuse)? Should the therapist withhold treatment until the forensic interviews are completed and the trial is over? On humanitarian grounds, many would argue against withholding treatment, particularly considering the slow pace of criminal justice proceedings: often children's sexual abuse cases may come to trial 1 to 3 years after the initial allegation.

Take the case of a child who has been removed from her home as a result of a report of sexual abuse and has been placed in emergency foster care, separated from her family, friends, and school. The child is greatly distressed and in need of immediate counseling. Are we to make this child languish in a strange family, community, and school for weeks, months, or years before providing mental health services?

In light of some research findings that children's reports are likely to be more accurate if interviews (which include therapy sessions) concerning the alleged abuse are held to a minimum until after the forensic interview takes place, when should the mental health professional begin therapy with the child? How can we avoid the twin dangers of, on the one hand, putting the child's emotional needs on hold until after the forensic interviews are completed, and, on the other hand, providing counseling that can be potentially damaging to the veracity of the child's report? We know of no easy answers.

Given the pressing needs of both sides in a criminal dispute to prepare, investigate, and often reinterview, no amount of child-friendly court procedures can totally alleviate some of the problems associated with children's testimony. Yet perhaps there are ways of providing therapeutic support that lessen the likelihood of tainting the child's report. Based on what we now know, it would be imprudent to use fantasy inductions, imagery play, and memory work during therapy sessions conducted before the completion of forensic interviews. These practices can be saved for after the legal resolution. Before that, perhaps therapy could be restricted to working on everyday coping strategies that cannot be challenged by the defendant's counsel as creating false memories. This would seem to be a reasonable compromise, one that provides needed mental health support to the child but minimizes potentially suggestive practices.

Although some might argue that it would be too restrictive and ultimately damaging to a child's development if therapists were to avoid potentially suggestive techniques, it could also be argued that employing such interventions simply constitutes too great a risk. On the one hand, if the defendant is innocent, such techniques could promote and reinforce false allegations. On the other hand, if the defendant is guilty, the use of such techniques may be invoked to discredit the child's testimony: defense attorneys may argue that the child's reports are the product of highly suggestive therapeutic practices. Finally, on the empirical side, we are unaware of any persuasive treatment-outcome validity research indicating that suggestive techniques are necessary in therapy to achieve a positive mental health outcome for children suspected of being abused. Therefore, until mental health professionals can demonstrate that these techniques are critical before the legal resolution of a case, the costs of using them would seem to outweigh their presumed benefits. Given this state of knowledge, therapists might consider limiting their interventions to nonsuggestive techniques until young clients have given sworn statements; such an approach may afford maximal protection for everyone, including the child.

## Implications for Recovered Memories in Adulthood

So far, we have addressed issues that are exclusively concerned with children's memories of childhood events. But what about an adult's retrieval of her childhood memories? Articles have appeared about the comedienne Roseanne Barr's alleged retrieval of memories of her abuse at the age of 6 months, and there are many other accounts of so-called repressed or dissociated memories of childhood abuse. What does the research on children's recollections have to say about the validity of such claims? This is a complicated issue, and we deal with it in some detail elsewhere (see Ceci and Bruck 1995). Here we provide only the basic syllogism and part of the argument.

When known abuse occurs during the first few years of life, but is never recalled, this does not logically lead to the conclusion that the memory was repressed. Rather, when events occur during this early period, or before the offset of infantile amnesia, we would expect these early experiences to be unrecallable, whether they are positive or negative. It may be beyond adult ability to resurrect the world of the 1-year-old or the 2-year-old, because the cognitive and neurophysiological architecture that was responsible for recording such memories in infancy is so unlike the architecture that guides the adult's retrieval of memories. As Sugar (1992) and others have argued, it may be possible for an adult to resurrect an image from the age of 18 months (e.g., of one's mother standing next to a pool of blood on the floor), but the interpretation given to that image at age 18 months may be one of undifferentiated anxiety, whereas the adult interpretation—that it was blood associated with the mother's miscarriage—is "back-propagated" from an advanced developmental architecture that was unavailable to the young child.

This presents a problem for those of us charged with helping clients retrieve memories of childhood events. How do we do it in a manner that avoids tainting the memory or, worse yet, completely constructing it?

Many therapists appear to have bought into the following set of assumptions: 1) childhood sexual abuse is traumatagenic, 2) it causes the memory to split off from the rest of cognitive and affective processing and as a result to be inaccessible until such time when the individual feels safe enough to make contact with the buried memory, and 3) the early trauma, though buried, nevertheless results in some symptoms that eventually bring the individual into therapy. As a result of these assumptions, there is a tendency to dig for such memories as answers to the current symptomatological riddle.

Putting aside the flimsy evidentiary basis for this chain of assumptions, we need to ask what the impact of digging will be, especially in light of the studies that were described earlier. Even if it is possible to resurrect memories of childhood abuse by using various forms of memory work—such as visually guided imagery, hypnosis, Amytal and Brevital interviews, repeated suggestions, role playing, self-empowerment training, and so on—it may also be the case that such techniques result in the construction of pseudomemories, particularly when they are used repeatedly over long periods of time. Given the legal implications of such recovered memories, it behooves a therapist to do everything possible to ensure that such "memories" are accepted as valid only when there is excellent evidence for doing so. There is no substitute for corroboration in its various forms. No symptom pattern, abreaction, or vivid imagery should suffice to convince us that the memory is real, at least not to the point of supporting a client's legal arguments. Roseanne Barr deeply believes her memories of abuse by her mother at age 6 months to be real; she can "see" the abuse vividly, and such abuse is consistent with her clinical presentation. Yet, if we had to testify about such memories, we would have to tell the court that they are almost surely pseudomemories, produced by repeated visualization exercises, both in and outside therapy. There is no credible scientific evidence that experiences in the first 6 months of life are accessible to conscious reconstruction during adulthood; there is considerable evidence that such "memories" can be fashioned out of memory work techniques.

Hence, although we must strive to uncover abuse, we must eschew interview processes that may promote false beliefs, fantasies, or fabrications—regardless of the nature of the initiating event. Earlier we argued that it is unethical for social scientists to institute experimental manipulations that might change the fundamental nature of children's emotionally salient autobiographical memories; in closing, we can extend this same argument to the case of constructing pseudomemories in therapy. It is just as indefensible for therapists or forensic interviewers to create such changes to one's autobiographies. The results of persistent erroneous suggestions and of failures to test alternative hypotheses can be lasting and haunting, as evidenced by the experiences and reactions of the child witnesses in the McMartin trials, described at the beginning of this report:

> No one who saw them will soon forget the frenzied faces of . . .
> former McMartin pupils [who] had spent their last six years—fully
> half their lives—instructed in the faith that they had been sub-

jected, at ages 4 and 5, to unspeakable sexual horrors; this belief they had come to hold as the defining truth of their lives and identities. It is not surprising that these children should have wept and raved when the verdict was handed down denying all that they believed in (Rabinowitz 1990, p. 63).

# References

Ackil JA, Zaragoza M: Developmental differences in eyewitness suggestibility and memory for source. J Exp Child Psychol 60:57–83, 1995

American Psychological Association: Statement on the use of anatomically detailed dolls in forensic evaluations. Washington, DC, APA Council of Representatives, 1991

Baker-Ward L, Gordon B, Ornstein PA, et al: Young children's long-term retention of a pediatric examination. Child Dev 64:1519–1533, 1993

Berry K, Skinner LG: Anatomically detailed dolls and the evaluations of child sexual abuse allegations: psychometric considerations. Law and Human Behavior 17:399–422, 1993

Binet A: La Suggestibilité. Paris, Schleicher Frères, 1900

Boat B, Everson M: The use of anatomical dolls among professionals in sexual abuse evaluations. Child Abuse Negl 12:171–186, 1988

Brown MR: Legal Psychology. Indianapolis, IN, Bobbs-Merrill, 1926

Bruck M, Ceci SJ, Rosenthal R: Amicus Brief to the Supreme Court of New Jersey in New Jersey v. Michaels. Psychology, Policy and the Law 1:1–51, 1995a

Bruck M, Ceci SJ, Francoeur E, et al: "I hardly cried when I got my shot": young children's reports of their visit to a pediatrician. Child Dev66:193–208, 1995b

Bruck M, Ceci SJ, Francoeur E, et al: Preschoolers' reports of genital touching. J Exp Psychol Applied 1:95–109

Ceci SJ, Bronfenbrenner U: On the demise of everyday memory: the rumors of my death are greatly exaggerated. Am Psychol 46:27–31, 1991

Ceci SJ, Bruck M: The suggestibility of the child witness. Psychol Bull 113:403–439, 1993a

Ceci SJ, Bruck M: The Child Witness: Translating Research Into Policy. Society for Research in Child Development Social Policy Reports 7, No 3, 1993b

Ceci SJ, Bruck M: America's Courtrooms in Jeopardy: A Scientific Analysis of Children's Testimony. Washington, DC, American Psychological Association, 1995

Ceci SJ, Ross D, Toglia M: Age differences in suggestibility: psycholegal implications. J Exp Psychol Gen 117:38–49, 1987

Ceci SJ, Leichtman M, Putnick M, et al: Age differences in suggestibility, in Child Witnesses, Child Abuse, and Public Policy. Edited by Cicchetti D, Toth S. Norwood, NJ, Ablex, 1993, pp 117–138

Ceci SJ, Crotteau M, Smith E, et al: Repeatedly thinking about nonevents. Consciousness & Cognition 3:388–407, 1994a

Ceci SJ, Loftus EW, Leichtman M, et al: The role of source misattributions in the creation of false beliefs among preschoolers. Int J Clin Exp Hypn 62:304–320, 1994b

Ceci SJ, Leichtman M, White T: Interviewing preschoolers: remembrance of things planted, in The Child Witness in Context: Cognitive, Social, and Legal Perspectives. Edited by Peters DP. Netherlands, Kluwer, in press

Clarke-Stewart A, Thompson W, Lepore S: Manipulating children's interpretations through interrogation. Paper presented at the biennial meeting of the Society for Research in Child Development, Kansas City, MO, April 1989

Cohen RL, Harnick MA: The susceptibility of child witnesses to suggestion. Law and Human Behavior 4:201–210, 1980

Conte JR, Sorenson E, Fogarty L, et al: Evaluating children's reports of sexual abuse: results from a survey of professionals. Am J Orthopsychiatry 78:428–432, 1991

Dawes R: The importance of alternative hypotheses and hypothetical counterfactuals in general social science. The General Psychologist, Spring, 2–7, 1992

Fivush R: Developmental perspectives on autobiographical recall, in Child Victims and Child Witnesses: Understanding and Improving Testimony. Edited by Goodman GS, Bottoms BL. New York, Guilford, 1993, pp 1–24

Gardner R: Sex Abuse Hysteria: Salem Witch Trials Revisited. Longwood, NJ, Creative Therapeutics Press, 1989

Goodman GS: Children's memory for stressful events: theoretical and developmental considerations. Paper presented at the biennial meeting of the Society for Research in Child Development, New Orleans, LA, March 1993

Goodman GS, Aman C: Children's use of anatomically detailed dolls to recount an event. Child Dev 61:1859–1871, 1990

Goodman GS, Clarke-Stewart A: Suggestibility in children's testimony: implications for child sexual abuse investigations, in The Suggestibility of Children's Recollections. Edited by Doris JL. Washington, DC, American Psychological Association, 1991, pp 92–105

Goodman GS, Wilson ME, Hazan C, et al: Children's testimony nearly four years after an event. Paper presented at the annual meeting of the Eastern Psychological Association, Boston, MA, April 1989

Goodman GS, Rudy L, Bottoms B, et al: Children's concerns and memory: issues of ecological validity in the study of children's eyewitness testimony, in Knowing and Remembering in Young Children. Edited by Fivush R, Hudson J. New York, Cambridge University Press, 1990, pp 249–284

Goodman GS, Batterman-Faunce JM, Kenney R: Optimizing children's testimony: research and social policy issues concerning allegations of child sexual abuse, in Child Abuse, Child Development, and Social Policy. Edited by Cicchetti D, Toth S. Norwood, NJ, Ablex, 1992

Gordon B, Ornstein PA, Clubb P, et al: Visiting the pediatrician: long-term retention and forgetting. Paper presented at annual meeting of the Psychonomic Society, San Francisco, CA, November 1991

Kendall-Tackett K: Professionals' standards of "normal" behavior with anatomical dolls and factors that influence these standards. Paper presented at the biennial meeting of the Society for Research in Child Development, Seattle, WA, April 1991

Leichtman MD, Ceci SJ: The effect of stereotypes and suggestions on preschoolers' reports. Developmental Psychology 31: 568–578, 1995

Lindsay DS, Gonzales V, Eso K: Aware and unaware uses of memories of postevent suggestions, in Memory and Testimony in the Child Witness. Edited by Zaragoza MS, Graham JR, Gordon CN, et al. Newbury Park, CA, Sage, 1995, pp 86–108

Lipmann O: Pedagogical psychology of report. Journal of Educational Psychology 2:253–261, 1911

Loftus EF: The reality of repressed memories. Am Psychol 48:518–537, 1993

Marin BV, Holmes DL, Guth M, et al: The potential of children as eyewitnesses. Law and Human Behavior 3:295–305, 1979

Mason MA: A judicial dilemma: expert witness testimony in child sex abuse cases. Journal of Psychiatry and Law 19:185–219, 1991

McGough L: Fragile Voices: The Child Witness in American Courts. New Haven, CT, Yale University Press, 1994

Melton G: Children as partners for justice: Next steps for developmentalists. Monographs of the Society for Research in Child Development 57:153–159, 1992

Messerschmidt R: The suggestibility of boys and girls between the ages of six and sixteen. J Gen Psychol 43:422–437, 1933

Ornstein PA, Baker-Ward L, Gordon B, et al: Children's memory for medical procedures. Paper presented at the biennial meeting of the Society for Research in Child Development, New Orleans, LA, March 1993

Ornstein PA, Gordon BN, Larus D: Children's memory for a personally experienced event: implications for testimony. Applied Cognitive Psychology 6:49–60, 1992

Otis M: A study of suggestibility in children. Archives of Psychology 11:5–108, 1924

Poole ME, Lindsay DS: Interviewing preschoolers: effects of nonsuggestive techniques, parental coaching, and leading questions on reports of non-experienced events. J Exp Child Psychol 60:129–154, 1994

Popper KR: Conjectures and Reflections. New York, Basic Books, 1962

Rabinowitz D: From the mouths of babes to a jail cell: child abuse and the abuse of justice. Harper's Magazine, May 1990, pp 52–63

Raskin D, Yuille J: Problems in evaluating interviews of children in sexual abuse cases, in Adults' Perceptions of Children's Testimony. Edited by Ceci SJ, Toglia MP, Ross DF. New York, Springer-Verlag, 1989, pp 184–207

Rudy L, Goodman GS: Effects of participation on children's reports: implications for children's testimony. Developmental Psychology 27:527–538, 1991

Sauer M: Decade of accusations. San Diego (CA) Union Tribune, D1–D3, August 29, 1993

Saywitz KJ, Goodman GS, Nicholas E, et al: Children's memories of a physical examination involving genital touch: implications for reports of child sexual abuse. J Consult Clin Psychol 59:682–691, 1991

Schooler JW, Gerhard D, Loftus EF: Qualities of the unreal. J Exp Psychol Learn Mem Cogn 12:171–181, 1986

Sherman I: The suggestibility of normal and mentally defective children. Comparative Psychology Monographs 2, 1925

Stern W: Abstracts of lectures on the psychology of testimony and on the study of individuality. Am J Psychology 21:270–282, 1910

Sugar M: Toddlers' traumatic memories. Infant Mental Health Journal 13:245–251, 1992

Terr L: Anatomically correct dolls: should they be used as a basis for expert testimony? J Am Acad Child Adolesc Psychiatry 27:254–257, 1988

Varendonck J: Les témoignages d'enfants dans un procès retentissant [The testimony of children in a famous trial]. Archives de Psychologie 11:129–171, 1911

Wolfner G, Faust D, Dawes R: The use of anatomical dolls in sexual abuse evaluations: the state of the science. Applied and Preventative Psychology 2:1–11, 1993

# RESOURCE APPENDIXES

*Sandra J. Kaplan, M.D. (Appendixes A–G)*
*Howard A. Davidson, J.D. (Appendix H)*

A     Selected Professional Practice Standards

B     Selected Position Statements of Professional
       Organizations

C     Selected Clinical Case Assessment and
       Management Protocols and Guidelines
          Child Sexual Abuse
          Child Physical Abuse and Neglect
          Partner Abuse and Domestic Violence
          Elder Abuse
          Adult Survivors of Child Abuse
          Family Violence

D     Selected Literature
          Child Abuse and Neglect
          Family Violence and Neglect: General
          Elder Abuse
          Adult Survivors of Child Abuse

E     Selected Victim Advocacy and Referral Resources
          Child Abuse and Neglect
          Child Sexual Abuse
          Partner Abuse and Domestic Violence
          Adult Survivors of Child Abuse
          Elder Abuse

F      Selected Prevention Resources
          Violence: General
          Adolescent Intentional Injury and Abuse
          Violence and Child Abuse and Neglect
          Child Sexual Abuse
          Adult Survivors of Child Abuse
          Elder Abuse
          Partner Abuse and Domestic Violence

G      Selected Mental Health Treatment Programs

H      Legal Appendix
          Suggestions for Improving the Legal and
              Judicial Process
          Legal References and Bibliography
          Legal Information Resources for Professionals

# APPENDIX A

## Selected Professional Practice Standards

1. Joint Commission on Accreditation of Health Care Organizations, 1 Renaissance Blvd., Oakbrook Terrace, IL 60181. Comprehensive Accreditation Manual for Hospitals, 1995

   ➤ Management and Administrative Services
   ➤ Alcoholism and Other Drug Dependence Services
   ➤ Emergency Services
   ➤ Special Care Units
   ➤ Hospital-Sponsored Ambulatory Care Services
   ➤ Medical Record Services

2. New York State Department of Health, Albany, NY. The Official Compilation Codes, Rules and Regulations of the State of New York, Title 10

   ➤ Part 405.19, Emergency Services, (c) General Policies and Procedures. (2)–(8), 4540.28–4540.29, H 12/31/88
   ➤ Part 405.9, Medical Facilities, (c) Sexual Offense Evidence. (1)–(6), pp 4533–4534 H 8/31/89
   ➤ Part 405.9, Title 10 Health, (d) Child Abuse and Maltreatment. p 4534 H 8/31/89
   ➤ Part 405.9, Chapter V Medical Facilities, (e) Domestic Violence. (f) Discharge, p 4534.1 H 2-28-90

3. State of New York Department of Health, Albany, NY, (212) 613-2440. Memorandum, Health Facilities Series H-9, D, and TC-6; Hospital Emergency Services Protocol: Identifying and Treating Adult Victims of Domestic Violence, Series 90-15, 3/28/90.

4. The University of the State of New York, The State Education Department, Division of Professional Licensing Services, Cultural Education Center, Albany, NY 12230. Coursework and Training in Identification and Reporting of Child Abuse and Maltreatment, PR 2 (H)-/5/90. Required for professional relicensure in New York State for psychologists, physicians, and educators.

# APPENDIX B

# Selected Position Statements of Professional Organizations

1. American Psychiatric Association, APA Library, 1400 K Street, N.W., Washington, DC 20005.

   ➤ Position Statement on Child Abuse and Neglect by Adults. Approved by the Board of Trustees, American Psychiatric Association, June 28, 1991. Document No. 910001
   ➤ Position Statement on Domestic Violence Against Women. Am J Psychiatry 151:4, 1994, p 630
   ➤ Position Statement on Elder Abuse, Neglect, and Exploitation. Am J Psychiatry 152:5, 1995, p 820

2. American Academy of Child and Adolescent Psychiatry, 3615 Wisconsin Ave., N.W., Washington, DC 20016. Corporal Punishment in Schools. Approved by Council of the AACAP, June 10, 1988

3. American College of Obstetrics and Gynecology, 409 12th St., N.W., Washington, DC 20024, (202) 638-5577. The Battered Woman, January 1989. ACOG Technical Bulletin No. 124

4. American Medical Association, 535 N. Dearborn St., Chicago, IL 60610, (312) 464-5066

   ➤ Public Health Policy Approach for Preventing Violence in America, Board of Trustees Report 34-A-95
   ➤ Campaign Against Family Violence: Annual Update, Board of Trustees Report 4-A-95
   ➤ Physicians and Family Violence: Ethical Considerations, Council Report, Report B (I-91)

➤ A Proposed AMA National Campaign Against Family Violence, Report G (I-91)
➤ Update on the AMA's National Campaign Against Family Violence, Report FF (A-92)
➤ Family Violence: Adolescents As Victims and Perpetrators, Report I of the Council on Scientific Affairs, Report (A-92)
➤ Physicians and Domestic Violence: Ethical Considerations. JAMA 267:3190–3193, 1992
➤ Violence Against Women: Relevance for Medical Practitioners. JAMA 267:3184–3189, 1992
➤ Alcohol, Drugs and Family Violence, Report A (A-93)
➤ Mental Health Consequences of Interpersonal and Family Violence: Implications for the Practitioner, Report B (A-93)

5. American Academy of Pediatrics, American Academy of Pediatrics, Division of Publications, 141 Northwest Point Blvd., P.O. Box 927, Elk Grove Village, IL 60009-0927, (708) 228-5005.

➤ Religious Exemptions from Child Abuse Statutes. Pediatrics 81, 1988
➤ Guidelines for the Evaluation of Sexual Abuse of Children, Committee on Child Abuse and Neglect. Pediatrics 87, 1991
➤ Public Disclosure of Private Information About Victims of Abuse, approved by the Council on Child and Adolescent Health. Pediatrics 84, 1988

6. American Medical Women's Association, 801 North Fairfax St., Alexandria, VA 22314

➤ Domestic Violence, National Council on Women in Medicine Newsletter, Summer/Fall 1991; complete position paper available upon request

7. Joint Commission of Accreditation of Health Care Organizations, 1 Renaissance Blvd., Oakbrook Terrace, IL 60181

➤ Organizations Manual, Emergency Medicine, 1992

# APPENDIX C

## Selected Clinical Case Assessment and Management Protocols and Guidelines

### Child Sexual Abuse

1. American Academy of Child and Adolescent Psychiatry, 3615 Wisconsin Avenue, N.W., Washington, DC 20016, (202) 966-7300.

   ➤ Guidelines for the Clinical Evaluation of Child and Adolescent Sexual Abuse. Approved by Council of the AACAP, June 10, 1988, modified December 14, 1990

2. American Academy of Pediatrics, Committee on Child Abuse and Neglect: Guidelines for the evaluation of sexual abuse of children. Pediatrics 87, 1991

3. American Medical Association, 535 N. Dearborn St., Chicago, IL 60610, (312) 464-5066. Diagnostic and Treatment Guidelines on Child Sexual Abuse (includes a listing of reporting agencies from various states), June 1992. AA22: 92-407 20M

4. American Professional Society on the Abuse of Children, 332 South Michigan Avenue, Suite 1600, Chicago, IL 60604, (312) 554-0166.

   ➤ Guidelines for Psychosocial Evaluation of Suspected Sexual Abuse in Young Children, 1990, pp 1–6
   ➤ Descriptive Terminology in Child Sexual Abuse Medical Evaluations, 1995, pp 1–8
   ➤ Use of Anatomical Dolls in Child Sexual Abuse Assessments, 1995, pp 1–12

5. Department of Psychiatry, University of North Carolina, Chapel Hill, NC 27514, (919) 967-2211. Boat B, Everson M: Using Anatomical Dolls: Guidelines for Interviewing Young Children in Sexual Abuse Investigations, 1986

6. U.S. Department of Justice, National Institute of Justice/Research in Action, 1-800-627-6872. Freeman K, Estrada-Mullaney T: Using Dolls to Interview Child Victims: Legal Concerns and Interview Procedures. Reprinted from NIJ Reports/SNI 207, January/February 1988

7. The C. Henry Kempe National Center for the Prevention and Treatment of Child Abuse and Neglect, University of Colorado School of Medicine, Denver, CO, (303) 355-9400. Jones DPH: Interviewing the Sexually Abused Child: Investigation of Suspected Abuse, 4th Edition, 1992

8. Department of Psychiatry, Case Western Reserve University School of Medicine, Cleveland Metropolitan General Hospital, Cleveland, OH, (216) 844-3420. White S, Strom G, Santilli G: Clinical Protocol for Interviewing Preschoolers With Sexually Anatomically Correct Dolls, 1985. No. 459-3745

# Child Physical Abuse and Neglect

1. American Medical Association, Council on Scientific Affairs: AMA diagnostic and treatment guidelines concerning child abuse and neglect. JAMA 254:796–800, 1985

2. American Medical Association, 535 N. Dearborn St., Chicago, IL 60610, (312) 464-5066. Diagnostic and Treatment Guidelines on Child Physical Abuse and Neglect (includes a listing of reporting agencies from various states), June 1992. AA22: 92-407, 20 M

3. State of New York Department of Social Services and Department of Health, Albany, NY, 1-800-342-3270, (518) 473-3170. Suspected Child Abuse and Maltreatment: Identification and Management in Hospitals and Clinics: Official Guidelines, 1991

4. American Professional Society on the Abuse of Children, 332 South Michigan Avenue, Suite 1600, Chicago, IL 60604, (312) 554-0166.

➤ Psychosocial Evaluation of Suspected Psychological Maltreatment in Children and Adolescents, 1995, pp 1–12
➤ Photographic Documentation of Child Abuse, 1995, pp 1–7

5. National Center on Child Abuse and Neglect, U.S. Department of Health and Human Services. Peterson MS, Urquiza AJ: The Role of Mental Health Professionals in the Prevention and Treatment of Child Abuse and Neglect. Washington, DC, U.S. Government Printing Office, 1993, pp 1–57

## Partner Abuse and Domestic Violence

1. American College of Obstetrics and Gynecology, Division of women's Health Issues, 409 12th St., N.W., Washington, DC 20024, (202) 638-5577. The Battered Woman, January 1989. ACOG Technical Bulletin No. 124
2. American Medical Association, 535 N. Dearborn St., Chicago, IL 60610, (312) 464-5066.

   ➤ Strategies for the Treatment and Prevention of Sexual Assault, October 1995. AF55:95-0742 10M
   ➤ Children's Safety Network: Domestic Violence: a Directory for Health Care Providers, 1995, pp 1–26

3. Jersey Battered Women's Service, Inc., 36 Elm Street, Morristown, NJ 07960, (201) 267-4763, (201) 455-1256. Brahaim R, Furness K, Holtz H, et al: Hospital Protocol on Domestic Violence, 1986
4. The Domestic Violence Project, 6308 8th Ave., Kenosha, WI 53143, (414) 656-8502. Fullin K, Fullin P, Cosgrove A: Screening Patients for Domestic Violence in Clinical Practice
5. National Coalition Against Domestic Violence, 1000 16th Street, N.W., Washington, DC 20005, (202) 638-6388, (703) 765-0339. Schecter S: Empowering Interventions with Battered Women— Guidelines for Mental Health Professionals
6. State of New York Department of Health, Albany, NY. State of New York Department of Health Memorandum Health Facilities Series: H-9, D, and TC-6, Hospital Emergency Services Protocol: Identifying and Treating Adult Victims of Domestic Violence, Series 90-15, March 28, 1990
7. National Center on Women and Family Law, 799 Broadway, Room 402, New York, NY 10003, (212) 874-8200. Zorza J, Schoenberg L: Improving the Health CCare Response to domestic Violence Through Protocols and Policies, 1994, pp A-1–A-2

## Elder Abuse

1. American Medical Association, Council on Scientific Affairs: Elder abuse and neglect. JAMA 257, 1987
2. American Medical Association, 535 N. Dearborn St., Chicago, IL 60610, (312) 464-5066. Diagnostic and Treatment Guidelines on Elder Abuse and Neglect (includes a listing of protective service programs from various states), November 1992. AA22: 92-698, 20M
3. Bloom J, Ansell P, Bloom M: Detecting elder abuse: a guide for physicians. Geriatrics 44, 1989
4. Carr K, Dix G, Fulmer T, et al: Practice concepts: an elder abuse assessment team in an acute hospital setting. Gerontologist 26, 1986
5. Department of Emergency Medicine, Akron General Medical Center, Northeastern Ohio Universities College of Medicine, Akron, OH, (216) 325-2511. Jones J, Dougherty J, Schelble D, et al: Emergency Department Protocol for the Diagnosis and Evaluation of Geriatric Abuse, June 17, 1988
6. Tomita S: Detection and treatment of elderly abuse and neglect: a protocol for health care professionals. Geriatrics 2:37–51, 1982

## Adult Survivors of Child Abuse

National Committee for the Prevention of Child Abuse, P.O. Box 94283, Chicago, IL 60690, (312) 663-3520. Brown P, Jones E: Help for Adult Survivors of Childhood Abuse

## Family Violence

1. American Medical Association, 535 N. Dearborn St., Chicago, IL 60610, (312) 464-5066. Diagnostic and Treatment Guidelines on Mental Health Effects of Family Violence, 1995. AF55: 95-0722 10M
2. American Bar Association Center on Children and the Law, 1800 M St., N.W., Washington, DC 20036. Waller AG: Handbook on Questioning Children: A Linguistic Perspective, 1994

# APPENDIX D

## Selected Literature

### Child Abuse and Neglect

Kempe Center Programs, Publications Catalog, 1990. C. Henry Kempe National Center for the Prevention and Treatment of Child Abuse and Neglect, University of Colorado Health Sciences Center, Department of Pediatrics, 1205 Oneida, Denver, CO 80220-2944, (303) 355-9400

Kessler DB, Hyden P: Physical, Sexual, and Emotional Abuse of Children (Clinical Symposia). CIBA-GEIGY 43, 1991

National Clearinghouse on Child Abuse and Neglect Information. P.O. Box 1182, Washington, DC 20013-1182, (703) 385-7565 or 1-800-FYI-3366. Various publications

U.S. Department of Justice, Office for Victims of Crime Resource Center, 1-800-627-6872. Various publications

U.S. Department of Health and Human Services: Catalog on Services and Publications, November 1993. USDHHS, P.O. Box 1182, Washington, DC 20013, (703) 385-7565

### Family Violence and Neglect: General

American Psychological Association: Violence and Youth: Psychology's Response, Vol I. Washington, DC, American Psychological Association, 1993

Family Violence Prevention Fund: News from the Homefront. The Family Violence Prevention Fund, 383 Rhode Island St., Suite 304, San Francisco, CA 94103, (415) 252-8900

Family Violence Research and Treatment Program: Family Violence Bulletin, Sexual Assault Bulletin, and Editors' Comments, Vol 9, Winter 1993. Family Violence Research and Treatment Program, 1310 Clinic Drive, Tyler, TX 75701, (903) 595-6600

## Elder Abuse

Gold DT, Gwyther LP: The prevention of elder abuse: an educational model. Family Relations 38:8–14, 1989

## Adult Survivors of Child Abuse

Brown P, Jones E: Help for Adult Survivors of Childhood Abuse. National Committee for the Prevention of Child Abuse, P.O. Box 94283, Chicago, IL 60690, (312) 663-3520

# APPENDIX E

## Selected Victim Advocacy and Referral Resources

### Child Abuse and Neglect

1. Child Abuse and Neglect Prevention Information Line, 1-800-342-7472
2. Missing Children Hotline, 1-800-FINDKID
3. National Runaway Switchboard, 1-800-621-4000
4. National Youth Crisis Hotline/Home Run-Runaway Hotline, 1-800-HIT-HOME
5. American Humane Association Children's Division, 9725 E. Hampden Avenue, Denver, CO 80231, 1-800-2ASK-AHA: Information on national reporting statistics, state child protection services policies, model programs
6. National Resource Center for Foster and Residential Care, Child Welfare Institute, P.O. Box 77364, Station C, Atlanta, GA 30357, (404) 876-1934
7. National Council on Child Abuse and Family Violence, 1155 Connecticut Ave., N.W., Suite 400, Washington, DC 20036, (202) 429-6695
8. National Center for Missing and Exploited Children, 2101 Wilson Blvd., Suite 550, Arlington, VA 22210, 1-800-843-5678
9. National Coalition Against Sexual Assault, c/o Fern Ferguson, President, Volunteers of America, 8787 State St., Suite 202, East St. Louis, IL 62203, (618) 271-9833
10. National Victims Resource Center, Office for Victims of Crime, Office of Justice Programs, U.S. Department of Justice, Washington, DC 20531, 1-800-627-6872, (202) 307-5933

## Child Sexual Abuse

National Resource Center on Child Sexual Abuse of the national Center on Child Abuse and Neglect, 2204 Whitesburg Drive, Suite 200, Huntsvile, AL 35801, (205) 534-6868

## Partner Abuse and Domestic Violence

1. National Coalition Against Domestic Violence, 1151 K Street, N.W., Room 409, Washington, DC 20037, (202) 638-6388
2. Center for Women Policy Studies, 2000 P Street, N.W., Suite 508, Washington, DC 20036, (202) 872-1770
3. National Victims Resource Center, Office for Victims of Crime, Office of Justice Programs, U.S. Department of Justice, Washington, DC 20531, 1-800-627-6872, (202) 307-5933
4. National Organization for Victim Assistance, 1757 Park Road, N.W., Washington, DC 20010, (202) 232-6682
5. New York State Coalition Against Domestic Violence, 79 Central Ave., Albany, NY 12206, (518) 432-4864
6. TDD (Telecommunications Device for the Deaf) National Domestic Violence Hotline, 1-800-873-6363
7. National Crime Prevention Council, 1700 K St., N.W., 2nd Fl., Washington, DC 20006-3817, (202) 466-6272
8. Marital Rape Information, University of Illinois at Urbana-Champaign, 415 Library, 1408 West Gregory Drive, Urbana, IL 61801, (217) 244-1024
9. The Family Violence Prevention Fund's Health Resource Center on Domestic Violence, 1-800-313-1310
10. National Resource Center on Domestic Violence, 6400 Flank Drive, Suite 1300, Harrisburg, PA 17112, 1-800-537-2238

## Adult Survivors of Child Abuse

National Committee for the Prevention of Child Abuse, P.O. Box 94283, Chicago, IL 60690, (312) 663-3520. Brown P, Jones ED: Help for Adult Survivors of Childhood Abuse

## Elder Abuse

1. National Aging Resource Center on Elder Abuse, 810 First Street, N.E., Suite 500, Washington, DC 20002-4205, (202) 682-2470
2. National Institute on Aging, National Institutes of Health, Public Health Service, U.S. Department of Health and Human Services, Gateway Building, Suite 533, Bethesda, MD 20892, (301) 496-3136. Older People in Society (publication)
3. National Committee for the Prevention of Elder Abuse, c/o Institute on Aging, Medical Center of Central Massachusetts, 119 Belmont St., Worcester, MA 01605

# APPENDIX F

# Selected Prevention Resources

## Violence: General

1. National Center for Health Education, 72 Spring St., Suite 208, New York, NY 10012, (212) 334-9470. Preventing Violence: Parents and Caregivers Can Make a Difference, 1995
2. Division of Injury Control, Center for Environmental Health and Injury Control, Centers for Disease Control, U.S. Public Health Service, Atlanta, GA. Earls F et al: Position paper and panel on violence prevention, presented at 3rd National Injury Control Conference, Denver, CO, 1991

## Adolescent Intentional Injury and Abuse

American Medical Association, Department on Adolescent Health, 515 N. State St., Chicago, IL 60610, (312) 464-5570. Gans J, Shook K: Policy Compendium on Violence and Adolescents: Intentional Injury and Abuse, 1993

## Violence and Child Abuse and Neglect

1. Teenage Health Teaching Module. Newton, MA, Educational Development Center: (617) 969-7100. Prothrow-Stith D: Violence Prevention: Curriculum for Adolescents, 1987
2. American Academy of Child and Adolescent Psychiatry, 3615 Wisconsin Avenue, N.W., Washington, DC 20016, (202) 966-7300. Facts for Families (series of five publications on children and family violence), 1992

➤ Child Abuse: The Hidden Bruises. No. 5
➤ Child Sexual Abuse. No. 9
➤ Children and TV Violence. No. 13
➤ Responding to Child Sexual Abuse. No 28
➤ Children and Firearms. No. 38

3. National Committee to Prevent Child Abuse, 332 S. Michigan Ave., Suite 1600, Chicago, IL 60604, (312) 663-3520

## Child Sexual Abuse

1. Committee for Children, 172 20th Avenue, Seattle, WA 98122, (206) 322-5050. Talking About Touching (publication)
2. Health Education Systems, Inc., Box GG, Palisades, NY 10964. Kraizer S: Safe Child Personal Safety Training Program (publication)
3. American Academy of Pediatrics, Division of Publications, 141 Northwest Point Blvd., P.O. Box 927, Elk Grove Village, IL 60009-0927, (708) 228-5005. Guidelines for Parents: Child Sexual Abuse: What It Is and How to Prevent It, 1990

## Adult Survivors of Child Abuse

National Committee for the Prevention of Child Abuse Catalog, P.O. Box 94283, Chicago, IL 60690, (312) 663-3520. Brown P, Jones ED: Help for Adult Survivors of Childhood Abuse

## Elder Abuse

1. National Aging Resource Center on Elder Abuse, 810 First Street, N.E., Suite 500, Washington, DC 20002-4205, (202) 682-2470
2. National Institute on Aging, National Institutes of Health, Public Health Service, United States Department of Health and Human Services, Building 31C, Room 5C32, Bethesda, MD 20892, (301) 496-3136. Older People in Society (publication)

# Partner Abuse and Domestic Violence

1. New York State Department of Social Services, Albany, NY 1989: (518) 473-3170. Fields MD, Lehman E: Handbook for Abused Women

2. American College of Obstetrics and Gynecology, 409 12th St., N.W., Washington, DC 20024, (202) 638-5577. Women's Health: The Abused Woman. APA 83, March 1993

3. Hunter House Publishers, P.O. Box 2914, Alameda, CA 94501, 1-800-266-5592. Creighton A, Kivel P: Helping Teens Stop Violence, 1992

4. Association of Trial Lawyers of America, 1050 31st St., N.W., Washington, DC 20007. Preventing Violence to Women: Integrating the Health and Legal Communities. Report of the Conference, June 1993

# $\text{A}$PPENDIX G

## Selected Mental Health Treatment Programs

1. Family Crisis Program of North Shore University Hospital-Cornell University Medical College, Sandra J. Kaplan, M.D., Department of Psychiatry, 300 Community Drive, Manhasset, NY 11030, (516) 562-3005
2. The Family Center, Presbyterian Hospital, Arthur H. Green, M.D., Columbia University Program for Abused and Neglected Children, 622 W. 168th St., Babies' Hospital, 6 North, Room 616, New York, NY 10032, (212) 305-6694
3. Therapeutic Nursery Program (Program for Abused and Neglected Children) (see above location)
4. Women's and Children's Program, North Shore University Hospital at Glen Cove, John E. Imhof, Ph.D., Department of Psychiatry DTEC Program for Substance Abusive Mothers and Their Children, St. Andrews Lane, Glen Cove, NY 11542, (516) 676-5000

# APPENDIX H

## Legal Appendix

### Suggestions for Improving the Legal and Judicial Process

There is a paramount but rarely met need for hospital-based and agency-based pediatricians, psychiatrists, psychologists, and other health and mental health care professionals to have ready access to their own institutional child abuse and family violence legal specialists for consultation and advice. This legal support should come from an attorney who either is on the staff of the facility or agency or is under contract to it. The lawyer should be an expert on child physical and sexual abuse, on partner abuse and domestic violence, and on legal issues related to reporting, investigation, confidentiality, and judicial intervention (both criminal and civil).

The following 12 recommendations are offered as suggestions for improving the medical-legal interface in family violence cases.

1. All hospital emergency rooms should have written protocols covering issues related to reporting, judicial system intervention, and when and how to obtain emergency legal consultation in family violence cases.
2. All hospital emergency room personnel, physicians, nurses, and other medical and mental health care professionals should receive training by a legal specialist about child and partner or spouse abuse statutory obligations and judicial interventions.
3. All states and large counties should be legally required to have

   ➤ Committees that review all unexplained and suspicious child fatalities, not just those reported to the child protective services (CPS) agency

➤ Multidisciplinary and interagency child protection case coordination teams, with clear legislative authority and direction (a model for this is Florida, where physicians are significantly involved in child protection teams)

➤ Multidisciplinary and interagency domestic violence case review and system improvement teams; these teams must have as members a knowledgeable physician, nurse, mental health professional, social worker, and attorney aware of all major civil and criminal court intervention issues related to family violence

4. State laws need to be expanded and clarified in defining complex concepts such as *emotional maltreatment, lack of adequate parental supervision of children, unlawful and excessive use of corporal punishment,* and *child endangerment due to parental drug abuse* (i.e., what can legally be done when a child is born addicted)

5. If mandatory child abuse reporting laws are going to be expanded, adding new categories of mandated reporters, as some states have done—such as domestic violence program personnel, substance abuse and addiction counselors, and marital and family therapists—there must be comprehensive training of these professionals regarding their legal obligations. This training can be mandated by law—as, for example, was done in New York for all hospital personnel and in New Mexico for all nurses. It is particularly important that those who work in drug and alcohol treatment programs be made aware of the effect of changes in federal law on drug and alcohol abuse treatment related to the confidentiality of patient information and records. These changes clarified the obligation to report suspected child abuse and neglect pursuant to the requirements of state law, despite federal law confidentiality provisions.

6. Laws should be enacted to mandate feedback to all professionals who are legally mandated reporters of child abuse and neglect. Such feedback should include information on what judicial system actions were taken as a consequence of the report. Professionals who have reported abuse or neglect should in addition be included as partners in all child maltreatment service and treatment plans developed by government child protection agencies.

7. Laws should be passed requiring that the full cost of medical, dental, and mental health examinations and evaluations pursuant to a report related to family violence be paid by

➤ a CPS agency, in cases involving allegations of intrafamilial child abuse or neglect

➤ a law enforcement agency or crime victim program, in cases involving allegations of a sex offense or other crime committed against a child or in cases that involve alleged domestic violence

8. Laws should clarify that all children and adults who have experienced intrafamily violence are eligible for, and should receive help in obtaining, crime victim compensation. States should create their own special funding mechanisms to add dollars to their funding pot for compensation programs for crime victims (such as special fines, property forfeitures, and special surcharges or penalty assessments).

9. Medical societies and other groups of health and mental health professionals should arrange to meet with juvenile, family, and criminal court judges to help develop new court case scheduling improvements designed to minimize the inconvenience, delays, and waiting periods that these professionals often experience in child abuse and family violence cases. Such approaches should consider

➤ Establishing routine use of on-call scheduling, in which pediatricians, psychiatrists, psychologists, or others agree to be available through a beeper system to come to the court for testifying within 30–45 minutes, thus avoiding needless hours of court waiting time

➤ Encouraging attorneys to hold pretrial case conferences that attempt to reach stipulated agreements on the qualifications of prospective health and mental health witnesses and other uncontested medical issues

10. There should be a formal mechanism created by which judges, attorneys, and health and mental health care professionals can communicate regularly about shared frustrations, inadequate resource allocations, vague and confusing expectations related to professional responsibilities, and the need to improve interagency coordination.

11. There should be careful consideration of a process that would develop better linkage of CPS, domestic violence shelters, and bat-

tered women's support programs, and the police. Attempts should be made to standardize and clarify interagency procedures and policies. For example, CPS intake and investigation workers should be routinely asking questions about adult domestic violence in the home, and police responding to partner abuse calls should be routinely asking questions about violence against children in the household.

12. All state laws should be clarified to provide explicitly that in all family violence cases, the legal preference is, whenever possible, to have the violent family member removed from the home rather than having the children placed in foster care or having the adult who was abused forcibly relocated. To this end, all courts with any authority in family violence cases should have the clear authority to issue removal, no-contact, and other necessary protective orders against violent adults in a family.

# Legal References and Bibliography

## ▍ Child Abuse and Neglect

Alexander GJ: Big Mother: The State's Use of Mental Health Experts in Dependency Cases. 24 Pac. L. J. 1465, 1993

American Bar Association: America's Children at Risk: A National Agenda for Legal Action. Washington, DC, American Bar Association, 1993

American Bar Association: Recommendations for Improving Legal Intervention in Intrafamily Child Sexual Abuse Cases. Washington, DC, ABA Center on Children and the Law, 1982

Bross DC, Krugman RD, Lenherr MR, et al (eds): The New Child Protection Team Handbook. New York, Garland Publishing, 1988

Bulkley J, Sandt C (eds): A Judicial Primer on Child Sexual Abuse. Washington, DC, American Bar Association Center on Children and the Law, 1994

Davenport KL: Due Process Claims of Abused Children Against State Protective Agencies: The State's Responsibility after DeShaney v. Winnebago County Department of Social Services. 489 U.S. 189, 1989; 19 Fla. St. U. L. Rev. 243, 1991

DeShaney v Winnebago County Department of Social Services, 489 U.S. 189, 1989

Duquette DN: Advocating for the Child in Protection Proceedings. Lexington, MA, Lexington Books, 1990

Dziech BW, Schudson CB: On Trial: America's Courts and Their Treatment of Sexually Abused Children. Boston, MA, Beacon Press, 1991

Fahn MS: Allegations of Child Sexual Abuse in Custody Disputes: Getting to the Truth of the Matter. 25 Fam. L. Q. 193, 1991

Feller JN, Davidson HA, Hardin M, et al: Working With the Courts in Child Protection. Washington, DC, National Center on Child Abuse and Neglect, 1992

Fischer v Metcalf, 543 So.2d 785 (FL 1989)

Horner TM, Guyer MJ: Prediction, Prevention, and Clinical Expertise in Child Custody Cases in which Allegations of Child Sexual Abuse Have Been Made. 25 Fam. L. Q. 217, 1991

Landeros v Flood, 551 P.2d 389 (CA 1976)

Levine M, Doueck HJ: The Impact of Mandated Reporting on the Therapeutic Process. Thousand Oaks, CA, Sage, 1995

Lowenstien SR: Incest, Child Sexual Abuse, and the Law: Concerns of Protecting Our Children From Abuse and the Integrity of the Family. 29 J. Fam. L. 791, 1990–1991

Melton GB, Barry FD: Protecting Children From Abuse and Neglect: Foundations for a New National Strategy. New York, Guilford, 1994

Myers JEB: Child Witness: Law and Practice. New York, Wiley Law Publications, 1987

Myers JEB: Evidence in Child Abuse and Neglect Cases, 2nd Edition. New York, Wiley, 1992

Myers JEB: Legal Issues in Child Abuse and Neglect. Newbury Park, CA, Sage, 1992

National Council of Juvenile and Family Court Judges: Resource Guidelines: Improving Court Practice in Child Abuse and Neglect Cases. Reno, NV, Spring, 1995

Nicholson EB, Bulkley J (eds): Sexual Abuse Allegations in Custody and Visitation Cases: A Resource Book for Judges and Court Personnel. Washington, DC, American Bar Association, 1988

O'Brien RC, Flanrey T: The Pending Gauntlet to Free Exercise: Mandating That Clergy Report Child Abuse. 25 Loy. L. A. L. Rev. 1, 1991

Puhlman ME: Family Law: Child Abuse Privilege Against Self-Incrimination. (Summary: The United States Supreme Court has held that a mother who is the custodian of a child pursuant to a court order may not invoke the Fifth Amendment privilege against self-incrimination to resist an order of the Juvenile Court to produce the child.) Baltimore City Department of Social Services v. Bouknight. 493 U.S. 549, 1990; 29 Duq L. Rev. 819, 1991

Ruddock EM: Something More Than a Generalized Finding: The State's Interest in Protecting Child Sexual Abuse Victims in *Maryland v. Craig* Outmuscles the Confrontation Clause. 8 Cooley L. Rev. 389, 1991

Smith GP: Incest and Intrafamilial Child Abuse: Fatal Attractions or Forced and Dangerous Liaisons? 29 J. Fam. L. 833, 1990–1991

Soler MI, Shotton AC, Bell JR: Representing the Child Client. New York, Matthew Bender, 1987

Tarasoff v Regents of the University of California, 551 P.2d 334 (CA 1976)

Thurman v City of Torrington, 595 F. Supp. 1521, 1984

Toth PA, Whalen MP, Berliner L, et al: Investigation and Prosecution of Child Abuse, 2nd Edition. Alexandria, VA, American Prosecutors Research Institute, 1993

U.S. v Foster, 113 S. Ct. 2849, 1993

U.S. Advisory Board on Child Abuse and Neglect: Child Abuse and Neglect: Critical First Steps in Response to a National Emergency. Washington, DC, U.S. Government Printing Office, 1990

U.S. Advisory Board on Child Abuse and Neglect: The Continuing Child Protection Emergency: A Challenge to the Nation. Washington, DC, U.S. Government Printing Office, 1992

U.S. Advisory Board on Child Abuse and Neglect: A Nation's Shame: Fatal Child Abuse and Neglect in the United States. Washington, DC, U.S. Government Printing Office, 1995

U.S. Advisory Board on Child Abuse and Neglect: Neighbors Helping Neighbors: A New National Strategy for the Protection of Children. Washington, DC, U.S. Government Printing Office, 1993

U.S. Advisory Board on Child Abuse and Neglect: Creating Caring Communities: Blueprint for an Effective Federal Policy on Child Abuse and Neglect. Washington, DC, U.S. Government Printing Office, 1991

Walker AG: Handbook on Questioning Children. Washington, DC, ABA Center on Children and the Law, 1994

Whitcomb D: When the Victim Is a Child: Issues for Judges and Prosecutors, 3rd Edition. Washington, DC, National Institute of Justice, 1992

Whitcomb D et al: The Child Victim as a Witness: Research Report. Washington, DC, Office of Juvenile Justice and Delinquency Prevention, 1994

Martin LH: Caseworker Liability for the Negligent Handling of Child Abuse Reports. 60 U. Cinn. L. Rev. 191, 1991

Adult Survivors of Childhood Sexual Abuse and Statutes of Limitations: A Call for Legislative Action. 26 Wake Forest L. Rev. 1245, 1991

Fitzpatrick TL: Innocent Until Proven Guilty: Shallow Words for the Falsely Accused in a Criminal Prosecution for Child Sexual Abuse. 12 U. Bridgeport L. Rev. 175, 1991

Rappaport JS: The Legal System's Response to Child Abuse: A "Shield" for Children or a "Sword" Against the Constitutional Rights of Parents. 9 N. Y. L. Sch. J. Hum. Rts. 257, 1991

Hagen AM: Tolling the Statutes of Limitations in Actions Brought by Adult Survivors of Childhood Sexual Abuse. 33 Ariz L. Rev. 427, 1991

Young CC: Abused Children: The Supreme Court Considers the Due Process Right to Protection. 29 J. Fam. L. 679, 1990–1991

Townsend EL: Maternal Drug Use During Pregnancy as Child Neglect or Abuse. 93 W. Va. L. Rev. 1083, 1991

Sailer CB: Qualified Immunity for Child Abuse Investigators: Balancing the Concerns of Protecting Our Children From Abuse and the Integrity of the Family. 29 J. Fam. L. 659, 1990–1991

# ▌Domestic Violence

American Bar Association: Domestic violence: the brutal truth about the American family. Family Advocate 17:3, Winter 1995

Balos B, Gomez I: Judicial Procedures in Misdemeanor Domestic Assault Cases: A Model Policy. 10 N. Ill. U. L. Rev. 259, 1990

Cahn NR: Civil Images of Battered Women: The Impact of Domestic Violence on Child Custody Decisions. 44 Vand. L. Rev. 1041, 1991

Davidson HA: The Impact of Domestic Violence on Children: Report to the President of the ABA. Washington, DC, American Bar Association Center on Children and the Law, 1994

Ensign DJ: Link Between the Battered Woman Syndrome and the Battered Child Syndrome: An Argument for Consistent Standards in the Admission of Expert Testimony in Family Abuse Cases. 36 Wayne L. Rev. 1619, 1990

Finn P: Statutory Authority in the Use and Enforcement of Civil Protection Orders Against Domestic Abuse. 23 Fam. L. Q. 43, 1989

Finn P, Colson S: Civil Protection Orders: Legislation, Current Court Practice, and Enforcement. Washington, DC, National Institute of Justice, 1990

Keith AM: Domestic Violence and the Court System. 15 Hamline L. Rev. 105, 1991

Konkol DL: Civil Restraining Orders. 63 Wis. Law. 10, 1990

Lemon NKD: Domestic Violence: The Law and Criminal Prosecution. San Francisco, CA, San Francisco Family Violence Project, 1990

Lengyel LB: Survey of State Domestic Violence Legislation. 10 Legal Refer. Serv. Q. 59, 1990

Lerman LG, Kuehl SJ, Brygger MP: Domestic Abuse and Mediation: Guidelines for Mediators and Policy Makers. Washington, DC, National Woman Abuse Prevention Project, 1989

Malinowski MJ: Federal Enclaves and Local Law: Carrying Out a Domestic Violence Exception to Exclusive Legislative Jurisdiction. 100 Yale L. J. 189, 1990

Minow M: Words and the Door to the Land of Change: Law, Language, and Family Violence. 43 Vand. L. Rev. 1665, 1990

National Council of Juvenile and Family Court Judges: Family Violence: Improving Court Practice, Recommendations from the NCJFCJ Family Violence Project. Reno, NV, National Council of Juvenile and Family Court Judges, 1990

Parnas RI: The American Bar Foundation Survey of the Administration of Criminal Justice and Past, Present, and Future Response to Domestic Violence. 69 Wash. U. L. Q. 107, 1991

Sonkin DJ: Domestic Violence on Trial: Psychological and Legal Dimensions of Family Violence. New York, Springer, 1987

U.S. Department of Justice: Attorney General's Task Force on Family Violence (Final Report). Washington, DC, U.S. Attorney General's Office, 1984

Voris MJ: Civil Orders of Protection: Do They Protect Children, the Tag-Along Victims of Domestic Violence? 17 Ohio N. U. L. Rev., 1991

Welch DM: Mandatory Arrest of Domestic Abusers: Panacea or Perpetuation of the Problem of Abuse? 43 DePaul L. Rev. 1133, 1994

# ▌ Elder Abuse

Bennett G, Kingston P: Elder Abuse: Concepts, Theories and Interventions. London, Chapman & Hall, 1993

Coleman N, Karp N: Recent State and Federal Developments in Protective Services and Elder Abuse. Journal of Elder Abuse and Neglect 1:51–63, 1989

Decalmer P, Ingman SR (eds): The Mistreatment of Elderly People. London, Sage, 1993

Eisenberg H: Combatting Elder Abuse Through the Legal Process. Journal of Elder Abuse and Neglect 3:65–96, 1991

Filinson R, Ingman SR: Elder Abuse: Practice and Policy. New York, Human Sciences Press, 1989

Garfield AS: Elder Abuse and the States' Adult Protective Services Response: Time for a Change in California. 42 Hastings L.J. 859, 1991

Johnson TF: Elder Mistreatment: Deciding Who Is At Risk. Westport, CT, Greenwood, 1991

Movsas TZ, Movsas B: Abuse Versus Neglect: A Model Approach to Understand the Causes of and Treatment Strategies for Mistreatment of Older Persons, 6 Issues L. and Med. 163, 1990

National Aging Resource Center on Elder Abuse: Summaries of National Elder Abuse Data: An Exploratory Study of State Statistics. Washington, DC, American Public Welfare Association, 1990

Pritchard J: The Abuse of Elderly People: A Handbook for Professionals. London, Jessica Kingsley, 1994

Rathbone-McCuan E, Fabian DR: Self-Neglecting Elders: A Clinical Dilemma. Westport, CT, Auburn House, 1992

Stiegel LA: Recommended Guidelines for State Courts in Handling Elder Abuse Cases. Washington, DC, ABA Commission on Legal Problems of the Elderly, 1995

U.S. General Accounting Office: Elder Abuse: Effectiveness of Reporting Laws and Other Factors. Washington, DC, U.S. General Accounting Office, 1991

U.S. House of Representatives, Select Committee on Aging: Elder Abuse: What Can Be Done? (congressional hearing) Washington, DC, Comm. Pub. No. 102-808, May 15, 1991

## ▌ General Materials

Hofford M (ed): Families in Court. Washington, DC, National Council of Juvenile and Family Court Judges, 1989

Kramer DT: Legal Rights of Children, 2nd Edition. Colorado Springs, CO, Shepard's/McGraw-Hill, 1994

Karp L, Karp CL: Domestic Torts: Family Violence, Conflict and Sexual Abuse. Colorado Springs, CO, Shepard's/McGraw Hill, 1989

---

# Legal Information Resources for Professionals

The following is a selected listing of law-focused organizations and publications that provide technical assistance, consultation, training, and information on the legal aspects of family violence.

1. ABA Center on Children and the Law, American Bar Association, 740 15th Street, N.W., Washington, DC 20005, (202) 662-1720

2. ABA Commission on Domestic Violence, American Bar Association, 740 15th Street, N.W., Washington, DC 20005, (202) 662-1737

3. ABA Commission on Legal Problems of the Elderly, American Bar Association, 740 15th Street, N.W., Washington, DC 20005, (202) 662-8685

4. Legal Counsel for the Elderly, American Association of Retired Persons, 601 E Street, N.W., Washington, DC 20049, (202) 434-2120

5. National Association of Counsel for Children, 1205 Oneida Street, Denver, CO 80220, (303) 322-2260

6. National Center on Elder Abuse and Neglect, American Public Welfare Association, 810 First Street, N.E., Suite 500, Washington, DC 20002, (202) 682-0100

7. National Center for the Prosecution of Child Abuse, National District Attorneys Association, 99 Canal Center Plaza, Suite 510, Alexandria, VA 22314, (703) 739-0321

8. National Center on Women and Family Law, 799 Broadway, Room 402, New York, NY 10003, (212) 874-8200

9. National Center for Youth Law, 114 Sansome Street, Suite 900, San Francisco, CA 94104, (415) 543-3307

10. National Committee for the Prevention of Elder Abuse, c/o Institute on Aging, The Medical Center of Central Massachusetts, 119 Belmont Street, Worcester, MA 01605, (508) 793-6166

11. National Council of Juvenile and Family Court Judges, University of Nevada, P.O. Box 8970, Reno, NV 89507, (702) 784-6012

# Index

Page numbers in **bold** type refer to tables or figures.

**A**

Abandonment, of children,
38
Abuse
cycle of, 140, 144–145, 150,
160–161, 187
definition of, 188, 189
elder. *See* Elder maltreatment
financial, 200–201
material, 189
medical, 191
partner, 129. *See* also
Domestic violence
legal definition of, 166–167
physical
definition of, 2, 188
in elders, 189–190, 198
psychological
definition of, 189
in elders, 190–191
ritualistic, 8–10
sadistic, 221–224
sexual. *See* Child sexual
abuse; Domestic
violence; Elder
maltreatment
spousal, 129
legal definition of, 166
Abusive relationships,
entrapment in, 150
Accommodation syndrome,
child sexual abuse, 134
Active neglect, 189

Adjustment disorder,
misdiagnosis of, 106
Adolescent abuse. *See* Child and
adolescent abuse
Adoptive Assistance and Child
Welfare Act (1980), 69
Adult-child conjoint supportive
therapy, 108
Adults Molested as Children,
109–110
Adult survivors of child
abuse/neglect, 209–236
in adult psychiatric
populations, 212–214
amnesia in, 227
assessment of, 223–224
borderline conditions in,
217–220
case example of, 218–219
case assessment/
management protocols
and guidelines for, 286
client confidentiality issues
in, 225
coexisting mental problems
in, 224
disclosure facilitation in, **226**
dissociative disorders in,
217–218, 220–223
case example of, 222–223
patient recognition of, 227
familial clustering of
symptoms in, 224

Adult survivors of child
  abuse/neglect *(continued)*
  historical perspective on,
    210–211
    Freud, 210–211
    post-Freudian theorists, 211
  history, sample, in, 225–226
  informed consent in, 225
  Klein/Kernberg/Mahler
    theories on, 219
  legal issues in, 233–236
    for abused/family
      members/offenders,
      233–235
    delayed discovery, 235–236
    expert witness testimony,
      236
    hypnosis use, 236
    judicial relief against
      abuser, 233
    litigation file by abused,
      234
    for mental health
      professionals, 235–236
    parental immunity, 233
    recollection validity,
      235–236
    statutes of limitations,
      234–235
    suggestibility, 236
  literature on, 288
  memory facilitation in,
    224–225
  political torture,
    resemblance to, 214
  posttraumatic stress disorder
    in, 215–217
    case examples of, 215–216
  posttraumatic symptoms in,
    223–225

  prevalence in adult
    populations, 211–214
  prevention resources for,
    294
  professions chosen by, 216
  recall of childhood
    experiences in, 219
  recovery in, 227
  remembering abuse in, 225
  research on, 230–233
    ascertainment problems in,
      230–231
    control populations in, 231
    cross-sectional studies in,
      232
    longitudinal follow-up
      studies in, 230
    minimization of abuse by
      abused, 230–231
    sampling in, 231
    therapy outcome studies
      in, 232–233
  self-destructive behavior in,
    218, 222
  stress, extreme or complex,
    in, 220
  successful treatment of, 219
  symptom clusters in, 213–214
  syndromes of maltreatment
    sequelae in, 214–223
  therapist role in treatment
    of, 219
  trauma theory and, 219–220
  treatment of, 226–230
    art and poetry therapy as,
      227
    group therapy as, 228
    hypnosis and Amytal
      interviews as, 228
    legal ramifications of, 228

patient family dynamics in,
229
play therapy as, 227
reporting to child
protective services in,
228
trauma-related symptoms
in, 229–230
victim advocacy and referral
resources for, 290
Advocacy, victim, 289–291
AIDS infection risk, in domestic
violence victims, 147–148
Alcohol abuse. *See also*
Substance abuse
in child maltreatment, 45
in child sexual abuse, 75
in domestic violence, 146
AMA Diagnostic and Treatment
Guidelines Concerning
Child Abuse and Neglect,
10–11
Amnesia, in adult survivors of
child abuse/neglect, 227
Amytal (amobarbital sodium),
in adult survivors of child
abuse/neglect, 228
Anger, at abuser, in child sexual
abuse, 112
Antisocial personality disorder,
in child/adolescent abuse
and, 7
Art therapy, 227
Assault
physical. *See* Child and
adolescent abuse,
physical
spousal, 129. *See also*
Domestic violence
verbal and emotional, 44

**B**
Battered child syndrome, xiii, 1,
18
Battered old person syndrome,
184
Battered woman syndrome, 173
as self-defense theory, 173
Batterers, treatment for, 174
Battering. *See also* Child and
adolescent abuse; Domestic
violence; Elder
maltreatment
assessment of, 152–160
battered old person
syndrome, 184
cycle of, 153, 160–161
definition of, 156
granny battering, 184
treatment for battered
partner in, 156–160
Behavior
modification, in child sexual
abuse treatment, 118
role models, in cycle of
abuse, 150
violent, in victims of child
abuse, 5
Blame and self-blame, in child
sexual abuse, 114
Borderline conditions
in adult survivors of child
abuse/neglect, 217–220
case example of, 218–219
Borderline personality disorder,
in adult survivors of child
abuse/neglect, 217

**C**
CAMDEX, 193
Candor, 64

CASA. *See* Court-Appointed
Special Advocate
Case management, cooperative
example: child abuse, 14–16
Case recognition training,
xvi–xvii
Child abuse. *See* Child and
adolescent abuse
Child Abuse Prevention and
Treatment Act (CAPTA), 19,
129
Child and adolescent abuse. *See
also* Adult survivors; Child
and adolescent emotional
maltreatment; Child and
adolescent neglect; Child
sexual abuse
in adult psychiatric
population, evidence of,
212–214
case assessment/
management protocols
for, 284–285
cost of, xiv–xv
definition of, xiv
definition of, legal, 26
dissociation caused by, 213
examination in, 10–11
failure to report, 27
*Fischer v. Metcalf,* case of
*Landeros v. Flood,* case of
investigation of/intervention
in, 20–26
by child protective
services, 20–26
Court-Appointed Special
Advocate (CASA) in,
24
culpability of nonabusive
parent in, 23

guardian ad litem
(GAL)/counsel in, 24
medical testimony and, 23
mental health evaluations
in, 23
mental health provider role
in, 24–25
multidisciplinary teams in,
25
protective jurisdiction in,
23
legal issues in
for mental health
professionals/
practitioners, 26–29
for victims/family
members/offenders,
18–26
legal literature on,
302–305
literature on, 287
partner abuse and, 149
physical, 1–29
abusers in, 3
age at onset of, 3
assessment of, 10–11
child treatment in, 12–13
confidentiality laws in, 25
cooperative management
treatment of, 14–16
corporal punishment as,
17–18
definition of, 2
domestic violence,
association with,
144–146
ecological model of, 4
effects in victims of, 4–6
etiology of, 4
fatalities from, 3–4

female victim
    preponderance in, 3
hospital child protection
    committees for, 17
hospital management of,
    14–16
imminent harm, likelihood,
    in, 22
intergenerational
    transmission of, 8
legal issues in, 18–29
litigation for, 26
mental health provider
    roles in, 16–17
parental psychopathology
    in, 7, 11, 16–17
parent treatment in, 12–13
prevalence of, 2–3
prevention of, 16
psychopathology of child
    in, 4–6
psychopathology of parent
    in, 5–6
psychotherapy for, 12
risk factors for
    psychopathology in,
    5–6
as ritualistic abuse, 8–10
social functioning/
    isolation of families
    in, 8
substance abuse in, 11,
    16–17
suicide in, 6–7
treatment of, 11–13
treatment outcome in,
    11–12
variables contributing to,
    11–12
victim behavior in, 1

physical abusers in, 3
prevalence of, xiv, 1
prevention resources for,
    293–294
reporting of, 18–22
    to child protective services,
        19
    duty to warn in, 28
    false, 27
    *Fischer v. Metcalf,* case, 27
    immunity law protection
        in, 27–29
    invasion of privacy and, 27
    to law enforcement,
        19–20
    *Landeros v. Flood,* case, 27
    laws on, 21–22
    privileged communications
        and, 28–29
    requirements in, 26–27
    *Tarasoff v. Regents of the
        University of
        California,* case, 28
severity vs. adult symptoms
    in, 213
as trauma, 209–210
victim advocacy and referral
    resources for, 289
Child and adolescent emotional
    maltreatment, 43–65. *See
    also* Child and adolescent
    neglect
abusers as victims of abuse
    in, 62
domestic violence as, 69
emotional abuse as, 43–45
    definition of, 43–44
    incidence of, **44**
    types of, 44–45
emotional neglect as, 45

Child and adolescent emotional
  maltreatment *(continued)*
  group therapy for victims of,
    57–58
  in-home services for parents
    at risk of, 70
  intervention in, 48–53
    with agency-referred
      families, 51
    diagnostic evaluations in,
      51–53
    in neglected/maltreated
      children, 54–58
    in neglectful families,
      49–53
    parental inability to care
      and, 54–55
    with self-referred families,
      50–52
    separation from parents as,
      54–55
    temporary, voluntary
      placement as, 55
    therapeutic goals for, 52–53
  intervention issues for
    clinicians in, 64
  legal issues in, 65–70
    physical neglect, 65–68
  parental psychological
    problems in, 62
  psychological effects on child
    of, 55–56
  with substance abuse,
    parental, 45–48
  therapeutic principles in,
    55–58
  treatment for, 58–61
    domestic violence
      witnesses in, 161–163
    family therapy as, 59–61
    respite care as, 58–59
    treatment for neglectful
      parents in, 61–64
      expressive, 63–64
      individual, 61–62
  in utero substance exposure
    as, 46–48
  from witnessing domestic
    violence, 148–149,
    150
Child and adolescent
  maltreatment
  legal issues in
    child protective
      intervention, 65–70
    for mental health
      professionals, 69–70
    for victims/family
      members/offenders,
      65–69
Child and adolescent neglect,
  37–43. *See also* Child and
    adolescent emotional
    maltreatment
  adult psychiatric evidence of,
    212–214
  assessment of, 41–42
    history taking in, 41–42
    physical exam findings in,
      41
    protocols in, 42
  case assessment/
    management protocols
    and guidelines for,
    284–285
  definition of, 37
  incidence of, 39
  legal issues in, 65–70
    educational neglect,
      68

for mental health
 professionals/
 practitioners, 69–70
for victims/family
 members/offenders,
 65–69
legal literature on, 302–305
literature on, 287
prevention resources for,
 293–294
psychopathology in
 of parents, 40–41
 of victims, 39–40
spouse abuse and, 41
treatment of, 42–43
 case example of, 42–43
 child victims of, 42
 parental perpetrators of, 42
types of, 37–39
 educational, 39
 emotional, 39
 physical, 38
victim advocacy and referral
 resources for, 289
Child custody and visitation,
 171–172
Childhood trauma, memories of,
 241–271
 age differences in
 suggestibility and,
 260–262
 child interviews
 believability of faulty
 reports in, 250–251
 critical factors in, 253
 increasing salience of
 techniques in,
 246–260
 influencing reports of,
 251–253

interviewer bias in, 247–248
perceptual details in,
 249–250
postevent suggestions and
 feedback in, 251–253
repeated suggestions in,
 248–251
resistance to erroneous
 suggestions in,
 251–253
source monitoring errors
 in, 256–260
stereotype induction in,
 248–251
suggestibility of
 anatomical dolls in,
 253–256
child testimony on, 241–242
child witnesses and, 242
current literature on,
 260–263
interview practice impact in
 abuse cases on, 263–264
mass-allegation day care
 cases, 241
recovered memories as,
 268–271
research vs. clinical practice
 in, 263–268
 anatomical doll use in,
 264–265
 authenticity of reports in,
 266–267
 impact of interview in,
 263–264
 source errors in, 265–266
suggestibility and, 242
 research on, 242–260
treatment and forensics
 conflict in, 267–268

Child protection committees, 17
Child protection teams, 14
Child protective intervention,
    65–70. *See also* Child
    protective services (CPS)
    bias against poor and
        minority families in, 67
    inadequate housing in, 66
    inadequate supervision in, 66
    parental refusal of medical
        treatment in, 67
    parental substance abuse in,
        66
Child protective services (CPS),
    19
    caseworker conditions in, 21
    in child sexual abuse, 74
    consultation with, 121
    reporting abuse of adult
        survivors to, 228
    role of, 18–20
Children's shelter, protective, 58
Child sexual abuse, 73–99. *See*
    *also* Adult survivors of child
    abuse/neglect; Incest;
    Incestuous family
    adjunctive treatments for,
        107–110
    conjoint supportive
        adult-child therapy,
        108
    environmental alterations,
        110
    family group therapy,
        107–108
    group therapy for abused
        child/supportive
        adult, 109
    individual therapy for
        supportive adult, 108

peer group therapy,
    108–109
pharmacotherapy, 110
self-help groups, 109–110
in adult patients, 209–236
    discriminators indicating,
        212–213
    psychiatric sequelae of,
        212–214
assessment of, 82–97
association with domestic
    violence of, 144–146
child advocacy in, 122–123
clinical case assessment/
    management protocols
    and guidelines for,
    283–284
clinical evaluation of, 85–88
    assessment of child in,
        85–88
    child credibility in, 86–87
    child memory and time
        sense in, 86–87
    child suggestibility in, 87
    guidelines for, 85
    qualifications of evaluator
        in, 85
    reliability of child in, 88
consultation with other
    professionals in,
    119–123
    child protective services,
        121
    legal system, 121–123
    pediatricians and
        family/ER physicians,
        120
    schools, 119–120
crisis help in, 106
definition of, 73

denial of, 76–77
diagnostic evaluation of, 106
example of disputed case of,
    92–97
expert witness testimony in,
    122
extrafamilial, 73–74
false allegations of, 88–97
  by child, 91–92
  confusion with sexual
      overstimulation by
      parent in, 90
  intentional, by parent, 91
  misinterpretation of
      caretaking in, 89
  misinterpretation of
      common
      psychological
      symptoms in, 90
  misinterpretation of
      normal sexual
      behavior in, 89
  misinterpretation of
      physical signs in child
      in, 90
  unintentional, 88–90
female victim preponderance
    in, 73
forensic consultation in, 121
guardian ad litem (GAL),
    appointing, 130
individual long-term
    psychotherapy for,
    110–117
  anger at abuser in, 112
  blame and self-blame in,
      114
  delayed consequences of
      abuse in, 116–117
  fault and blame in, 114

fear of homosexuality in,
    113
  goals of, 111–112
  leaving home as, 113–114
  man-hating and fear of
      men in, 113
  power imbalance in, 112
  retaliation/recurrence
      fears in, 114–115
  sexualized behavior and
      talk in, 115–116
  treating omnipotent
      children with, 112
intervention in, 105–123
intrafamilial, 73–74
  guidelines for legal
      intervention in,
      129–130
legal issues in, 97–99
  children as reliable
      witnesses, 131–133
  child sexual exploitation
      laws, 129
  court testimony, child, 99
  court testimony, mental
      health professional, 99
  criminal laws, 127–128
  incest definition and laws,
      128
  *Maryland v. Craig,* case,
      131
  mental health expert
      witnesses, 133
  for mental health
      professionals/
      practitioners, 98–99,
      133–134
  out-of-home care setting,
      131
  privacy issues, 98–99

Child sexual abuse *(continued)*
  professional reporting
    responsibilities, 133
  recent legislative reforms,
    120–131
  sexual psychopath/
    dangerous offender
    statutes, 128–129
  testimony about child
    witness credibility,
    133
  treatment and prevention,
    127–134
  treatment plan for abused
    child and abuser, 99
  for victims/family
    members/offenders,
    97–98, 127–133
  videotaped/closed circuit
    TV child testimony,
    131
  legal literature on, 302–305
  literature on, 287
  multiple personality disorder
    with, 80
  pedophilia and, 76
  pharmacotherapy for, 110
  physical evaluation of, 82–85
    examination in, 83–85
    findings of acute
      trauma/penile
      penetration in, 84
    history taking in, 82–83
    sample interview for, 83
  posttraumatic stress disorder
    in, 78–79, 106
  prevalence of, 74–75
  prevention of, 123–127
    advice from abusers on,
      126–127

  day care programs for, 125
  locales for programs in,
    124–126
  by on-the-spot child
    training, 126
  parental involvement in
    programs for, 125
  program content in, 124
  rationales for, 123–124
  role of child self-esteem in,
    127
  school-based programs for,
    125–126
  by teaching children to
    deter, 125
prevention resources for, 294
psychological sequelae of,
    77–82
  depression and suicidal
    behavior, 79–80
  hysterical and dissociative
    symptoms, 80
  impaired peer
    relationships, 80–81
  paranoid reactions and
    mistrust, 79
  poor school performance,
    81
  poor self-image, 79
  sexual behavior
    disturbances, 81–82
  substance abuse, 81
research on, 77
treatment of, 105–123
treatment of abusers in,
    117–119
  behavior modification
    treatments, 118
  comprehensive programs,
    118–119

cost-benefit analysis, 117
efficacy, 117
group therapy, 118
penile plethysmography,
117–118
treatment of children in,
106–117
treatment of supportive
adults in, 106–117
underreporting of, 74–75
victim advocacy and referral
resources for, 290
Child sexual abuse
accommodation syndrome,
134
Child sexual abuse syndrome,
134
Child witness credibility, in
child sexual abuse cases,
131–133
Clinical case assessment
guidelines, 283–286
Cocaine abuse. *See also*
Substance abuse
in child maltreatment, 45
in domestic violence, 146
infant addiction to, 45
in utero exposure to, 46
Committee on Family Violence
and Sexual Abuse, xiii
Confidentiality, 64
breach of, in child abuse
cases, 25
Confinement, close, 44
Conflict resolution, nonviolent,
166
in elder maltreatment, 183
Conflict Tactics Scale, 2
Consultation-liaison service,
196–197

Corporal punishment, 17–18
as child abuse, 22
definition of, 17
prevention of, 17
"reasonable" forms of, 22
in schools, xviii, 18
Council on Children,
Adolescents, and Their
Families, xiii
Countertransference, 64
Court-Appointed Special
Advocate (CASA), 24
Covert sensitization, 118
Crime victim compensation
program, 172–173
Crisis intervention
in child sexual abuse, 106
in domestic violence, 157
Cults, child/adolescent abuse
in, 9
Custody, and child abuse, 38
Cycle of abuse, 140, 150
of children, 144–145
cycle of battering behavior
and, 160–161
in elder maltreatment, 187
Cycle of battering, 153, 160–161
Cycle of dependency, in
domestic violence, 150

**D**
Damaged goods syndrome, 79
Daughters and Sons United
(DSU), 57
Day care cases, mass allegation,
241–242
Delayed discovery, 235–236
Dependency, cycle of, 150
Depression
child/adolescent abuse and, 7

Depression *(continued)*
  child sexual abuse and, 79–80
  in domestic violence, 146,
    147
  in elder maltreatment, 183,
    187
Diagnosis training, xvi–xvii
Diagnostic Interview for
  Children and Adolescents
  (DICA)
  in child sexual abuse, 80
  in physical abuse of children,
    5
Dissociative disorder
  in adult survivors of child
    abuse/neglect,
    217–218, 220–223
  in child and adolescent
    abuse, 213
  in child sexual abuse, 80
  in ritually abused children,
    9
  in sadistic abuse, 221–224
    case example of, 222–223
Dissociative disorder
  in adult survivors of child
    abuse/neglect
    history, sample, for,
    225–226
    patient recognition of,
    227
Dolls, anatomically detailed
  arguments against use of, 254
  doll play in abused vs.
    nonabused children and,
    254–255
  practice vs. research
    concerns in use of,
    264–265
  suggestibility of, 253–256

  use in child abuse
    interviews/testimony of,
    246
Domestic violence, 139–175.
  *See also* Family violence
  abuser psychosocial
    characteristics in, 148
  assessment of, 152–160
  association with child abuse,
    144–146
  battered woman syndrome in,
    173
  behavior role models in, 150
  case assessment/
    management protocols
    and guidelines for, 285
  case example of, 161–163
  child emotional
    maltreatment and, 69
  community prevention of,
    163, 165–166
  concurrent child and partner
    abuse in, 149
  conflict resolution training
    for, 166
  couple violence in, 143–144
  crime victim compensation
    program for, 172–173
  cycle of abuse in, 140, 148,
    150
  cycle of dependency in, 150
  definition of, xiv, 139
  depression in, 146, 147
  discrimination against
    women and, 140
  drug overdose/suicide
    attempts in, 147
  dynamics of, 149–150
  entrapment in abusive
    relationships in, 150

evaluation and treatment of
professional education, 164
research, 164–165
services, 165
expert testimony on, 173
family background in, 145
female assaultive behavior in,
143
female response pattern in,
146–148
historical perspective on,
139–140
in homosexual relationships,
144
impact of abuse in, 146–148
intervention by mental
health professionals in,
163–166
jealousy in, 148
legal definition of, 166–167
legal issues in, 166–175
arrest powers, 168
assault and battery, 168
avoidance and mishandling
of cases, 167
battered woman syndrome,
173
child custody and
visitation, 171–172
community response,
167–168
criminal justice system role
in, 167
custody and visitation
cases, 171–173
diversion agreements, 169
duty to warn, 173–174
expert testimony, 173
law enforcement response,
168–169

legal response,
appropriate, 167
mandatory arrest laws, 168
marital rape, 169
mediation, court-ordered,
174–175
for mental health
professionals/
practitioners,
172–175
privacy and confidentiality,
173–174
probable cause, 168, 171
repeat offenders, 169
restraining orders,
enforcement, 171
restraining orders,
enforcement, cases
in, *Thurman v. City of
Torrington* and *U.S. v.
Foster,* 171
restraining orders and
protection from
abuse, 170–171
role of legal system, 167
substance abuse, 169, 174
suicide risk, 174
*Tarasoff v. Regents of the
University of
California,* case, 174
treatment programs for
batterers, 174
for victims/family
members/offenders,
166–172
legal literature on, 305–306
physical signs and history in,
152–156
cycle of battering and,
153

Domestic violence *(continued)*
  interview for,
    behavior/emotional
      status, 154–156
  interview for,
    clinician-patient,
      153–154
  physical injury pattern as,
    152–153
  posttraumatic stress disorder
    in, 165
  power imbalance in, 175
  predictors of future violence
    in, 148
  during pregnancy, 145
  prevalence of, xiv, 140–144
    against females, 139–140,
      142
    husband-to-wife violence
      in, 142
    wife-to-husband violence
      in, 142–143
  prevention of, 165–166
  prevention resources for, 295
  rape-trauma syndrome and,
    146–147
  repeated assault risk in, 166
  risk factors for, 145–146
  role of mental health
    professionals in,
      150–152
  rule of thumb in, 140, 167
  sexual assault in, 144
  social isolation in, 146
  substance abuse in, 146, 166
  suicide risk in victims of, 156
  symptoms and disorders with,
    146–149
  in assaulted partners,
    146–148

  in assaulting partners, 148
  in child witnesses, 148–149
  temporary separation in, 157
  therapeutic interventions in,
    156
  traumatic bonding in, 150
  treatment for battered
    partner in, 156–160
  behavioral training, 158
  couple therapy, 159
  crisis intervention, 157
  parenting therapy, 159–160
  pharmacotherapy, 158
  psychotherapy, 157
  psychotherapy, group,
    159
  psychotherapy, individual,
    157–158
  treatment of
    child/adolescent
      witnesses in, 161–163
  treatment of violent partners
    in, 160–163
  cycle of battering behavior
    and, 160–161
  underreporting of, 147, 151
  victim advocacy and referral
    resources for, 290
  Victims of Crime Act and,
    172–173
  Workshop on Violence and
    Public Health
      recommendations on,
        164–166
Drug abuse. *See* Substance abuse
Duty to warn, 173–174

E
Ecological model, 4
Ecological view of child, 11

Education for the Handicapped
Act (EHA), 47
Elder abuse. *See also* Elder
maltreatment
agencies for, 198
definition of, xiv, 201
laws against, 184, 188
prevalence of, xiv
programs for, 198
Elder Abuse, Prevention,
Identification and
Treatment Act (1985),
188
Elder Abuse Reporting Act,
189
Elder Assessment Instrument
(EAI), 188
Elder maltreatment, 181–203
assessment of, 193–194
case assessment/
management protocols
and guidelines for, 286
case example of, 194–196
case histories of, 185–187
conflict resolution in, 183
consultation-liaison service
for, 196–197
cycle of abuse in, 187
definitions of terms in,
188–191
depression and isolation in,
183, 187
elder abuse laws and, 184,
188
Elder Abuse, Prevention,
Identification and
Treatment Act (1985)
and, 188
Elder Abuse Reporting Act
and, 189

Elder Assessment Instrument
(EAI) for, 188
epidemiology of, 183
etiologies of, 185–187
evaluation of, 192–193
financial abuse/exploitation
as, 200–201
forcible intervention in, 200
government economics and,
184–185
history of recognition of,
184–185
incapacity issues in, 200
incidence of, 185
involuntary protective
services in, 201
issues in study of, 181–183
risk factors, 182–183
spousal abuse, 182
women as targets, 182–183
lack of financial incentives
for, 185
legal issues in, 197–203
case reporting laws, 198,
199
confidentiality, 203
criminal charges, 198
determination of
competence, 202
guardianship and
conservatorship
actions, 202
law enforcement response,
198
legislative changes needed,
203
for mental health
professionals/
practitioners,
202–203

Elder maltreatment *(continued)*
   presumption of mental
      capacity, 202–203
   programs and agencies, 198
   restraining orders, 198–199
   victim court testimony, 199
   for victims/family
      members/offenders,
      197–202
   legal literature on, 306–307
   literature on, 288
   multidisciplinary team to
      treat, 193
   National Aging Resource
      Center on Elder Abuse,
      199
   National Committee for the
      Prevention of Elder
      Abuse and Neglect, 199
   National Guardianship
      Association, 200
   nursing home ombudsman
      program for, 201–202
   in nursing homes and
      institutions, 201–202
   Older Americans Act, 199,
      201–202
   power imbalance in, 183, 192
   prevention of emotional
      abuse in, 193
   prevention resources for, 294
   public policy response to, 199
   research on, 186–187
   risk factors for, 187, 193
   role of psychiatrist in,
      192–197
   self-neglect as, 201
   spousal abuse in, 21
   state laws on, 193–194,
      197–198

   Subcommittee on Health and
      Long-Term Care (1990),
      183–184, 185–186
   substance abuse in, 183, 186
   treating maladaptive feelings
      in, 194
   underreporting of, 184
   victim advocacy and referral
      resources for, 291
   Washington State Medical
      Association
      classifications of,
      189–191
      exploitation, 191
      medical abuse, 191
      neglectful behavior, 191
      physical abuse, 189–190
      psychological abuse, 190
Elder neglect, 201
Emotional abuse, 43–45. *See
   also* Child and adolescent
   emotional maltreatment
   incidence of, **44**
Emotional assault, 44
Emotional maltreatment. *See*
   Child and adolescent
   emotional maltreatment
Empathy, teaching of, xviii
Environmental alterations, in
   child sexual abuse, 110
Examination, physical, in
   child/adolescent abuse,
   10–11
Expert witness testimony
   in adult survivors of child
      abuse/neglect, 236
   in child sexual abuse, 122
Exploitation
   definition of, 188, 191
   in elders, 191

financial, 201
sexual, of children, 129
Expressive therapy, 63–64
Expulsion, of child from home,
38

**F**
Fabrication, 259
Family Preservation and Support
Services, 69–70
Family therapy, 59–61
Family violence
assessment of, xvi–xvii
case assessment/
management protocols
and guidelines for, 286
case recognition and
diagnosis of, xvi–xvii
cost of, xiv–xv
definition of, xiv, 188
education about, xvii–xviii
education and research on,
xiii
legal definition of, 166
literature on, 287
prevalence of, xiv
prevention of, xvii–xviii
protection from, xvi
recognition of, xiii
reduction strategies for, xv
rehabilitation programs for,
xvii
risk factors for, xv–xvi
statutes on, 128
treatment efficacy in, xvi–xvii
underdiagnosis of, xiii
Fatalities, from child/adolescent
abuse, 4
Federal Adoption Assistance and
Child Welfare Act (1980), 20

Federal Drug and Alcohol Abuse
Treatment Law, 70
Fetal alcohol syndrome, 45
Financial abuse, 200–201
Financial exploitation, 201
Firearms
control of, xvii–xviii
homicide/suicide and, xvi
Foster care, for child abuse, 22
Foster grandparent program, 58
Foster homes, 59

**G**
GAL. *See* Guardian ad litem
Geriatric Depression Scale, 193
Grandparent, foster, 58
Granny battering, 184
Group home living, 113–114
Group therapy
for adolescent emotional
maltreatment, 57–58
for adult survivors of child
abuse/neglect, 228
for child sexual abuse, 118
child, 109
child/supportive adult, 109
family, 107–108
parent groups, 108–109
peer, 108–109
self-help groups,
109–110
for domestic violence, 159
Guardian ad litem (GAL), 24
in child sexual abuse, 130
Guardianship and
conservatorship, 202
Guidelines, clinical case
assessment, 283–286
Guilt, in child, in sexual abuse,
79, 106

**H**
Hachinski scale, 193
Hamilton Rating Scale for
    Depression, 193
Harm, imminent, 22
Harm, physical, 199
Health care, child
    delay in, 38
    refusal of, 38
Health care provider roles, xv
Heterophobia, in child sexual
    abuse, 113
Homophobia, in child sexual
    abuse, 113
Hypnosis
    in adult survivors of child
        abuse/neglect, 228
    validity of, in adult
        recollection of child
        abuse/neglect, 236
Hysteria, in child sexual abuse,
    80

**I**
Incapacity, in elders, 200,
    202–203
Incest. *See also* Child sexual
    abuse; Incestuous family
    in childhood, witnesses of,
        224
    definition of, 73
    laws on, 128
    legal definition of, 128
    prevalence of, 211–212
Incestuous family
    alcohol abuse in, 75
    denial of abuse in, 76–77
    patriarchal family structure
        in, 75–76
    pedophilia and, 76

    psychodynamics and
        psychopathology of,
        75–77
    role confusion in, 76
Injury and abuse, intentional, in
    adolescent
    prevention resources for, 293
Insomnia, in child witnesses of
    domestic violence, 149
Interviewing
    of children
        anatomically detailed doll
            use in, 246
        impact in abuse cases of,
            263–264
        influencing, 251–253
        interviewer bias effect in,
            247–248
        repeated suggestions in,
            248–251
        source monitoring errors
            in, 256–260
        stereotype induction in,
            248–251
        suggestibility of
            anatomically detailed
            dolls in, 253–256
    effect of, on child
        suggestibility, 246–260
    increasing salience of
        techniques of, 246–260
    interviewer bias in, 246–247
Isolation, social
    of abused adolescent, 7
    in domestic violence, 146
    in elder maltreatment, 183

**J**
Jealousy, in domestic violence,
    148

**K**
Kempe, C. Henry, 1, 18

**L**
Lability
child/adolescent abuse and, 7
in domestic violence victims, 147
Laws
Child Abuse Prevention and Treatment Act of 1974 (CAPTA), 19
on child abuse reporting, 18–22
Learned helplessness, 150
Legal and judicial process, improving, 299–302
Legal issues. *See also* under specific topics
information resources for professionals, 307–308
suggestions for improving legal and judicial process, 299–302
Literature, selected, 287–288

**M**
Male phobia, in child sexual abuse, 113
Management protocols and guidelines, 283–286
Man-hating, in child sexual abuse, 113
Marijuana, in child maltreatment, 45
Marital rape, 144. *See also* Domestic violence
Masturbatory satiation, 118
Material abuse, 189

Mediation, court-ordered, in domestic violence, 174–175
Medical abuse
definition of, 191
in elders, 191
Memory
adult
of childhood abuse/neglect, 224–225
of childhood trauma, 241–271
in children, 242, 261
recovered, in adults, 268–271
Mental health provider roles, xv
Mental health treatment programs, 297
Miller, Alice, 216
Mini-Mental State examination, 193
Mistrust, in child sexual abuse, 79
Molestation. *See* Child sexual abuse
Monitoring
reality, 257
source, 256–260
Multiple personality disorder (MPD)
in child sexual abuse, 80
in ritually abused children, 9

**N**
National Aging Resource Center on Elder Abuse, 199
National Center on Child Abuse and Neglect, 74
National Center on Elder Abuse and Neglect, 183

National Committee for the
   Prevention of Elder Abuse
   and Neglect, 199
National Guardianship
   Association, 200
National Incidence Studies of
   Violence in America, 2, 3
National Incidence Study, 74
Neglect. *See also* Child and
   adolescent neglect; Elder
   maltreatment
   active, 189
   definition of, 189, 201
   elder, 191, 201
   passive, 189
Nursing home ombudsman
   program, 201–202

**O**
Older Americans Act, 199,
   201–202
Older Americans Resources and
   Services (OARS)
   questionnaire, 193
Omnipotence, 111

**P**
Paranoid reactions, in child
   sexual abuse, 79
Parental immunity, 233
Parent competency
   enhancement/education, 16
Parenting therapy, 159
Parents United, 109–110, 125
Partner abuse, 129. *See also*
   Domestic violence
   appropriate legal response to,
   167
   legal definition of, 166–167
Passive neglect, 189

Peer relation impairment, in
   child sexual abuse, 80–81
Penile penetration, signs of, in
   child, 84
Penile plethysmography,
   117–118
Pharmacotherapy. *See* under
   specific types of
   abuse/maltreatment
Physical abuse
   definition of, 188
   in elders, 189–190, 198
   suicide with, 6–7
Physical harm, 199
Play therapy, 227
Poetry therapy, 227
Poisonous pedagogy, 214
Position statements of
   professional organizations,
   281–282
Posttraumatic stress disorder
   (PTSD)
   in adult survivors of child
      abuse/neglect, 215–217
   cases, 215–216
   in child sexual abuse, 78–79,
      106, 110
   in domestic violence, 165
   symptoms of, 209–210
Posttraumatic symptoms
   in adult survivors of child
      abuse/neglect, 223–225
   history, sample, for,
      225–226
Power imbalance
   in child sexual abuse, 112
   in domestic violence, 145,
      150, 159, 175
   in elder maltreatment, 183,
      192

Practice standards, 279–280
Pregnancy, domestic violence in, 152
President's Child Safety Partnership, 8
Prevention resources, 293–295
Probable cause
    in domestic violence arrests, 168, 171
    U.S. v. Foster case and, 171
Professional practice standards, 279–280
Protection from abuse orders
    in domestic violence, 170–171
    enforcement of, 171
Protection of Children Against Sexual Exploitation Act of 1977, 129
Protocols, management, 283–286
Pseudomemories, 270
Pseudoritualistic abuse, 9
Psychiatric population, adult
    discriminators of childhood sexual abuse in, 212–213
    incidence of childhood abuse/neglect in, 212–214
Psychological abuse
    definition of, 189
    in elders, 190–191
Psychopathological ritualism, 9
Psychopathology
    of abused children, 4–5
    of abusive parents, 7
    of child abusers, 4–6
    of neglected children, 39–40
    of neglectful parents, 40–41

R
Rape, marital, 144. See also Domestic violence
Rape-trauma syndrome, 146–147
Reality monitoring, 257
Recovered memories, 268–271
Recurrence, fear of, in child sexual abuse, 114–115
Referral resources, 289–291
Reliability, of children's reports, 260
Respite care, 58–59
Restraining orders
    in domestic violence, 170–171
    in elder maltreatment, 198–199
    enforcement of, 171
Retaliation, fear of, in child sexual abuse, 114–115
Ritualism, psychopathological, 9
Ritualistic abuse, 8–10
    caution in care of, 9–10
    definition and subtypes of, 8–9
    effects of, 9
    prevalence of, 9
Role models, nurturing, xviii
Rule of thumb, 140, 167

S
Sadistic abuse, 221–224. See also Satanic abuse
    behavioral signs and histories of, 221
SADS-L. See Schedule for Affective Disorders and Schizophrenia, Lifetime Version

Safe houses, 59
Sand-tray play, 227
Satanic abuse, 8. *See also*
     Ritualistic abuse; Sadistic
     abuse
Schedule for Affective Disorders
     and Schizophrenia, Lifetime
     Version (SADS-L), 147
School performance
     impairment, in child sexual
     abuse, 81
Select Committee on Aging,
     184, 185
Self-destructive
     behavior/mutilation
     in adult survivors of child
          abuse/neglect, 212,
          218, 222
     in child abuse, 6
Self-image, in child sexual
     abuse, 79
Severe Violence Index (Conflict
     Tactics Scale), 2
Sex offenders. *See also* Child
     sexual abuse; Domestic
     violence; Elder
     maltreatment
     convicted, registration and
          employment
          requirements for, 97
     juvenile, 120
     treatment for, 98
     statutes on, 128–129
Sexual abuse. *See* Child sexual
     abuse; Domestic violence;
     Elder maltreatment
Sexual assault, 144
Sexual behavior disturbance, in
     sexually abused children,
     81–82

Sexual exploitation, of children,
     129. *See also* Child sexual
     abuse
Sexualized behavior and talk, in
     child sexual abuse, 115–116
Sexually dangerous offender
     statutes, 128–129
Sexually transmitted diseases
     (STDs), in child sexual
     abuse, 85
Sexual psychopath statutes,
     128–129
Shame, in child sexual abuse, 79
Shelters
     for maltreated children, 58
     for runaway teenagers, 59
Social isolation
     in domestic violence, 146
     in elder maltreatment, 183
Socioeconomic disadvantage, in
     domestic violence, 145
Sons and Daughters United,
     109–110, 125
"Soul murder," 214
Source monitoring
     definition of, 257
     errors in, 265–266
          in children's report of
               abuse, 256–260
          as confusions, 257
          as fabrications, 259
Special education, inattention
     to, 38
Spousal assault, 129
Spouse abuse, 129
     child neglect and, 41
     legal definition of, 166
Standards, professional
     practice, 279–280
Statutes of limitations, 234–235

Steele, B.F., 1
Stigmatization, in child sexual
    abuse, 79, 109
Stress, extreme or complex, 220
Study of the National Incidence
    and Prevalence of Child
    Abuse and Neglect, 44
Subcommittee on Health and
    Long-Term Care (1990),
    183–184, 185–186
Substance abuse
    child abuse/neglect and, 7,
        45–48, 212
    child protective intervention
        with, 66
    in domestic violence, 146,
        166, 169, 174
    in elder maltreatment, 183,
        186
    parental, child safety
        concerns in, 70
    prior to birth of child,
        interventions for, 66–67
    as risk factor for child abuse,
        11
    in sexually abused children,
        81
    in utero exposure to, 46–48
        child behavior with, 46–47
        prevalence of, 46
        treatment for, 47–48
Suggestibility
    in adult recollections of child
        abuse/neglect, 236
    in children, 242
        age differences in, 260–261
        age vs. accuracy in, 243
        anatomically detailed dolls
            and, 246
        early studies on, 243

increasing salience of
    events and, 244–246
increasing salience of
    interviewing and,
    246–260
new paradigms for,
    243–244
research on, 242–260
resistance to, 261–263
in sexual abuse cases, 87
in older children and adults,
    261–262
Suicide
    in adolescent abuse, 6–7
    in child sexual abuse,
        79–80
    in domestic violence, 147,
        156
    duty to warn and, 174
    maternal risk factors for, 6
    physical abuse and, 6
Supervision, child, 38

T
Testimony, by children, 131,
    241–242. *See also* Expert
    witness testimony; Witness,
    child
    closed circuit TV, 131
    videotaped, 131
Trauma
    from child maltreatment,
        209–210
    signs of, in child abuse, 84
Traumatic bonding, 150
Treatment programs, mental
    health, 297
Triggers, of abuse memories,
    215
Truancy, child, 38

**U**
U.S. Advisory Board on Child
    Abuse and Neglect, 21

**V**
Validity
    of adult recollections of child
        abuse/neglect, 235–236
    of child recollections of
        abuse/neglect, 241–271
Verbal assault, 44
Victim advocacy and referral
    resources, 289–291
Victims of Crime Act, 172–173
Violence
    domestic, 139–175
    exposure to, xviii
    prevention resources, 293
    severe, 2

**W**
Washington State Medical
    Association elder abuse
    classification, 189–191
Weapons control, xvii–xviii
Witness, child, 242
    credibility of, 131–133
    in domestic violence,
        148–149, 161–163
    interview techniques for,
        246–260
Workshop on Violence and
    Public Health
    recommendations
    on evaluation and treatment,
        164–165
    on prevention, 165–166